ENVIRONMENTAL EPIDEMIOLOGY

Volume 1

Public Health and Hazardous Wastes

Committee on Environmental Epidemiology

Board on Environmental Studies and Toxicology

Commission on Life Sciences

NATIONAL RESEARCH COUNCIL

NATIONAL ACADEMY PRESS
Washington, D.C. 1991

363 · 728
N 279
v. 1

NATIONAL ACADEMY PRESS • 2101 Constitution Ave. • Washington, D.C. 20418

NOTICE: The project that is the subject of this report was approved by the Governing Board of the National Research Council, whose members are drawn from the councils of the National Academy of Sciences, the National Academy of Engineering, and the Institute of Medicine. The members of the committee responsible for the report were chosen for their special competencies and with regard for appropriate balance.

This report has been reviewed by a group other than the authors according to procedures approved by a Report Review Committee consisting of members of the National Academy of Sciences, the National Academy of Engineering, and the Institute of Medicine.

National Research Council (U.S.). Committee on Environmental Epidemiology.
  Environmental epidemiology / Committee on Environmental Epidemiology, Board on Environmental Studies and Toxicology. Commission on Life Sciences, National Research Council.
    p. cm.
  Includes bibliographical references and index.
  Contents: v. 1. Public health and hazardous waste.
  ISBN 0-309-04496-0 (v. 1)
  1. Environmental health. 2. Epidemiology. I. Title.
  [DNLM: 1. Epidemiologic Methods. 2. Hazardous Waste—adverse effects. 3. Refuse Disposal. WA 788 N275e]
  RA565.N323 1991
  363.72'87—dc20
  DNLM/DLC
  for Library of Congress   91-28051
                                                                        CIP

Cover photograph: LES MOORE/UNIPHOTO

Printed in the United States of America

The National Academy of Sciences is a private, non-profit, self-perpetuating society of distinguished scholars engaged in scientific and engineering research, dedicated to the furtherance of science and technology and to their use for the general welfare. Upon the authority of the charter granted to it by the Congress in 1863, the Academy has a mandate that requires it to advise the federal government on scientific and technical matters. Dr. Frank Press is president of the National Academy of Sciences.

The National Academy of Engineering was established in 1964, under the charter of the National Academy of Sciences, as a parallel organization of outstanding engineers. It is autonomous in its administration and in the selection of its members, sharing with the National Academy of Sciences the responsibility for advising the federal government. The National Academy of Engineering also sponsors engineering programs aimed at meeting national needs, encourages education and research, and recognizes the superior achievements of engineers. Dr. Robert M. White is president of the National Academy of Engineering.

The Institute of Medicine was established in 1970 by the National Academy of Sciences to secure the services of eminent members of appropriate professions in the examination of policy matters pertaining to the health of the public. The Institute acts under the responsibility given to the National Academy of Sciences by its congressional charter to be an adviser to the federal government and, upon its own initiative, to identify issues of medical care, research, and education. Dr. Samuel O. Thier is president of the Institute of Medicine.

The National Research Council was organized by the National Academy of Sciences in 1916 to associate the broad community of science and technology with the Academy's purposes of furthering knowledge and advising the federal government. Functioning in accordance with general policies determined by the Academy, the Council has become the principal operating agency of both the National Academy of Sciences and the National Academy of Engineering in providing services to the government, the public, and the scientific and engineering communities. The Council is administered jointly by both Academies and the Institute of Medicine. Dr. Frank Press and Dr. Robert M. White are chairman and vice chairman, respectively, of the National Research Council.

The project was supported by the Agency for Toxic Substances and Disease Registry, U.S. Public Health Service, Department of Health and Human Services.

Preface

In response to a request from the Agency for Toxic Substances and Disease Registry (ATSDR), the Board on Environmental Studies and Toxicology in the Commission on Life Sciences of the National Research Council (NRC) convened the Committee on Environmental Epidemiology. The Board charged the Committee to review current knowledge of the human health effects caused by exposure to hazardous-waste sites and to suggest how to improve the scientific bases for evaluating the effects of environmental pollution on public health, including specifically the conduct of health assessments at Superfund sites. This first report of the committee examines and evaluates the published scientific literature on health effects that could be linked with exposure to hazardous-waste disposal sites, and develops recommendations about major data gaps that need to be remedied in order to advance the field.

With additional support from the Environmental Protection Agency, a second report of the committee will identify research opportunities and issues in methodology for environmental epidemiology and will select and evaluate a sample of non-peer-reviewed reports on the subject of the epidemiologic study of hazardous wastes. This literature includes such sources as state health department reports and relevant technical evaluations from judicial decisions that have been subject to extensive review, but are not available in the peer-reviewed literature. To the extent feasible, the second report also will assess newly available reports from Eastern Europe and Asia that may be relevant.

In light of the paucity of information readily available, the Committee struggled with its charge early on. We developed the policy of looking at peer-reviewed, published studies of persons exposed at hazardous-waste sites, and also examining those studies involving environmental exposures similar to those that might be found at such sites.

The chapters reflect the consensus of the committee. We are grateful to a number of colleagues who provided drafts and critiques of sections of the report for the Committee, including Drs. Diane Wagener, Director of Environmental Epidemiology at the National Center for Health Statistics; Claire Weinberg, National Institute of Environmental Health Sciences; Peter Infante, Health Standards Division, the Occupational Safety and Health Administration; Ken Cantor, Environmental Epidemiology Branch, National Cancer Institute; Lynn Goldman, Public Health Administrator, State of California; and Marvin Schneiderman, Senior Scientist, NRC. In preparing this report, we have met with citizen groups, industry representatives and state officials (including the National Governors' Association Task Force on Environmental Epidemiology), all of whom provided valuable suggestions. Dr. Barry Johnson, Assistant Administrator for the Agency for Toxic Substances (ATSDR), provided helpful recommendations and guidance at the outset of the study, as did a number of members of that agency. Dr. Dorothy Canter of EPA assisted us in gathering relevant agency information and navigating through the bureaucratic maze.

Linda Miller Poore provided able research and administrative support and document supervision, and Paulette Adams managed document preparation and meeting organization. Most importantly, the committee acknowledges its enormous debt to Dr. Devra Davis, Scholar in Residence, National Research Council, who not only ably fulfilled the role of project director, but contributed substantially to the drafting and revision of all chapters in the report. Without her skills and input, the report would have lacked much, and our task could never have been completed in the timely manner it has been.

Finally, as chairman, I should like to thank all of the members of the committee for their expertise, input and support throughout our deliberations.

ANTHONY B. MILLER, *Chairman*
Committee on Environmental
Epidemiology

Contents

Tables

Figures

ENVIRONMENTAL EPIDEMIOLOGY

Summary

P ART OF OUR MODERN HERITAGE is the increasing volume of waste created by all industrial societies. Today, there also is unprecedented concern over the potential consequences for public health and the environment of exposure to wastes that are deemed hazardous under a variety of regulatory regimes. According to recent opinion polls, the American public believes that hazardous wastes constitute a serious threat to public health. In contrast, many scientists and administrators in the field do not share this belief. On the basis of its best efforts to evaluate the published literature relevant to this subject, the committee cannot confirm or refute either view. A decade after implementation of Superfund, and despite congressional efforts to redirect the program, substantial public health concerns remain, and critical information on the distribution of exposures and health effects associated with hazardous-waste sites is still lacking.

Without doubt, however, substances toxic to humans and several animal species abound in hazardous-waste sites. Human health studies have shown that serious health effects cannot be ruled out. Indeed, they have occurred at a few hazardous-waste sites. Since the earliest days of industrialization, substantial volumes of waste have been produced and sometimes disposed of both at specific sites and through broader distribution in ways that could create problems for later generations. In the U.S. more than 6 billion tons of waste is produced annually—nearly 50,000 pounds per person. One recent EPA survey found that more than 40 million people live within four miles and about 4 million within one mile of a Superfund site. Residential proximity itself, however, does not mean that exposures and health risks are occurring, only that the potential for exposure is increased.

At the request of the Agency for Toxic Substances and Disease Registry (ATSDR), the National Research Council (NRC) convened the Committee on Environmental Epidemiology to review current knowledge of the human health effects caused by exposure to substances emanating from hazardous-waste sites and to clarify and suggest how to improve the scientific bases for evaluating the effects of environmental pollution on public health, including specifically the conduct of health assessments at hazardous-waste sites. With additional support from the Environmental Protection Agency, the committee is preparing a second volume that will examine relevant information from state health departments, and selected unpublished studies from other sources that are relevant to this field.

This first report of the committee reviews and assesses the published scientific literature on health effects that could be linked with exposure to substances from hazardous-waste disposal sites and makes recommendations about major data gaps that need to be filled as scientists go on to answer important questions in the field. A second volume will review state-generated reports and studies emerging from other countries and will recommend research opportunities for the field of environmental epidemiology.

ORGANIZATION OF THE REPORT

This report is organized into two broad sections; it contains eight chapters overall. The first section—Chapters 1, 2, and 3—introduces the study of the public health impact of exposure to hazardous-waste sites; discusses the role of state, local, and federal regulations in shaping the development of studies in this area; and sets forth the complexity of assessing exposures to hazardous materials.

The introductory chapter defines environmental epidemiology and discusses conventional views of statistical significance and guidelines for inferring causation based on epidemiologic evidence. After that, the principles of statistical inference are evaluated in the context of constraints associated with the litigious and controversial world of hazardous-waste sites and toxic torts. Toxic torts is a rapidly growing field of litigation that involves legal claims of injuries allegedly caused by exposure to toxic chemicals. The relatively small number of studies published reflects the difficulties of conducting valid studies of this complex issue, the tendency of courts to seal records of resolved disputes on these matters, and the meager resources committed to such studies.

In recognition of the role of government agencies in generating information, Chapter 2 discusses relevant federal and state laws, regulations, and programs for assessing and remediating hazardous-waste sites. Chapter 3 discusses available data on materials commonly found at listed hazardous-waste sites and notes some problems in estimating human exposures to these agents.

The remainder of the report reviews the published literature and considers the problems of obtaining epidemiologic information about specific routes of exposure to hazardous wastes. Chapters 4, 5, and 6 review evidence on health effects associated with toxic pollution of air, water, and soil and food, respectively, noting those few studies on hazardous-waste sites and other relevant studies of adverse health effects of materials found at such sites. Chapter 7 describes important developments in the study of biologic markers as they relate directly to the environmental epidemiology of hazardous-waste sites. Chapter 8 identifies data gaps in the areas discussed in preceding chapters, summarizes the literature reviewed in this report, and recommends that a six-part program in environmental epidemiology be developed to inform policy decisions about risks to public health presented by hazardous-waste sites.

SECTION ONE:
PUBLIC HEALTH AND HAZARDOUS WASTES: THE CONTEXT

Chapter 1: Introduction

In recent years the term "environmental epidemiology" has seen extensive use, although it has not been well defined. In Chapter 1, the Committee on Environmental Epidemiology therefore adopts the following definition:

Environmental epidemiology is the study of the effect on human health of physical, biologic, and chemical factors in the external environment, broadly conceived. By examining specific populations or communities exposed to different ambient environments, it seeks to clarify the relationship between physical, biologic or chemical factors and human health.

Real world constraints impede the ability to estimate health effects associated with exposures to hazardous wastes. The committee relies on a combination of evidence from different sources to reach conclusions in accordance with its mandate to estimate health effects associated with hazardous wastes.

• Knowledge of *potential exposures* is derived from studies that characterize the substances found at hazardous-waste sites.
• Knowledge of *health risks* to humans from potential exposures can be obtained from a variety of sources. For some chemicals such knowledge will be available from published studies of occupational risks, usually involving higher exposures than those in the general environment. For others, especially for airborne and waterborne exposures, knowledge of health risks will come from studies of the general effects of the pollutants and from clinical reports, case-comparison studies, and animal studies, and it can be extended to circumstances where such pollutants are emitted from hazardous-waste sites.
• Knowledge of *symptomatology* or *disease occurrence* has in some instances been derived from studies of populations exposed to hazardous-waste sites. Often, these reports have not described exposures accurately, or they have failed completely to identify a specific causal factor. Nevertheless, with the knowledge that is available about exposure elsewhere, and from the knowledge that some of these exposures can result in the observed symptomatology or diseases found in excess in those exposed to hazardous-waste sites, sufficient indirect evidence of causality can sometimes be inferred.

The world of epidemiology, like that of any human science, seldom permits elegant inferences to be drawn about causation. The object domain of epidemiology consists of numerous uncontrollable aspects, with considerable variations. To make a reasonable inference of causation in environmental epidemiology, eight basic characteristics of the findings should be considered: the strength, specificity, and consistency of the association, the period of exposure, the relationship between the dose and the response, the effects of the removal of the suggested cause, the biologic plausibility of the association, and the overall coherence of the findings.

The advent of meta-analysis as a technique that pools related studies offers an important opportunity to strengthen the inferences that can be drawn from epidemiologic research. Potentially misleading conclusions can be drawn from single studies because of insufficient sample size, inadequacies of exposure determination, or publication and other biases. Meta-analysis reduces these problems and can lessen the danger of misinterpretation because it allows for combining relevant studies. Meta-analysis is limited by lack of routine publication of negative findings, and interpretation must be tempered by the awareness that reporting and publication biases can distort the sample of studies available for pooling.

Chapter 2: State and Federal Context for Environmental Epidemiology of Hazardous Wastes

Chapter 2 discusses how federal and state environmental policies have largely shaped the development of environmental epidemiology as it pertains to the study of hazardous-waste sites in the U.S. First, scientists working for state and federal agencies perform most of such studies. Second, federal and state regulations determine the nature and limitations of available data on environmental contamination related to hazardous-waste sites. Third, federal and state agencies are continuously involved in the process of defining which chemicals found in the environment are of concern for human health and the levels at which action should be taken to protect human health.

The legislation that produced these state and federal programs was clearly intended to protect human health. Congress and the states enacted the legislation which created Superfund in the early 1980s in response to public concern about the effect of hazardous-waste sites on the health of nearby communities—concerns that persisted and escalated through the decade as the dimensions of the problem continued to expand. ATSDR was also established by this legislation to provide health assessments and other relevant information on hazardous-waste sites. These programs have not allayed public concerns. Public opinion surveys consistently rank hazardous-waste sites among the most serious environmental risks and the environment as an issue of great public concern. Hazardous-waste sites are a major public health management issue in every state. Half of the U.S. population and 95 percent of the rural population relies on groundwater as the main source of drinking water. Each year thousands of wells are closed because of hazardous-waste contamination. According to a number of polls, the public fears hazardous waste, wants it cleaned up, and is willing to pay the enormous sums currently spent on Superfund because of the belief that this program will protect public health.

Chapter 2 questions how so much effort and money could have been spent with such a moderate yield in knowledge. It reviews federal and state legislation, policies, and programs that determine how hazardous-waste sites are evaluated; what information on exposure and health effects is collected; how the data are analyzed and used in setting priorities and planning remediation programs; and what proportion of hazardous-waste-control budgets is spent on assessing population exposures and risks. It also discusses the nature and extent of environmental epidemiology carried out by federal and state agencies, and recommends a program for the field that will generate needed information.

The intent of Congress in enacting legislation on hazardous-waste sites was clear. As set forth in the legislative history of the Comprehensive Environmental Response, Compensation, and Liability Act (CERCLA), passed in 1980 and generally known as Superfund, the goals of the bill included

> [establishment of] an inventory of inactive hazardous-waste sites in a systematic manner, establishment of priorities among the sites based on relative danger, a response program to contain dangerous releases from inactive hazardous-waste sites, acceleration of the elimination of unsafe hazardous-waste sites, and a systematic program of funding to identify, evaluate and take responsive actions at inactive hazardous-waste sites to assure protection of public health and the environment in a cost-effective manner.

In essence, Congress wanted to know how much environmental contamination has been caused by hazardous-waste sites and how serious a threat this is to human health. It also wanted to ensure that the sites that presented the worst problems would be dealt with first. The actual health risks to communities living around specific hazardous-waste sites were to be identified, so that the information could be used in making decisions about remediation. Finally, Congress's intent was that the remediation programs would do the most possible, with limited resources, to protect the health of the public.

These objectives are in fact the traditional elements of a public health strategy: The discovery and preliminary assessment of as many sites as possible to describe the universe of potential exposures; the priority ranking of sites by a defined protocol, to identify and act on those most urgently requiring attention; the collection and use of data on current human exposures and health effects early in the triage and evaluation processes; and the development of remediation programs with direct and continuous attention to the public health effects of releases from the sites. Analyses of the limited federal and state regulatory support for environmental epidemiology reveal, however, that the intent of Congress in creating Superfund has not been realized, in that the public health consequences of exposures to substances from hazardous-waste sites have not been adequately assessed.

Moreover, there is little reason to believe that current procedures identify the most important abandoned hazardous-waste sites, from the point of view of public health. Decisions have been made not to list some sites on the National Priority List (NPL) of Superfund even though those sites have never been fully characterized. The congressional Office of Technology Assessment (OTA) notes that efforts to assess candidate NPL sites typically relegate public health concerns to a minor role; the process as a whole is directed at remediation, rather than at the assessment of public health risks.

The absence of a comprehensive national program to identify and evaluate hazardous-waste sites makes it difficult to assess fully the nature and magnitude of the problem for the health of the public. Similar difficulties attend efforts to estimate the public health effects of exposures to other potentially hazardous materials, such as unregulated nonconventional pollutants that can result from agricultural practices and industrial processes. The current regulatory system has failed to devise a protocol for managing hazardous-waste sites that incorporates the essential components of public health policy. Not only is it possible that the public residing in some of these neighborhoods is imperiled, but the conditions for development of environmental epidemiology programs and methods are so adverse as to impede useful scientific investigations of many important questions.

As the committee's review of federal programs concludes, there is no comprehensive national inventory of hazardous-waste sites, no site discovery program, no minimum data set on potential human exposures, no adequate system for the early identification of sites for which immediate action to protect public health or continued surveillance of health effects could be necessary, and no validation or evaluation of the components of the site assessment process. The Environmental Protection Agency (EPA) and the ATSDR are instituting some improvements in each of these areas, but these improvements are largely limited to sites proposed for or already on the NPL.

A six-part environmental epidemiology program needs to be developed to improve the bases for policy decisions about hazardous-waste sites.

• Establish an active and coordinated system of site discovery for hazardous-waste sites, based in EPA and providing technical assistance to other federal and state programs. An aggressive site discovery program, in combination with improved assessments and triage of sites for interim and final remediation, will restore the original congressional intent to protect the health of the public from exposure to hazardous-waste sites.

• Define a revised approach to site assessments that integrates epidemiologic determinations of population exposures, health effects, and the necessity of interim and final remediation or other actions into a continuum of site evaluation. Establish protocols and criteria for the revised preliminary assessment of all sites, with triggers for interim remediation or other action, such as relocation, and require that all sites undergo a revised preliminary assessment within one year of discovery.

• Establish a comprehensive national inventory of hazardous-waste sites that will track the status of all sites through assessment and remediation or closure and include health hazard assessments. Use the inventory to ensure that sites are not deferred or placed in closure status without a revised preliminary assessment as described above.

• Rigorously evaluate the data and methodologies used in site assessment, including the characterization of potential and actual releases of contaminants to groundwater, surface water, air, and soil that result in human exposure. Evaluate the methodologies for estimating which populations are exposed to hazardous-waste-site emissions, and use this information in preliminary assessments and in deciding how to protect the public health. Evaluate compliance with public health recommendations for the protection of exposed populations and site remediation.

• Improve and expand research in environmental epidemiology to illuminate the distribution and severity of exposures, risks, and health effects associated with hazardous-waste sites. Authorize ATSDR to direct responsible parties to conduct research to fill data gaps on critical substances. Expand the ATSDR mandate to establish an extensive program of applied research, including exposure registries linked to priority substances, and further the development of surveillance methods such as community health data bases, biologic monitoring, and sentinel events, that is, events that may signal environmental health problems.

• ATSDR, the National Institute of Environmental Health Sciences (NIEHS), and other relevant agencies should expand cooperative agreements with states and develop a comprehensive program of technical assistance for state and local agencies. They also should provide funding for competitive research grants and contracts in environmental epidemiology.

Chapter 3: Dimensions of the Problem: Exposure Assessment

Chapter 3 notes that exposure assessment is a crucial, and often inadequate, component of studies in environmental epidemiology. In order to establish causal relationships between exposure to chemical and physical agents from hazardous-waste sites and adverse consequences to human health, obtaining valid measures or estimates of exposure is essential.

The field of exposure assessment entails numerous techniques to measure or estimate the contaminant, its source, the environmental media of exposure, avenues of transport through each medium, chemical and physical transformations, routes of entry to the body, intensity and frequency of contact, and its spatial and temporal concentration patterns. It also includes estimations of total exposure to different compounds and mixtures. Exposure assessment has proved difficult, because epidemiologic research typically involves retrospective studies. Records of ambient pollutant concentrations can sometimes provide a surrogate for exposure, but these surrogates are not always available, and direct measures of past exposures have not usually been recorded and must be estimated with models.

Within the past decade, estimates of the number of potential NPL sites have grown dramatically. OTA concludes that there could be as many as 439,000 candidate sites. These sites include mining waste sites, leaking underground storage tanks, pesticide-contaminated sites, federal facilities, radioactive release sites, underground injection wells, municipal gas facilities, and wood-preserving plants, among others. As of December 1988, one ATSDR report concluded, 109 NPL sites (11 percent of the total) were associated with a risk to human health because of actual exposure (11 sites) or probable exposure (98 sites) to hazardous chemical agents that could cause harm to human health. Chiefly on the basis of exposure assessments, these sites were placed in the categories of "urgent public health concern" or "public health concern."

Repositories of potentially dangerous substances can be found at a number of hazardous-waste sites that have been generated by a wide range of activities. Information about the materials generally reflects the data requirements of environmental engineering and site remediation, rather than public health considerations. Accordingly, whether the materials pose a risk to public health cannot readily be determined in the absence of more detailed information about potential human exposures.

The focus of many studies has been on site-specific characterization, even though pollutants do not respect such boundaries. Given the potential for movement of materials in groundwater and air and the importance of multiple routes of exposure, efforts need to proceed to estimate plume characteristics and groundwater staging to improve the ability to anticipate the movement of pollutants and ultimately to prevent greater exposures. Similarly, exposure from domestic water is not limited to ingestion, but includes airborne exposures from materials released during showering, bathing, or cooking. Therefore, estimates of exposure from domestic water need to be expanded to take into account the role of airborne exposures.

The best estimates are that groundwater is the major source of drinking water for about 50 percent of the U.S. population. In California, groundwater provides drinking water to nearly 70 percent of the population. Millions of tons of hazardous materials are slowly migrating into groundwater in areas where they could pose problems in the future, even though current risks could be negligible. For instance, plumes of chemicals, including many nonconventional pollutants (NCPs) that are not currently regulated, are moving down the canyon from the Superfund site at Stringfellow Pits in California and may pose important problems in the future.

There is evidence that NCPs are a potentially important source of hazardous exposure. Some preliminary toxicologic studies suggest that NCPs have important biologic properties, environmental persistence, and mobility. Additional studies are needed to characterize the mixture of materials deposited as hazardous wastes and to give better estimates of their potential transport and fate in the environment. In the broadest sense these unidentified, unregulated substances represent a risk of unknown magnitude. The absence of evidence of their risk is solely the result of the failure to conduct research; it should not be misconstrued as demonstrating that NCPs and "inert" pesticide components are without risk.

SECTION TWO:
HAZARDOUS WASTES IN AIR, WATER, SOIL, AND FOOD; BIOLOGIC MARKERS

Chapter 4: Air Exposures

Chapter 4 notes that although there is an extensive body of literature on the epidemiology of air pollution, there is little information about airborne exposures from hazardous-waste sites. To improve the scientific basis for studying those potential effects, methodological approaches to the study of air pollution are reviewed and discussed in terms of their applicability to the study of hazardous wastes. Also, relevant studies on airborne exposure to materials similar to those found at hazardous-waste sites are assessed, along with some evidence of exposures from hazardous-waste sites or other related exposures, such as might occur with the sick building syndrome.

Many approaches have been taken to the study of air pollution epidemiology. The methods can be used in the study of hazardous wastes, but their successful application will vary. Thus, studies of trends over time in air pollution and disease patterns have produced a growing body of literature that has associated day-to-day fluctuations in air pollution with daily fluctuations in mortality across a wide range of exposures with no evidence of thresholds. It is not likely to be worthwhile to conduct such studies at hazardous-waste sites, especially because the pollutants are complex and because there are no long-term records, such as exist for a number of monitored air pollutants.

Cross-sectional studies provide epidemiologic snapshots of a given area at one point in time. Recent computer technology has permitted maps to be drawn that show comparative mortality data from different regions of the U.S., Canada, and other industrial countries. Such maps can show county-wide cancer and other mortality data by decade, for example, as a hypothesis-generating tool to detect geographic variations in these diseases and to infer possible causes. Of more relevance to hazardous-waste studies are small-scale comparisons of adjacent counties or ZIP codes, where differences could be better highlighted. The study of health effects that have shorter latency than most cancers—such as birth defects, neurologic effects, and other acute and chronic effects—increases the likelihood that a connection can be drawn between environmental exposures and disease.

Cross-sectional community studies typically compare communities with different levels of air pollution or populations that live different distances from a hazardous-waste site. All such studies have several problems: Measurement error occurs because of the assumption of the same exposure for every subject within a group. There can be undetected differences between communities for risk factors, such as illness, tobacco use, or occupational exposures. There can be "recall bias" if one group knows it is in the high-exposure category. There is little standardization of the equipment used to measure exposure in different locations.

In spite of these difficulties, successful community studies have been done on air pollution patterns. In contrast to purely descriptive studies, which lack information on potential confounders, community studies generally contain data on nonpollution risk factors. A few studies have involved materials like those which occur at hazardous-waste sites. Excesses of the rare cancer angiosarcoma occurred in residents near a vinyl chloride manufacturing plant. Another study found increased rates of birth defects in children whose parents lived near such plants.

Longitudinal analyses also have been developed for the epidemiologic study of air pollution. These have some direct bearing on the study of hazardous wastes, and they include long-term studies of actively exposed persons, prospective studies of a distinct group, and follow-up studies of exposed children. Here, problems of execution relate to the emotional turmoil that usually surrounds suspicion of exposure to hazardous wastes, the difficulty of following residents who might have moved away, and the climate of distrust that sometimes arises after the discovery of a hazardous-waste site. In addition, because the courts often seal resolved lawsuits, potentially valuable information on long-term consequences of exposure is unavailable for scientific review and analysis. The committee's second report will discuss this further.

Although few studies directly assess airborne exposures to hazardous wastes, the committee finds persuasive evidence that health effects can occur from such exposures. Review of the relevant animal literature on compounds known to occur at hazardous-waste sites, along with the few epidemiologic studies, shows that a wide range of effects may occur, including such serious diseases as cancer, birth defects, and neurologic disease. Studies of populations near hazardous-waste sites have detected complaints of neurobehavioral symptoms. Although it might be concluded that recall bias explains the differences in such subjectively reported symptoms, the real possibility nevertheless exists that the symptoms complained of are more sensitive as indicators of significant exposure than are more severe diseases that have long latencies, such as cancer and other chronic diseases.

The constellation of self-reported symptoms in persons living near some hazardous-waste sites shows remarkable consistency in populations with similar exposures in different countries. These symptoms have recently been provoked in double blinded tests using subjects who might or might not have previously reported symptoms. Those exposed to odorless test agents developed neurobehavioral symptoms, further strengthening the argument that there is a physiologic basis to some of the complaints.

Symptom reports appear to be sensitive indicators of adverse health effects. Simultaneous use of air monitoring and diary records could reduce the problem of recall bias, which is especially troubling in situations where people suspect ill effects could be produced by their exposures. These methods are particularly valuable when small changes in pollutant levels cannot be detected by the subjects in a study. The committee believes that further studies of acute symptoms linked to monitoring data, based on concurrent exposure measurements, are likely to reveal that reported symptoms are not completely explained by recall bias. The current data base clearly indicates the importance of continued use of these techniques.

Chapter 5: Domestic Water Consumption

Water is the key medium of concern in most hazardous-waste sites. Chapter 5 reviews evidence on the possible impact on health of waterborne exposures that could emanate from hazardous-waste sites, and it discusses several abandoned hazardous-waste sites in the U.S., such as Love Canal, New York, and Woburn, Massachusetts. Contamination of groundwater and aquifers occurs where the waste dumps are poorly constructed or managed, or where wastes have been disposed of improperly, sometimes over long periods.

Few studies have been conducted directly on populations exposed to water contaminated with hazardous wastes. Accordingly, this chapter reviews evidence about some compounds commonly found at hazardous-waste sites that have been shown to cause adverse effects in humans exposed to these materials through the use of domestic water. Epidemiologic evidence on the risk to health from contaminated water from hazardous-waste sites or from other sources of contamination, such as pesticide runoff, has largely been derived from ecologic (descriptive) studies, and therefore is seldom conclusive as to cause. The ecologic studies that involve broad-scale comparisons of available data are unable to control for important confounding variables such as smoking, occupational exposures, dietary factors, or other relevant exposures.

A number of descriptive and case-control studies indicate that drinking water can include by-products of domestic water chlorination that pose increased risks of cancer. Some chlorination by-products, particularly halogenated hydrocarbons or trihalomethanes (THMs), occur in greater quantities in drinking water if large amounts of organic matter are present. Two THMs, chloroform and carbon tetrachloride, have been commonly found in the chemical mixtures at some toxic dump sites at levels above those permitted in drinking water. The by-products of chlorination can include dichloroacetic acid and trichloroacetic acid, which are metabolites of trichloroethylene (TCE), one of the most common contaminants at Superfund sites. Of course, chlorinated water and its by-products do not come from hazardous-waste sites. Still, studies of the impact of these materials on public health are relevant to this report, insofar as exposures can occur in connection with hazardous-waste sites.

The largest individual- and population-based case-control study of cancer and exposure to contaminated drinking water was performed in 1978 in 10 areas of the U.S. by researchers from the National Cancer Institute. Their results showed the risk of bladder cancer increased with intake of beverages made with tap water. In particular, women and nonsmokers of both sexes who consumed chlorinated surface water at rates above the median for 60 or more years had rates of bladder cancer that were more than three times the rates of those who had not consumed surface water. The gender difference could be due to the fact that men are subject to other, more important risk factors for bladder cancer.

In New Jersey, descriptive studies have linked exposures to hazardous-waste sites to increased cancer risks. These studies have related cancer mortality at the county and municipal levels to environmental variables, including the location of chemical toxic-waste-disposal sites, and presumed contamination of water and air. One analysis of age-adjusted female reproductive organ and breast cancer mortality showed significant positive associations between breast cancer mortality and proximity to toxic disposal sites among whites in 21 New Jersey counties. The clusters of excess cancer mortality were confined for the most part to the highly urban and industrial northeastern part of the state. Such descriptive investigations provide, at best, suggestive evidence.

Other evidence linking consumption of industrially polluted, domestic water use with cancer is provided by an unusually strong cohort study of residents of North Carolina, who consumed raw, industrially polluted river water from 1947 to 1976. Residents had rates of all forms of cancer that were more than twice those expected, at times corresponding to the expected latency for cancer. Moreover, once exposure ceased, rates returned to the expected level, adjusting for latency.

The study of adverse reproductive effects on males and females exposed to hazardous-waste sites remains surprisingly sparse. Nonetheless, several important reports have found adverse reproductive effects associated with use of contaminated domestic water. In a case-control study it was found that women in the Mount Gambier area of South Australia who consumed principally groundwater had nearly a threefold increase in the risk of bearing malformed children who had defects of the central nervous system compared with women who drank only rainwater. The children of parents who regularly used water that contained nitrate at more than 15 parts per million had four times more central nervous system defects. It was recognized, however, that other, as-yet-undetected chemicals could have been responsible for the excess.

Despite the serious problems that must be overcome in developing reliable data on the connection between birth defects and environmental contamination, several lines of evidence point to a causal nexus between exposure to TCE and cardiac congenital anomalies. Both animal and human studies have found that exposure to TCE increases the risk of some cardiac anomalies. Persons living in a small valley of Tucson, Arizona, who consumed contaminated water were three times more likely to produce offspring with congenital heart disease. A limited number of reports in the peer-reviewed scientific literature have linked spontaneous abortion, low birth weight, and birth defects to the consumption of domestic water or to other environmental exposures. A variety of other health effects, including liver and neurologic disease, have also been associated with waterborne exposure to substances from hazardous-waste sites. Some studies have detected increased rates of neurologic deficits in persons with chronic exposures to contaminants such as TCE.

Several factors lead us to conclude that contamination of domestic water supplies with a number of hazardous chemicals, such as those that could be encountered at hazardous-waste sites, is injurious to human health, although the magnitude of the risk cannot be determined. Some of the common by-products of chlorination also occur as contaminants at Superfund sites, such as dichloroacetic and trichloroacetic acid, metabolites of TCE. Moreover, exposures are not limited to ingestion, but include those due to volatization of hazardous gases and dermal absorption.

There is also evidence from epidemiologic studies that neurologic, hepatic, and immunologic function can be damaged by exposure to domestic water contaminated with some toxic chemicals. The long-term consequences of the abnormalities detected, however, are largely unknown and must be the subject of further research, on which the committee will comment in more detail in its next report.

Chapter 6: Soil and Food as Potential Sources of Exposure at Hazardous-Waste Sites

Soil provides a usually unrecognized source of exposure to contaminants. Models indicate that adults can be exposed directly or indirectly, through the food chain, and that children incur greater exposures per unit of body weight. Home gardening and ingestion of subsistence or recreational fish can be important sources of these contaminants. In addition, commercial shellfish and finfish may also be contaminated. Epidemiologic studies of hazardous-waste sites need to incorporate broader consideration of soil and food as routes of exposure.

It is difficult to identify completely the routes of exposure when ill health effects are suspected from hazardous-waste sites, as Chapter 5 notes. The same problem of determining precisely who is exposed exists for exposure through ingestion of soil as it does for exposure through domestic water use, in that direct ingestion does not constitute the sole route. Soil ingestion suffers from an additional complexity. Except among small children, it is unusual for soil to be ingested directly, although adults do ingest small amounts of soil nonetheless. Unless a chemical is extremely potent, the exposure is particularly direct (as with certain occupations), or there is extensive dust contamination of food and residences, exposure due chiefly to contaminated soil is unusual. However, contaminated soil and domestic water can act as vehicles for contamination of plant or animal foods that are subsequently ingested—as is the case for mercury and pesticide contamination of fish and heavy metal or pesticide contamination of fruits and vegetables. The questions of the effects of pesticide residues on foods and the subsequent health risks for children are the subject of study for another NRC committee, and are not considered here.

A recent report from the Institute of Medicine documents the extent to which fish may bioconcentrate lipophilic pollutants from the surrounding water. Persons that consume fish taken from contaminated waters have average blood levels of polychlorinated biphenyls (PCBs) that are several times those found in other general population groups, in ranges that extend into concentrations typically found in industrially exposed workers. In the U.S., mercury contamination of fish is especially prevalent in the Great Lakes region. Although advisories have been issued to pregnant women, nursing mothers, and women who intend to have children, no such advisory has been developed for men who may wish to reproduce, despite evidence that sperm are also vulnerable to subtle toxic effects.

The routes of exposure to PCBs are not well characterized, despite the ubiquity of this compound and its occurrence at some level in most persons tested in the U.S. PCBs also occur at many Superfund sites. Studies from a number of research institutions confirm that exposure to background levels of PCB below both the relevant standards for occupational exposure and those for food contamination produces developmental deficits in children. In addition, studies of Japanese children exposed to higher levels of PCBs prenatally and through lactation indicate higher rates of abnormalities of lungs, skin, nails, teeth, and gums, low birthweight, and reduced growth. In investigations of a number of species, perinatal exposure to PCBs causes similar effects. However, humans appear to be particularly sensitive. Other studies have indicated that exposure to PCBs occupationally or through transformer fires is linked to a range of neurobehavioral and functional problems, including muscle pain, skin color changes, nervousness, or sleep problems.

Because of the difficulties of determining relevant exposures and health outcomes, studies of sentinel animals can provide some hypothesis-generating results. Wild mice trapped in Love Canal, New York, showed weight loss and impeded development associated with areas of the greatest contamination. Similar studies of wildlife and of domestic animals could provide useful indicators of, or sentinels for, potential exposure at hazardous-waste sites, especially for playgrounds or other sites that have been used for recreation that involves frequent contact with soil.

Chapter 7: Biologic Markers in Studies of Hazardous-Waste Sites

Chapter 7 draws on emerging developments in molecular biology to describe a conceptual framework for using biologic markers in the study of hazardous-waste sites. This chapter reviews studies of biologic markers in persons exposed to materials such as those commonly encountered at hazardous-waste sites, along with the few studies of persons directly exposed at sites. Examples of markers of exposure, effect, and susceptibility are provided and methodologic or other important considerations in their use are presented. Important ethical and legal issues are involved in the use of biologic markers in studies at hazardous-waste sites.

As defined by the NRC Committee on Biologic Markers, a biologic marker is any cellular or molecular indicator of toxic exposure, adverse health effects, or susceptibility. It is useful to classify biologic markers into three types—exposure, effect, and susceptibility—and to describe the conditions (normal exposure, disease, or susceptibility) that each kind of marker represents. A biologic marker of exposure is an exogenous substance or its metabolites or the product of an interaction between a xenobiotic agent and some target molecule or cell that is measured in a compartment within an organism. A biologic marker of effect is a measurable biochemical, physiologic, or other alteration within an organism that, depending on magnitude, can be recognized as an established or potential health impairment or disease. A biologic marker of susceptibility is an indicator of an inherent or acquired limitation of an organism's ability to respond to the challenge of exposure to a specific xenobiotic substance.

Biologic markers have been used occasionally in epidemiologic studies of hazardous-waste sites, predominantly as indicators of effect. An array of dermatologic, behavioral, and neurological symptoms have been identified that might provide markers of exposure to toxic chemicals, or early indicators of effect. Not counting symptoms or frank signs of morbidity, changes in liver enzymes, which indicate liver function, are among the most commonly used, presumably because of their nonspecificity and ease of analysis. Sometimes these effects are transitory, as was shown in a study of persons with increases in the liver enzyme alkaline phosphatase who had been exposed to chlorinated chemicals in domestic water in Hardeman County, Tennessee.

Other multiphasic tests to find markers of exposure or effect in blood and urine also have been used, but to a lesser extent. For example, serum cholesterol, gamma-glutamyl transpeptidase (an indicator of enzyme induction in the liver), and blood pressure have been studied as markers of effect in residents of Triana, Alabama, who were exposed to PCBs chiefly from subsistence eating of contaminated fish. Eighty to 90 percent of the population in Triana had levels of PCB within the range found in other community groups. For those with elevated levels, results indicated that PCB was positively associated with measures of blood pressure and other indicators, independent of age, sex, body mass, and social class. Similar findings have been reported in studies of workers exposed to PCBs in capacitor manufacturing.

Researchers also have studied markers of neurologic function in persons from Woburn, Massachusetts, some six years after exposure to TCE ceased, and in others with similar exposure. In Woburn, TCE levels in domestic water had been from 30 to 80 times higher than the recommended EPA Maximum Contamination Level of 5 parts per billion (ppb). Exposed and control subjects were studied with a neurobehavioral evaluation protocol that included clinical tests, nerve conduction studies, blink reflex measurements, and extensive neuropsychological testing. The highly significant differences in a variety of neuropsychologic tests indicate that neurotoxic effects occurred in those who had been exposed.

Although they are not commonly thought of as constituting markers, the results of neurobehavioral tests can provide a diverse range of measures of toxic exposures and effects. A battery of neurobehavioral tests has been applied to the study of persons exposed to materials that occur at hazardous-waste sites. A comprehensive review of developing techniques in neurobehavioral assessment found consistent and significant neurobehavioral effects and a range of other subtle neurological alterations in persons exposed to metals, solvents, and insecticides, with some indication of greater effects in those with higher estimated exposures. These findings corroborate studies that reveal that TCE inhalation induces a range of neurotoxic effects in rodents.

Although the risk of cancer provides a central focus for much research on markers, risks to human reproduction offer another focal point for which much shorter time periods between exposure and evidence of a related health effect are involved. Several studies have revealed that workplace exposures to hazardous materials, as well as consumption of alcohol, drugs, and tobacco, influence both the ability of males and females to reproduce and the health of their offspring. Whether environmental exposures could also create such effects on reproductive function needs to be studied further.

A series of studies using refined and automated measures of sperm concentration and sperm head morphology has recently found significant effects on male reproductive capacity related to exposures to pesticides. Studies of Vietnam veterans noted that those who served in Vietnam were twice as likely to have lowered sperm concentrations and significantly different sperm morphology, with longer axis length and greater head circumference. The number of children fathered by both groups was comparable. Whatever the mechanism, a variety of characteristics of sperm have been detected and found to change with exposures to pesticides and other toxic chemicals, including those encountered at hazardous-waste sites or through other channels. Markers of exposure or effect can include changes in sperm shape, concentration, pH, viability, velocity, and motility.

CONCLUSIONS

Whether Superfund and other hazardous-waste programs actually protect human health is a critical question with respect to federal and state efforts to clean up hazardous wastes. To answer this question requires information on the scope of potential and actual human exposures to hazardous wastes and about the health effects that could be associated with these exposures. Based on its review of the published literature on the subject, the committee finds that the question cannot be answered. Although billions of dollars have been spent during the past decade to study and manage hazardous-waste sites in the U.S., an insignificant portion has been devoted to evaluate the attendant health risks. This has resulted in an inadequate amount of information about the connection between exposure and effect.

A decade after implementation of Superfund, and despite congressional efforts to redirect the program, substantial public health concerns remain, and critical information on the distribution of exposures and health effects associated with hazardous-waste sites is still lacking. Whether for the purposes of environmental epidemiology or for the protection of public health, the nation is failing to adequately identify, assess, or prioritize hazardous-waste-site exposures.

In spite of the complex limitations of epidemiologic studies of hazardous-waste sites, several investigations at specific sites have documented a variety of symptoms of ill health in exposed persons, including low birth weight, cardiac anomalies, headache, fatigue, and a constellation of neurobehavioral problems. It is less clear whether outcomes with a long delay between exposure and disease also have occurred, because of complex methodological problems in assessing these outcomes. However, some studies have detected excesses of cancer in residents exposed to compounds, such as those that occur at hazardous-waste sites.

Although current public health burdens from hazardous-waste sites appear to be small, the future risk might be greater insofar as many of the substances involved are highly persistent, and other materials already in the groundwater can migrate into areas where exposure potential is greater. In some cases, unnecessary or inappropriate remediation might create more of a hazard than would be caused by leaving such materials undisturbed.

Despite the lack of adequate data with which to characterize the effects of hazardous wastes on public health in general, the committee does find sufficient evidence that hazardous wastes have produced serious health effects in some populations. We are concerned that populations may be at risk that have not been adequately identified, because of the inadequate program of site identification and assessment.

To improve the ability to evaluate health effects associated with exposures to hazardous-wastes sites, a number of important data gaps and resource constraints need to be remedied, as this report illustrates. There is a need to make public health assessments an early priority in the routine evaluation of hazardous-waste disposal sites and a need to create mechanisms for sharing this information and epidemiologic investigations of these sites nationwide. There must be adequate support for state and local health department investigations of hazardous-waste sites. Better measurements or estimates of human exposure are needed from a variety of sources, including abandoned hazardous-waste disposal sites, and other point sources such as leaking storage tanks, and from agricultural and industrial practices that may produce nonconventional pollutants. Monitoring of sentinel health events, and increased use of disease registries and vital statistics systems will be required to assess the public health impacts of all of these sources of exposures.

Although the effect on large populations of very low levels of toxic pollutants is unknown, measures must now be taken to protect future public health. According to a number of previous assessments from the NRC, a substantial risk of contamination of the groundwater is not being averted by current remediation practices. Moreover, the Institute of Medicine recently noted that pollution of lakes and rivers increases contamination in fish. It should be recognized that if exposure becomes general and almost uniform, current epidemiologic techniques will not be able to ascertain any related health effects. There is a window of opportunity to initiate studies in areas where groundwater pollution has remained high and localized. There is also an important opportunity for prevention that could forestall major public health problems in the future.

The legislative mandates, policies, and programs of the federal and state agencies that currently manage hazardous-waste sites are inadequate to the task of protecting public health. The distribution and frequency of exposures of specific populations near specific hazardous-waste sites cannot be ascertained, because the needed data have not been gathered.

Our report indicates that the nation is not adequately identifying, assessing, or ranking hazardous-waste site exposures and their potential effects on public health. We are currently unable to answer the question of the overall impact on public health of hazardous wastes. Until better evidence is developed, prudent public policy demands that a margin of safety be provided regarding potential health risks from exposures to substances from hazardous-waste sites. We do no less in designing bridges and buildings. We do no less in establishing criteria for scientific credibility. We must surely do no less when the health and quality of life of Americans are at stake.

Public Health and Hazardous Wastes: The Context

1

Introduction

ASTE HAS BEEN A PRODUCT OF human activity since the dawn of human history. In the early stages of industrial development, workplace wastes were generated on site and swept, sent, or poured "away." Occasionally, "away" meant literally out of the door and into the street or into local stoves or community incinerators. Later, waste materials were sold as fill for uneven ground and spread over large expanses of unsettled land that was subsequently urbanized. Waste oils were used as dust suppressants; unneeded products were poured down drains, or directly or indirectly dumped into streams, rivers, lakes, and oceans. Recognition that such wastes were potentially hazardous usually came long after they had been generated and distributed.

During the nineteenth century, improvements in basic sanitation, housing, nutrition, and sewage treatment substantially improved life expectancy throughout the industrial world by reducing deaths from such infectious diseases as tuberculosis, diphtheria, and pertussis (McKeown, 1976). Attention in the twentieth century has shifted to chronic illnesses, such as some kinds of cancer (NCI, 1990) and neurologic disease (Lilienfeld et al., 1989), that have become more common in industrial societies than before. Questions have come to be raised about the possible relationship of industrial waste and other aspects of modern life to chronic diseases.

Part of our modern heritage is the increasing volume of waste created by all industrial societies. There also is an unprecedented concern over the potential consequences for public health and the environment caused by exposure to wastes that are deemed hazardous under a variety of regulatory regimes. Since the earliest days of industrialization, substantial volumes of wastes have been produced and sometimes disposed of in ways that could create problems for later generations. In the U.S. more than 6 billion tons of waste is produced annually—nearly 50,000 pounds per person (OTA, 1989). Some analyses indicate that in the U.S. racial and ethnic minorities are more likely than are non-minorities to live in areas where abandoned hazardous-waste dumps or operating waste disposal facilities are located (Bullard, 1990). One study noted that in communities with two or more commercial waste disposal facilities, the average minority percentage of the population was more than three times that of communities without such facilities (Commission for Racial Justice, 1987).

In many industrial countries, a number of highly publicized episodes of pollution have made it clear that pollutants can migrate in complex and not completely understood ways. Accordingly, a variety of laws now require that public policy should provide for better waste disposal practices. The legacy of past practices, however, provides a series of difficult challenges to policy makers and scientists regarding how to analyze the public health and environmental effects of old methods of disposal, how to set appropriate policies to reduce harm in the future, and how much resources should be devoted to these issues.

At the request of the Agency for Toxic Substances and Disease Registry (ATSDR), the National Research Council (NRC) convened the Committee on Environmental Epidemiology to review current knowledge of the human health effects caused by exposure to hazardous-waste sites and to suggest how to improve the scientific bases for evaluating the effects of environmental pollution on public health, including specifically the conduct of health assessments at Superfund sites. With additional support from the Environmental Protection Agency (EPA), the Committee also is examining the role of state health departments in generating relevant information on this topic. This first report of the committee reviews and assesses the published scientific literature on health effects that could be linked with exposure to hazardous-waste disposal sites, and makes recommendations about major data gaps that need to be filled as scientists go on to answer important questions in the field.

A second report of the committee will identify research opportunities and issues in methodology for the general field of environmental epidemiology and will evaluate selected non-peer-reviewed reports on the subject of the epidemiologic study of hazardous wastes. This literature includes such sources as state health department reports and selected technical reports from the legal literature. While not accessible in the peer-reviewed literature, such reports can also be found in recent court decisions in which evidence about hazardous-wastes sites has been extensively reviewed and is at issue. To the extent feasible, the second report also will evaluate emerging reports from a variety of newly available international sources that bear on these questions, such as those from Eastern Europe (Environment and Health in Developing Countries, 1991).

This first report, to be consistent with the sponsors' requests, focuses on an evaluation of the published literature on the health effects of exposures from hazardous-waste sites. Because of this limited scope and also because a number of other NRC committees are concerned with environmental issues, the Committee on Environmental Epidemiology is excluding from its consideration dietary factors and the effects of radiation, including the hazards of exposure to radon, low-level radioactive waste contamination, and electromagnetic fields.

The first section of this chapter defines environmental epidemiology. The second section discusses conventional views of statistical significance and principles for inferring causation based on epidemiologic evidence. After that, the principles of statistical inference are evaluated in the context of constraints associated with the litigious and controversial world of hazardous-waste sites and toxic torts. Toxic torts are among the fastest growing field of litigation involving legal claims of alleged injuries caused by exposure to toxic chemicals. The next section describes the historical context for the committee's work. The chapter concludes with an outline of the rest of this volume.

ENVIRONMENTAL EPIDEMIOLOGY

In recent years the term "environmental epidemiology" has seen extensive use, although it has not been well defined. For example, Report 27 in the Environmental Health Criteria series, published under the joint sponsorship of the United Nations Environment Program, the International Labor Organization, and the World Health Organization, was entitled *Guidelines on Studies in Environmental Epidemiology* (WHO, 1983). The report considered "[The use of] . . . epidemiological methods for assessing the effects of environmental agents on human health." Similarly, neither a compendium published as *Environmental Epidemiology* in 1986 (Kopfler and Craun, 1986) nor a didactic volume with the same title (Goldsmith, 1986) presented a definition of the field of environmental epidemiology. The recently established International Society for Environmental Epidemiology devised a definition in its charter in 1988: epidemiologic studies on the effects of environmental exposures of human populations.

The Committee on Environmental Epidemiology has adopted the following definition:

Environmental epidemiology is the study of the effect on human health of physical, biologic, and chemical factors in the external environment, broadly conceived. By examining specific populations or communities exposed to different ambient environments, it seeks to clarify the relationship between physical, biologic or chemical factors and human health.

One challenging question that confronts environmental epidemiologists is how to estimate the health effects associated with *past* patterns of disposal of hazardous chemicals and effects that could occur in the *future* as a result of continued or projected exposure from failures to clean up sites, or from proposed remediation plans. Investigating these problems is technically difficult, time consuming, and expensive (Ozonoff and Boden, 1987). As part of its project on environmental epidemiology, the committee elected to focus first on an evaluation of available scientific and technical literature that concerns the health effects of exposure to materials found in and issuing from hazardous-waste sites. In using this focal point, the committee has not restricted itself to sites officially listed under various state and federal laws, but has undertaken a broad review of available evidence on the human health effects that could be linked to exposures from materials at sites where disposal of hazardous wastes has taken place.

The committee's members acknowledge that the published literature regarding toxic chemical waste disposal sites is limited and uneven and that profound methodological and practical problems attend the field, as others have noted (Grisham, 1986). However, the committee members believe that a deliberate and systematic assessment of current knowledge will provide a useful foundation for their later work in developing and extending the intellectual framework of the larger field of environmental epidemiology.

EPIDEMIOLOGIC RESEARCH

In general, epidemiologists conduct two major types of studies to assess relationships between suspected risk factors and disease: descriptive and analytic. Descriptive studies portray disease patterns in populations according to person, time, and place and include time-series analyses and prevalence studies that analyze large sets of data and are usually used to generate hypotheses. Analytic studies include case-control (retrospective) and cohort (prospective) studies and typically test hypotheses. In case-control studies, comparable series of cases of a disease and controls drawn from the same population are investigated to determine past exposures that could have resulted in the development of the disease. In cohort studies, comparable series of exposed and unexposed persons are followed to ascertain the incidence of disease or mortality caused by disease in association with the exposure. This traditional delineation between descriptive and analytic studies has fostered the notion that distinct research principles apply to each type of study. In fact, both descriptive and analytic studies can generate and test hypotheses.

It is readily apparent that studies of hazardous-waste sites pose some special practical and ethical challenges. Long-term cohort studies of continued exposures cannot ethically be conducted on persons who have reasons for assuming they are at risk of chronic disease as a consequence of exposure. For instance, persons living near most hazardous-waste sites have in common a measured or estimated exposure to toxic substances in the area. Researchers cannot both verify this exposure and expect people to remain near the sites and continue to be exposed. Moreover, at many sites, citizens groups and neighbors have provided the first information about the existence of a suspected health problem associated with exposure to hazardous wastes. Once suspicions are expressed publicly, residents often leave the area if they can, and the study becomes mired in public fears and expectations. Who can be expected to wait patiently for scientists to gather and analyze data when they fear for their own and their children's safety—even if these fears later prove unfounded?

Because all the major methods of epidemiology are essentially observational and nonexperimental, drawing inferences about causation is considerably more difficult than it is for those controlled experiments that use random samples and controls. People move around, eat different foods, engage in different social and recreational activities, have different genetic backgrounds, and live their lives with the full diversity of the human experience. Yet, all of these factors can directly or indirectly influence their health at any given time. To sort out the relative role of such factors, epidemiologists, like other scientists who study human events, must rely on inductive methods for drawing inferences about their data.

The committee acknowledges that experimental (e.g., toxicologic) studies and epidemiologic studies each have their strong points and that they complement each other with respect to making causal inferences. To a large extent, all empirical scientists rely on inductive methods. Moreover, while one can frame and often answer precise questions experimentally, experimental constraints may make it very difficult to generalize from them. In this regard, continued support for epidemiologic studies constitutes a linchpin of public health research.

CAUSAL INFERENCE

As we expect to describe more fully in the second report, an optimal investigation of potential adverse health effects from hazardous-waste sites would proceed from an adequate assessment of past as well as current exposures to chemicals at a site (see Chapter 3 of this report) to the formulation of testable hypotheses of effects to be studied in a specific population. Then, an assessment would be made of adverse health effects in exposed and unexposed persons and would take account of all potential confounders. No study that fits this ideal has been published, and it seems unlikely that any such study could be conducted in the immediate future.

Accordingly, the committee must rely on a combination of evidence from different sources to reach any conclusion in accordance with its mandate to estimate health effects associated with hazardous wastes. Figure 1-1 illustrates the types of information on which the committee has relied.

A. Knowledge of *potential exposures* is derived from studies that characterize the substances present in or migrating from hazardous-waste sites. As discussed more fully in Chapter 3, these must be described in terms of their toxicity—including their carcinogenicity and other effects studied experimentally in animals; and where the knowledge is available, effects studied on humans. Information about the nature of toxic substances is derived from the general scientific literature.

B. Knowledge of *health risks* to humans from potential exposures can be obtained from other sources, including, sometimes, related epidemiologic studies involving analogous exposures. For some chemicals such sources will include published studies of occupational risks, usually involving higher exposures than those in the general environment. For others, especially for airborne exposures, it will come from studies of the general effects of specific pollutants and may be extended to circumstances where such pollutants are emitted from hazardous-waste sites.

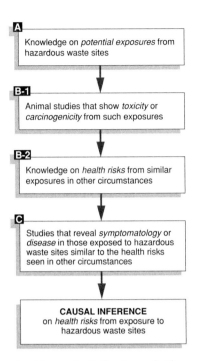

FIGURE 1-1 Sources of evidence for inferring whether exposures from hazardous-waste sites cause an impact on public health.

C. Knowledge of *symptomatology* or *disease occurrence* has in some instances been derived from studies of populations exposed to hazardous-waste sites. Often, these have not described exposures accurately, or they have failed completely to identify a specific causal factor. Nevertheless, with the knowledge that is available about exposure elsewhere, and from the knowledge that some of these exposures can result in the observed symptomatology or diseases found in excess in those exposed to hazardous-waste sites when compared to suitable controls, sufficient indirect evidence of causality might have been accumulated to justify remedial action for purposes of protecting public health.

In adopting the above framework, the committee does not follow the approach traditionally used by epidemiologists in deriving inferences of causality (Hill, 1953; USDHHS, 1976). Historically, discussions on causality have proceeded once a statistically significant relationship between a potential causal factor and a disease has been found, as is discussed below. However, what constitutes the best means of evaluating statistical significance itself is evolving, as are the grounds for inferring causation in some circumstances. Small numbers, rare events, or small populations are often involved in hazardous-waste sites. Consequently, the committee does not adhere strictly to conventional approaches to establishing causality only after a finding of statistical significance has been made. Before detailing the committee's reasons for relying on an inferential approach in developing an understanding of causation in environmental epidemiology, it is useful to consider the function and limits of statistically significant findings in studies of the health effects of hazardous wastes.

STATISTICAL SIGNIFICANCE

The requirement that a finding be statistically significant has been a convention of epidemiologic research. If results have a likelihood of only 5 percent or less of occurring by chance, then they are usually considered statistically significant, as measured by a number of customary tests, such as p and t values. Under some circumstances, this stipulation can stifle innovations in research when studies that fail to meet the conventional criteria for a positive finding are prematurely dismissed. Thus, a study of a common disease in a small number of people might not achieve a level of statistical significance, even though a causal association could, in fact, exist.

Several analysts maintain that the indiscriminate application of tests for statistical significance to epidemiologic studies has discouraged advances in research and conferred undue importance on negative findings. Rothman (1986) argues that conventionally applied tests of statistical significance, such as p values, are inadequate and subject to extensive misinterpretation. He favors the broad application of confidence intervals, so that results are depicted as ranging over a set of possible values, viz., there is a 90 percent chance that a given finding falls between some high value and some low value. Ahlbom et al. (1990) describe two general categories of negative studies that can result from an overreliance on traditional tests of statistical significance: those that actually suggest that a given exposure lacks an effect of a detectable size on the studied disease risk, and those that might miss such an effect because of inadequate sample size, random error, or because systematic error biases the study toward finding no such effect. Random error increases the chance that inaccurate measures of the effect will imply that there is no difference between those exposed and unexposed. Discussions of negative studies must recognize the importance of the size and detectability of the effects being missed.

According to some philosophers of science, the hypothesis that a given exposure has no effect on increasing the risk of a particular disease can be rejected (Buck, 1975), but can never be proved (Bunge, 1963). Greenland (1988) has criticized this strict application of philosophy for its failure to meet the requirements of epidemiology regarding public health. Several analysts have noted that an inductive approach can be more appropriately applied to epidemiologic study, considering epidemiologic study a measurement exercise with which relevant measures of effect are estimated (Miettinen, 1985).

Even the inductive approach to causation in epidemiology is vulnerable to random or systematic error. Where the size of a study is small, random error can overwhelm a finding. Whether the level of statistical significance exceeds or fails to meet the 0.05 level does not necessarily bear on whether the effect parameter is biologically important or is equal to the null value, that is, does not differ significantly from what is expected to occur by chance. A better indication of the statistically plausible range of values can be provided by identifying the estimated confidence interval, that is, the range within which there is a 90 percent chance that the true value is contained. The confidence interval brackets the interval or range of values that may occur and provides a clearer indication of the significance of a study than does strict application of p values and other measures of statistical significance.

Systematic error in classifying disease or exposure produces invalid results. Error arising from a misclassification of exposure can occur under a number of conditions, including the following: if the exposure measurement is random or subject to error; if an invalid or systematically inaccurate proxy for exposure is used, such as distance from a hazardous-waste site independent of relevant wind patterns or sources of domestic water; if a biologically inaccurate indication of exposure is applied, such as the use of a point-in-time exposure intensity rather than a cumulative dose; or if people either do not know the amount of exposure or exaggerate it. The problem of reconstructing exposures is especially subject to recall bias. Recall bias occurs where persons who have learned that they may be at risk from an exposure associate nonspecific health problems with the exposure or develop a health problem that they seek to attribute to the exposure and then "remember" specific symptoms better than do nonexposed persons. Error also can be introduced through misclassification of disease. For instance, including persons who do not, in fact, have a given disease along with those who do have the disease, produces low specificity in the results.

Ahlbom et al. (1990) warn that over-interpretation of epidemiologic results can occur when results that show no effect are believed to prove no effect, even though they are actually inconclusive. Among the factors that can contribute to this over-interpretation of negative studies are failure to achieve statistical significance, too small a sample size, the poor assessment of exposure, the presence of confounding factors, and the lack of known biologic mechanisms that may account for the particular relationship between exposure and disease.

CAUSATION IN EPIDEMIOLOGY

The world of epidemiology, as that of any human science, seldom permits elegant inferences to be drawn about causation. The object domain of epidemiology consists of numerous uncontrollable aspects, with considerable variations in precedents, so that we cannot vary only one factor at a time. With human sciences, causation usually must be inferred, and is never proved absolutely.

> Human minds seem to be more credulous than skeptical, and most people need protection against being gulled. Undue skepticism, however, can be as dangerous as credulity to scientific progress and the improvement of health. Only judgment can prevent the hypercritical rejection of useful results. (Susser, 1973, p. 141)

Susser's statement reminds us that the judgment of experts is a critical component for interpreting any findings in epidemiology. A fundamental dilemma for epidemiologic research on hazardous-waste sites, or any other topic involving multiple causes and results, derives from the fact that the statistical correlation of variables does not necessarily indicate any causal relationship among them, even where tests of statistical significance may be met. Mere coincident occurrence of variables says nothing about their essential connection. Moreover, partial correlations between variables that exclude other relevant variables can be misleading.

To estimate the relationship between exposure and health status it is necessary to include relevant variables or their appropriate proxies, to the extent that these can be determined. Efficient use of that information requires the choice of a functional form that is compatible with the health-related practices and decisions of the individuals who are under study. No matter how carefully such proxy variables are estimated, causal inference should not be equated with statistical inference. Nor can statistical expertise alone establish causation. In order to facilitate the inference of causation from statistical information, contemporary epidemiologists have developed guidelines based on the view that absolute truth cannot be determined scientifically

(Mill, 1865). The relative likelihood that a finding is true must be inferred from careful, systematic, and repeated observations of recurring phenomena. Thus, association can be proved beyond a reasonable doubt, but not refuted, while causation can be refuted, but cannot be proved.

To make a reasonable inference of causation in environmental epidemiology, eight basic characteristics of the findings should be considered: the strength, specificity, and consistency of the association; the period of exposure; the biologic gradient or the relationship between the dose and the response; the effects of the removal of the suggested cause; the biologic plausibility of the association (Hill, 1953; USDHHS, 1986), including how well it coheres with other findings.

Strength of the Association

How great is the risk of disease apparently induced by a given factor (exposure)? This is often expressed as relative risk (RR), standard mortality ratio (SMR), odds ratio (OR), or standard fertility ratio (SFR), each of which compares the risk of disease incurred by exposed persons with that of unexposed persons. The greater the RR, SFR, or SMR, the stronger the inferred link for exposed individuals. Of equal concern for public health, however, is the attributable risk, which might be much harder to detect, study, and estimate in environmental epidemiology, given the problems of evaluating baseline rates for a disease of interest. An RR of 3 for a lifetime that affects 1 of 100 persons in a small population produces a much smaller impact on public health than does a lifetime RR of 1.1 that affects several million persons.

Epidemiologists have long appreciated that high RRs are relatively easy to detect. Thus, evidence linking lung cancer and cigarette smoking is strong; active smokers have a tenfold or greater risk of contracting lung cancer than non-smokers do. In contrast, evidence linking lung cancer and passive smoking is less firmly established; a variety of studies (NRC, 1986a) place the RR between 1.2 and 2.0, with the 95 percent confidence interval for a summary of the case-control studies ranging from 0.9 to more than 2.

The difficulty with the use of this criterion of the strength of the association in environmental epidemiology is that misclassification of exposure can greatly attenuate the strength of a relatively weak observed association. Other sources can contribute to a specific chemical exposure, and the same health effect can be caused by different pollutants. Most of the results of concern are common, chronic diseases, for which the baselines—their normally expected rates—are not clearly established. It is possible to validate a true elevation in a rate only if it can be demonstrated that an event is unusual (or improbable); this implies that the researcher drawing the inference has a good grasp of what is usual (Rothenberg et al., 1990). For instance, the assessment of time trends in birth defects or reproductive health must contend with the lack of well-established national and regional information about rates of major birth defects and spontaneous abortion. Moreover, the system used to code and classify minor and major birth defects can differ from one place to the next. Evaluating the occurrence of spontaneous abortions requires information about regional and cultural variations in rates and kinds of contraceptives used, rates of elective abortion, and genetic-screening tests that can provide the basis for such procedures. In areas where proportionally more pregnancies are voluntarily terminated, reported rates of spontaneous abortion might be lower.

For multiply caused diseases the strength of association measured depends on many factors, including the power of the overall study to detect an effect. Power is a statistical measure of the potential of the study to find an association. It varies with the inverse of the square root of size of the population studied and the expected relative risk of the disease. In order to detect significant patterns, rare diseases are best studied in larger populations. More common diseases can be studied in smaller populations. However, to the extent that multiple causes are involved, as they are with most chronic diseases, larger populations are generally required in order to obtain significant results in studies of more common diseases as well. Refining the measures of diseases and the assessment of exposure can improve the power of a study to detect an association. "Strong" associations are not more biologically correct then "weak" associations. They may be less readily dismissed as confounding, however, and are more readily detected.

Cancer clusters and spontaneous abortion clusters are among the most commonly reported events linked to exposure to hazardous-waste sites. These clusters also rank as among the most difficult outcome for which causation can be inferred. In part, this is because both outcomes reflect multiple causes and because it is difficult to determine the relevant regional baseline rate. Also, for cancer, the latent period (between exposure and onset of disease) is often long.

Neutra (1990) notes that because of the small populations exposed at many hazardous-waste sites, the observed rates of occurrences for diseases studied in a given cluster often must be at least 20 times greater than expected to support an inference of causation. Today, one of three people in the U.S. will develop some form of cancer; one in four will die of it (NCI, 1990). The expected rate of spontaneous abortion is estimated to be as much as one in four of all pregnancies (NRC, 1989). Therefore, clusters of cancer, spontaneous abortion, or other common diseases can easily arise by chance. Assessing whether a given cluster of these common health problems could be linked to environmental exposure requires either the study of very large numbers of persons or the finding of extraordinarily elevated rates. Further, most hazardous-waste sites involve potential or actual exposures of only small numbers of persons. Because many of them no longer live in the area when a cluster is identified, tracking down all who potentially could have contributed to a cluster is extremely difficult.

Another problem relates to the fact that analyses of health effects possibly linked with exposures from hazardous-waste sites usually involve making implicit multiple comparisons, which results in increased rates of disease due to chance alone. "When eager environmental epidemiologists check to see if cancer registry data suggest that a particular waste site has increased the incidence of any one of the 80 types of cancer with a p value of 0.01 or less, . . . we know that there is a 0.99 probability of escaping an increase in all of these cancers. . . . So there is a better-than-even chance that the risk of some kind of cancer will be elevated around the site" (Neutra, 1990, p. 5). Multiple comparisons are being made in an implicit manner, in that only the single type of cancer that is elevated becomes the subject of public concern and study, rather than each type of cancer separately or all cancers combined. In the state of California 55 percent of the 5,000 census tracts will have at least one type of cancer elevated because of chance alone. Hence, there are potentially 2750 false-positive clusters to investigate each decade.

Finally, for many hazardous-waste sites, there usually are no data on relevant exposures that could have occurred several decades earlier, given the long and indefinite period for development of many forms of cancer. This and the other considerations described in this section explain why the observed strength of an association between pathology and exposure to hazardous wastes can be weak, even though the link may be causal.

Specificity of the Association

Specificity implies that a putative cause induces a specific disease. However, a one agent-one disease model has been shown not to apply for many diseases, such as lung cancer, in which multiple causes are involved. Further, many agents, such as cigarette smoke, produce different diseases, making the determination of their relative role more difficult (Lilienfeld and Lilienfeld, 1980).

Specificity also is diminished when diseases are inappropriately grouped together, or inaccurately classified, obscuring important differences. Thus, a proposed study of vinyl chloride-exposed workers in 1973 would have failed to detect the real effect of increased cancer, because it lumped the relatively rare form of cancer involved, namely angiosarcoma of the liver, into the category of all cancer. This particular study included over 10,000 workers in 37 plants, the majority of the industry at the time. In preparing the analysis of this group, the researchers calculated the SMRs in which the expected numbers of deaths from specific causes were derived from national mortality statistics for all cancers combined. This aggregation of cancer would have obscured the extraordinary finding that one fifth of all recorded incident cases of angiosarcoma for the U.S. in a single year occurred in this group of highly exposed vinyl chloride workers (Utidjian, 1988). Subsequent studies that used appropriate classifications of disease detected significant excesses of angiosarcoma and brain cancer in exposed workers (Utidjian, 1988). Excesses of angiosarcoma have also been detected in residents living near a vinyl chloride manufacturing plant in New York (Brady et al., 1977).

Where a given factor is related to many diseases, its specific causal association with a single disease can prove difficult to demonstrate. Thus, vinyl chloride emissions have also been tied to clusters of birth defects, but the study lacked sufficient power and the findings were not significant (Rosenman et al., 1989). In general, hazardous wastes have been linked in toxicological studies to a wide range of diseases, some of which have long latencies and many of which have multiple causes. Moreover, the common nature of many of the health problems suspected to be caused by exposure to hazardous-waste sites makes the identification of their specific causes problematic. Here again, the problem of multiple comparisons occurs, in that the study of a number of different diseases in different locations will randomly produce some elevations due to chance alone.

Consistency of the Association

Does the relationship between exposure and disease occur regularly in independently conducted studies? To revert to the example of passive smoking and lung cancer, although the RR might be 2.0 or less, this elevated risk was reported consistently in more than 30 different studies conducted in six countries (NRC, 1986a). Even where statistical significance is not attained in all studies, their results may be combined, so long as they comply with sound methods. Data may be pooled to determine whether a particular effect is linked to a particular exposure. However, such pooling does not readily allow estimation of the size of that effect. To facilitate syntheses of different studies, general criteria need to be developed for evaluating their overall compliance with basic standards of good epidemiologic practice (CMA, 1991). To bolster the finding of consistency, a number of studies that meet these criteria of good epidemiologic practice can be grouped for meta-analyses. This grouping allows for statistical pooling of results in different studies (Chalmers et al., 1987). Such groupings of studies are feasible, provided that the studies are selected or excluded from the group solely on the basis of their conforming to stringent methodologic criteria for what constitutes good epidemiologic practice, independently of their results. Similarly, repeated findings of clusters in time and space of exposure and effect strengthen the plausibility of the inferred relationship.

Consistency of findings in different populations and in different countries especially strengthens a finding of causation. It is unlikely that the same relationship would occur by chance alone in different populations, unless, of course, the studies were subject to the same biases. Assessing the consistency of an association in the arena of hazardous wastes is also hampered by the diversity of exposures. In principle, studies can be conducted in several communities where there have been varying levels of exposure after those exposures are reasonably well defined. Estimates can be roughly correlated with degrees of exposure, after controlling for confounding by other variables (Neutra, 1990, citing Robbins, 1988).

Many hazardous-waste sites entail multiple exposures to a mixture of chemicals. Further, the multicommunity approach assumes that the high-exposure communities are homogeneous as to the risk they convey to the public. This assumption could be unwarranted if major differences in industrial hygiene and disposal practices are involved. Unfortunately, consistency is not easily achieved for studies of hazardous-waste sites; we do not have enough data to be able to determine for which sites similar health effects might be anticipated, as is illustrated in Chapter 3. This is because of the lack of data on potential exposures that would permit characterization of sites in similar groupings of exposures to single or multiple chemicals. In this regard, insisting upon consistency between studies could pose an unreasonable burden where other factors mitigate the actual and potential exposures incurred.

Temporality

Does exposure occur at a reasonable interval before the development of the symptoms or disease of interest? The amount of time
between exposure and onset of disease should comply with the underlying biological concept of the disease at hand. For tobacco-in-
duced lung cancer, the latency between exposure and disease often is
25 years or more, although a few cases occur within 10 years of first
exposure (Doll and Peto, 1978). Theoretically, higher doses shorten
latency. For diseases of shorter latency, periods of hours of acute exposure can be involved. In general, the period of observation should be
consistent with the hypothesized relationship, taking into account that
variable latencies may be involved. With diseases of long latency, accurate recall or reconstruction of exposures remains a serious problem.

For studies of hazardous-waste sites, the temporality requirements
of inferring causation could prove difficult to pin down, given the
mobility and the diversity of the study population and the lack of
models of many chronic diseases in the human populations. Despite
this, studies of diseases with short latencies can sometimes provide
useful information. For example, Vianna and Polan (1984) reported
that the peak in low birth weight in children born to women who
were residents of Love Canal, New York, occurred during the time of
greatest estimated exposure to contaminants at that site.

Biologic Gradient or Relationship Between Estimated Exposure and Disease

In general, the greater the exposure, the stronger the effect. The
relationship between dose (either estimated or measured) and response should be logical and uniform. The risk of contracting lung
cancer increases with the number of cigarettes smoked. Although
dose usually equals the concentration integrated over time, there are
some important exceptions in which dosing patterns can be more
important than overall dose. For instance, early and high exposure
to alkylating agents, such as ethylene oxide, could produce a greater
response than continual low exposure to the same quantity over a
long period of time (Vesselinovitch, 1969).

Also, timing of exposure and host condition can be critical. Exposures to toxic chemicals in infancy and childhood or exposures of
persons who are already compromised by some pre-existing chronic
disease can produce a stronger effect than that found in healthy adults.
It is well known that exposures to some toxic agents during the first
trimester of pregnancy are critical for many teratologic and reproductive effects. Thus, there can be long-term and permanent effects

from short-term exposure, such as that resulting from a single episode of exposure that occurs at the critical time in pregnancy, and other windows of vulnerability exist for neurodevelopmental effects (NRC, 1989). Such time- and dose-dependent exposure also could be involved in the development of other chronic diseases, such as learning and behavioral disabilities caused by exposure to lead.

For studies of hazardous-waste sites where common diseases with multiple causes are found, the finding of a dose-response relationship can be obscured by the operation of multiple causal factors and the absence of valid estimates of exposure. As Neutra (1990) notes, we can rarely reconstruct the individual exposures accurately, especially because they can stem from periods several decades past. In the absence of detailed measurements of exposure, we are forced to assume that people in a given neighborhood endured comparable and uniform exposures, even where that is not likely to have been the case.

Effects of the Removal of a Suspected Cause

Where an assumed causal relationship exists, removal of the suspected cause in individuals should reduce or eliminate the suspected effect, unless the effect is irreversible. Thus, those who stop smoking reduce their risk of contracting lung cancer. At the population level, reductions in cigarette smoking among men and women in the United Kingdom and among men in the U.S. have resulted in reduced rates of lung cancer (NCI, 1990). Where different causes contribute to a single disease, this principle will be relevant only for the specific causal factor removed.

The above considerations explain why it is not easy to evaluate the *effects of removal* of an exposure at many hazardous-waste sites. Despite these problems, after the fact analyses have been produced that permit some causal inferences regarding a few studies. Thus, allowing for a five-year latency, no new cases of leukemia have occurred in families in Woburn, Massachusetts, since those families stopped using contaminated wells (R. Clapp, Center for Environmental Health Studies, JSI, personal communication, 1991). Similarly, in the Lipari Landfill study by the state of New Jersey (NJDOH, 1989) and at Love Canal, after exposure from hazardous materials declined, birth weights returned to normal (Goldman et al., 1985; Vianna and Polan, 1984).

Biological Plausibility

Does the association make sense in terms of the current understanding of basic human biology? Animal studies or other experimental evidence can enhance the credibility of epidemiologic findings by indicating mechanisms of disease or by corroborating the basic association between exposure and disease (Davis, 1988). However, the absence of such information does not necessarily invalidate a causal association. The underlying mechanisms for many modern diseases are not readily apparent. Thus, the precise mechanisms by which cigarette smoking induces lung cancer are unknown, although the causal relationship is clear (Doll and Peto, 1978).

CHALLENGES IN THE STUDY OF HAZARDOUS-WASTE SITES

Among the major challenges for this field are the small populations and small numbers of events usually involved in such studies and the consequent lack of significance of findings, even when the confidence interval is used. The advent of meta-analysis offers an important opportunity to strengthen the inferences that can be drawn from epidemiologic research (Chalmers et al., 1987). Potentially misleading conclusions can be extracted from single studies because of insufficient sample size, inadequacies of exposure determination, or publication and other biases. Meta-analysis can combine data from a variety of studies and reduce the danger of misinterpretation because it allows for pooling of all available information (Greenland, 1990). Meta-analyses must be carried out properly if they are to supply useful information. Retrospective combinations of research must be approached with caution. Searches for primary studies must be as exhaustive as possible. Biases must be minimized by blinding the evaluators of the methods of the studies with regard to the authors, institutional sources, and findings of the original studies. Opportunities for bias in the original research must be tabulated and used to temper conclusions. The statistical methods must be logical and reliable. The interpretation of meta-analyses must also be tempered by the awareness that reporting and publication biases can distort the sample of studies available for pooling. The future widespread application of meta-analytic techniques to studies of hazardous-waste sites will require recognition of deficiencies in primary research and consequent improvements in the gathering and reporting of data in a way that will facilitate meta-analysis later.

Another challenge to environmental epidemiology is the major effect that emerging case and tort law wield on the subject matter. In most tort cases, a plaintiff must demonstrate by a preponderance of the evidence that his or her version of the facts is correct. The number of lawsuits that request monetary payment in compensation for injury induced by exposure to toxic substances has skyrocketed in the past two decades (Black, 1990). A substantial number of tort cases involve listed Superfund sites and other hazardous-waste disposal sites. Because courts have sealed disputes on these matters that have been resolved, some potentially relevant information is not routinely available to the scientific community regarding the health effects associated with exposures from hazardous-waste sites.

As a number of legal theorists have noted, the requirements for inferring causation in law and for inferring them in science differ in several important ways (Henderson, 1990). Chief among these is that science, by conventional practice, infers causation where a statement has a 5 in 100 chance of being false. However, in the law, a "but for" showing can be sufficient to establish causation. That is, it is acceptable to establish that a causal agent was more probably than not a substantial factor in producing a given result. Indeed, some case law specifically denies the need to make a statistically significant showing of a relationship to imply causation, and it allows that damages can be awarded so long as an expert can testify that in his or her opinion a cause-and-effect relationship is more likely than not to exist between the substances involved and the injuries incurred (Davis, 1985). The fact that a few courts have ruled that fear of contracting a disease such as cancer is a compensable harm, per se, further complicates the arena. These legal trends will continue to have a major influence on the field of environmental epidemiology and on the public demand for studies of the health effects associated with exposures to hazardous-wastes sites.

One important difference of focus is apparent. In epidemiology we want to know whether a population of exposed persons has an increased risk, and by what proportion their mean risk is elevated. In law, what matters is whether a specific individual's disease was more probably caused than not caused by the specific exposures encountered. In fact, epidemiology cannot answer questions about the causes of illness in a specific individual. However, such evidence can indicate the likelihood that particular exposures are linked with specific diseases. A risk in a specific individual is in practice assigned from the experience of the group (NRC, 1984).

Like most environmental sciences, epidemiology derives a substantial part of its current support from renewed concern about the consequences of environmental factors for public health and the environment. Unfortunately, the intense public arena in which epidemiology operates can have a chilling effect on the ability of scientists to assess the health effects of a particular hazardous-waste site if that site is the subject of active litigation. The pressures of environmental laws, lawsuits, and news media disclosures about suspected contamination or outbreaks of disease substantially impair the ability of epidemiologists to obtain unbiased information on past exposure. Experts who are privy to the discovery process may acquire useful information, but this information may not be available in the peer-reviewed literature on which most scientists rely. In response to these pressures, the legal arena is fundamentally shifting its use of the definitions of causation applied to epidemiologic study and to environmental issues broadly conceived. The recent proliferation of mass exposure cases, such as the Agent Orange litigation, and the class action lawsuits and courtmaster reviews on asbestos, the Dalkon Shield, and DDT contamination, are forcing a fundamental reassessment not only of traditional causation standards, but of the underlying concept of causation (Schuck, 1991). Where case law previously resisted reliance on probabilistic and statistical information, such as that generated by epidemiologic studies, recent decisions have accepted this line of evidence.

The Committee on Environmental Epidemiology recognizes that, whether in law or science, the inference of causation must be understood as a process that involves judgment and interpretation. Because the basic mechanisms of most modern chronic diseases are not well understood, analysts are forced to interpret observational data to find clues about etiology. Despite the immense public interest in the effect of hazardous wastes on public health, rather few empirical data are available. Nevertheless, public health policy requires that decisions be made despite the incomplete evidence, with the aim of protecting public health in the future.

HISTORICAL CONTEXT OF THE STUDY

Lethal episodes of severe air pollution, such as those in Donora, Pennsylvania in 1948; London in 1952; and the Meuse Valley in 1930, raised public consciousness about environmental epidemiology. The London episode led directly to the British Clean Air Act in the 1950s. The environmental decade of the 1970s included the passage of a host of laws intended to address, prevent, or control such major environmental pollution problems in the United States. Subsequently, incidents at Love Canal; Michigan feed contamination with the fire retardant chemical polybrominated biphenyls (PBBs); the James River; the Hudson River pollution with the pesticide kepone; Times Beach, Missouri; Bhopal, India; and most recently burning Kuwaiti oilfields and oil spills have provided the global village with vivid images of devastating pollution.

In response to concerns spawned by several of these earlier episodes, Congress passed laws that included requirements for scientific assessments at the very frontiers of the environmental sciences (Davis, 1985). Thus, under terms of the Toxic Substances Control Act, the EPA was charged with developing policies to control new and existing chemicals. To effect this control, EPA must incorporate evidence on whether agents pose or could pose an unreasonable risk of causing significant adverse health effects, including birth defects, neurological disease, synergistic effects, environmental effects, and other not-well-specified harms to public health and the environment. To make such assessments, EPA relies on a series of risk assessment models that use animal and other experimental data to estimate effects on humans. Unfortunately, many important synthetic and natural chemicals have not been adequately tested and most have not been tested at all. Risk assessment techniques are highly speculative, and almost all rely on multiple assumptions of fact—some of which are entirely untestable (NRC, 1983; 1986b). The anticipatory, preventive intention of these environmental laws has resulted in their heavy reliance on experimental models and theoretical inferences.

As recognition mounted that past disposal practices had contaminated neighborhoods near disposal sites, Congress promulgated the Superfund law (the Comprehensive Environmental Response, Compensation, and Liability Act, CERCLA, Public Law 96-510, 94 Statute 2767) in 1980 to provide a short-term remedy for abandoned hazardous-waste sites. The precise number of these sites is unknown, although estimates go as high as the tens of thousands—an issue discussed in more detail in Chapter 2. Reauthorizing amendments in 1986 further strengthened the provisions of the Superfund law to address the issue of assessing health effects of persons exposed to hazardous wastes.

In 1980, a Congressional Research Service report for the Senate Committee on Environment and Public Works noted that in many cases adequate data on the extent of contamination and its effects on public health and the environment could not readily be obtained (CRS, 1980). A decade later, the congressional Office of Technology Assessment reiterated that conclusion, faulting the regulatory process and the failure to seek scientific and technical studies of many key questions, including the health effects attendant to exposure to hazardous wastes (OTA, 1989).

AGENCY FOR TOXIC SUBSTANCES AND DISEASE REGISTRY

The original Superfund law, in 1980, established ATSDR as a new agency of the Public Health Service within the U.S. Department of Health and Human Services. The agency's "mission is to prevent or mitigate adverse human health effects and diminished quality of life resulting from environmental exposure to hazardous substances" (Johnson, 1988, p. 10132).

ATSDR did not come into operating existence until 1983, after a lawsuit was filed jointly by the Environmental Defense Fund, the Chemical Manufacturers Association, and the American Petroleum Institute (Siegel, 1990). When ATSDR was still in the early stages of development, Congress expanded the agency's responsibilities with the passage of the Superfund Amendment and Reauthorization Act of 1986 (SARA, Public Law No. 99-499, 100 Statute 1613) (Johnson, 1990). ATSDR is required to conduct health assessments of every site listed on, or proposed for inclusion on, the NPL; establish a priority list of hazardous substances found at CERCLA sites; produce toxicological profiles for each substance on this list; and undertake various research and health studies related to hazardous substances.

As its charter indicates, ATSDR can rely on a broad spectrum of evidence in conducting health assessments at a hazardous-waste site. This spectrum encompasses experimental models of chemical structure and activity patterns, in vitro test systems, whole-animal long-term and short-term studies, and clinical studies and epidemiologic investigations of potentially exposed persons. The animal and experimental models on which site assessments can depend are designed to anticipate human and environmental effects. Their results affect decisions that can cost tens of millions of dollars. Validation and development of these models are the subject of intense debate, reflecting both technical problems and their substantial impact.

Animal studies and other experimental models of toxicity should remain important to the development of environmental policies, because new materials cannot be studied with the tools of epidemiology. Moreover, many recently introduced compounds of interest, such as the new generation of pesticides, are of such recent vintage that it will not be possible to obtain evidence on their chronic effects in humans for a decade or more. Further bolstering the importance of animal and other experimental studies is the fact that all of the 52 compounds known to cause cancer in humans also produce it in animals. However, evidence of the carcinogenicity of only 9 of these compounds was first demonstrated in animals, and later confirmed in humans (Rall, 1991). For the remaining 43 compounds, evidence that humans were at increased risk of contracting cancer was subsequently confirmed in animal studies. Reliance on results from improved animal and other experimental studies remains an important tool for preventing chronic disease in humans.

Efforts to validate experimental models that predict health effects on humans are always faced with a paradox. Animal models and computer-based algorithms are generated in an effort to anticipate human health effects—ultimately, to prevent their occurrence—and to suggest appropriate remedies. Requiring epidemiologic confirmation of the validity of animal and other models is often not possible and may be questioned ethically. In addition, the exposures can be self-limiting; people often move away once they become aware or afraid that they face exposure or once they become symptomatic. Moreover, people have prior exposures to other substances that affect their uptake and response to later exposures to hazardous-waste-site contaminants.

OVERVIEW OF THIS VOLUME

Because the basic mechanisms of many modern chronic diseases are not well understood, analysts must interpret observational data to find clues about etiology and also must rely on experimental observations. Table 1-1 summarizes published studies that the Committee reviews for this report on the health effects linked with exposures from hazardous-waste disposal sites. The relatively small number of studies published to date reflects the difficulties of conducting valid studies of this complex issue, the tendency of courts to seal resolved disputes in this area, and the meager resources committed to such studies. The first section of this report presents the Committee's framework of the field of environmental epidemiology as applied to the study of exposures from hazardous-waste sites and discusses the governmental context under which most relevant data are generated. Chapter 2 discusses relevant federal and state legislation and programs for assessing and remediating hazardous-waste sites. Chapter 3 discusses available data on common materials at listed hazardous-waste sites and notes a number of secondary problems in estimating human exposures to these agents. The remainder of this report assesses problems of obtaining epidemiologic information about hazardous-waste exposures through the air, water, and other media. Chapters 4 and 5 review evidence on the health effects associated with hazardous-waste pollution of air and water. Chapter 6 assesses studies on soil and food pollution, noting those few studies on hazardous-waste sites and other relevant studies of adverse health effects of materials found at such sites. Chapter 7 describes important developments in the field of biologic markers as they relate directly to studies of the environmental epidemiology of hazardous waste. Chapter 8 identifies data gaps in the areas discussed in preceding chapters and summarizes our findings.

Our next report will complete the review of selected state health

TABLE 1-1 Summary of Studies of Residential Exposure to Hazardous-Waste Sites

Study Location and Year of Publication	Study Design and Period of Observation	Number and Type of Subjects	Exposure Measure	Major Health End Points	Reported Outcome
Tucson, AZ 1990 Goldberg et al.	Case-control 1969-1987	Children with congenital heart disease: 246 families, contact with contaminated water area (CWA) Referent: 461 families no contact with CWA	Child conceived and first trimester spent in Tucson Valley	Congenital cardiac lesion	Significant association between parental exposure to CWA and increased proportion of congenital heart disease among live births
Fresno County, CA 1988 Wong et al.	Restrospective follow-up 1978-1982	Birth ratio among 45,914 females in census tracts grouped by DBCP levels Referent: internal	Surrogate: residence in Fresno County	Decreased birth rate due to male infertility	No difference
Stringfellow Site Glen Avon, CA 1988 Baker et al.	Cross-sectional 1983	403 households Referent: 203 households	Proximity to site	Self-reported health problems	Weak to moderate positive associations: ear infection, bronchitis, asthma, angina pectoris, and skin rash

Santa Clara County, CA 1985 CA Dept. of Health Services	Retrospective follow-up 1980-1981 1981-1982	1980-1981: Pregnancies in one census tract served by contaminated water Referent: Pregnancies in one census tract not served by contaminated water 1981-1982: live births in a 7 census tract study area served by contaminated water Referent: live births in the rest of the county	Surrogate: residence in households served by contaminated water at the time of chemical leak	1980-1981: pregnancy outcomes 1981-1982: congenital cardiac defects	1980-1981: significant excess of spontaneous abortions and congenital malformations 1981-1982: excess incidence of cardiac defects within and outside the study area. No support for an association with the chemical leak
Santa Clara County, CA 1989 Swan et al.	Retrospective follow-up 1981-1983	106 babies with diagnosis of cardiac anomaly, born in county during period county exposed to contaminated water Referent: babies born in unexposed area and during unexposed time	Surrogate: residence in households served by contaminated water	Cardiac anomalies	Increased prevalence of cardiac anomalies but temporal distribution suggests solvent leak not responsible

TABLE 1-1 *Continued*

Study Location and Year of Publication	Study Design and Period of Observation	Number and Type of Subjects	Exposure Measure	Major Health End Points	Reported Outcome
Galena, KS 1990 Neuberger et al.	Retrospective follow-up 1980-1985	White residents of Galena exposed to heavy metal mining Superfund site Referent: Two unexposed towns	Residence in towns for at least 5 years prior to 1980	Age and sex-specific illnesses	Significant associations of stroke, anemia, hypertension, heart disease, skin cancer with exposure
Lowell, MA 1987 Ozonoff et al.	Cross-sectional 1983	1049 potentially exposed Referent: 948 presumably unexposed	Surrogate: residence in households within a given distance from site	Self-reported health problems	Increased prevalence of minor symptoms, irregular heart beat, fatigue, bowel complaints
Woburn, MA 1986 Lagakos et al.	Case-control 1964-1983	20 childhood leukemia cases Referent: 164 children resident in Woburn	Surrogate: residence in households served by contaminated wells	Childhood leukemia	Significant association with estimated exposure
Woburn, MA 1986 Lagakos et al.	Retrospective follow-up 1960-1982	4936 pregnancies among Woburn residents 5018 residents 18 or younger Referent: internal	Surrogate: residence in households served by contaminated wells	Adverse pregnancy outcomes; childhood disorders	Association with perinatal deaths; eye/ear anomalies, CNS anomalies; association with kidney/urinary tract infection

Woburn, MA 1988 Feldman et al.	Clinical case-control 1987(?)	28 members of 8 families with suspected neurotoxicity due to chronic exposure to TCE contaminated water Referent: 27 subjects evidencing no sign of neurologic disease or exposure to neurotoxins	Surrogate: residence in households served by contaminated wells	Blink reflex measurement as indicator of neurotoxic effects of TCE exposure	Significant differences in blink reflex function when means were compared
Rutherford, NJ 1980, Burke et al. Halperin et al.	Case-control 1973-1978	13 leukemia cases, 9 Hodgkin's cases Referent: 25 sixth graders and 17 community controls (leukemia); 17 age-sex-race matched cases from random digit dialing (Hodgkin's)	Surrogate: residence in the area	Possible etiologic risk factors for leukemia and Hodgkin's	Reduced prevalence of rubella vaccination in leukemia cases. Excess of prior vaccinations and tonsillectomies in Hodgkin's cases
Hyde Park, NY 1981 Rothenburg	Cross-sectional 1979	246 persons working in the area Referent: 492 persons from HANES National Survey	Surrogate: employment in plants near site	Health problem, urine and blood tests	Increased prevalence of hiatus hernia and other minor gastrointestinal problems

TABLE 1-1 *Continued*

Study Location and Year of Publication	Study Design and Period of Observation	Number and Type of Subjects	Exposure Measure	Major Health End Points	Reported Outcome
Love Canal, NY 1981 Janerich et al.	Retrospective follow-up (census tract) 1955-1977	700 census tract residents Referent: NY state population	Surrogate: proximity to dump site	Cancer: 1. liver 2. lymphomas 3. leukemias	Incidence: no increase
Love Canal, NY 1984 Heath et al.	Cross-sectional 1982	45 residents in houses potentially contaminated by organic chemicals Referent: 46 residents in adjacent census tract	Surrogate: testing of chemicals (two years before) in the house of exposed	Cytogenic: 1. SCE 2. chromosomal aberrations	No difference
Love Canal, NY 1984 Vianna and Polan	Retrospective follow-up 1941-1978	174 live births in swale areas near dump site Referent: 1. 443 live births in the rest of Canal area 2. all live births in upstate NY	Surrogate: proximity to dump site and at least 5 months residence	Low birth weight	Elevated incidence among exposed
Love Canal, NY 1985 Paigen et al.	Cross-sectional 1980	523 children residents of L.C. neighborhood Referent: 440 children of adjacent census	Surrogate: proximity to dump site	Health problems: seizures, learning problems, hyperactivity, eye irritation, skin rash, abdominal	Increased prevalence

53

Location/Year/Author	Study type	Population/Referent	Surrogate	Outcome measure	Results
Love Canal, NY 1987 Paigen et al.	Cross-sectional 1980	172 children born and 75% of life in Love Canal area Referent: 404 children born in adjacent census tract	Surrogate: proximity to dump site	Anthropometric measurements	Increased prevalence of shorter stature
Hamilton, Ontario 1987 Hertzman et al.	Retrospective follow-up Workers: 1965-1980 Residents: 1976-80	Workers: 197 workers at site Referent: 235 nonlandfill outdoor workers from Hamilton Wentworth Region; Residents: 614 households within 750 m of edge of dumpsite Referent: 636 households in same air pollution region as landfill site	Workers: outdoor employment on or adjacent to site; Residents: long/short-term residence in area during 1976-1980	Self-reported health outcomes	Workers: clusters of respiratory, skin, narcotic, and mood disorders; Residents: confirmed association between landfill site exposure and mood, narcotic, skin, and respiratory conditions
Clinton County, PA 1984 Budnick et al.	Mortality 1950-1979	Clinton County and three adjacent counties, PA Referent: 1. State of Pennsylvania 2. U.S.A.	Surrogate: residence in the area	Bladder cancer mortality	Increased bladder cancer mortality in male resident population after 1970

TABLE 1-1 *Continued*

Study Location and Year of Publication	Study Design and Period of Observation	Number and Type of Subjects	Exposure Measure	Major Health End Points	Reported Outcome
Clinton County, PA 1986 Logue and Fox	Cross-sectional 1983	179 long-term residents in the area near waste site Referent: 151 residents of surrounding communities	Surrogate: residence in the area	Self-reported health problems	Increased prevalence of skin problems and sleepiness
Dauphin County, PA 1985 Logue et al.	Cross-sectional 1983	65 potentially exposed Referent: 64 presumably unexposed	Surrogate: residence in households with past contamination of water with TCE	Self-reported health problems	Increased prevalence of eye irritation, diarrhea, and sleepiness
Hardeman County, TN 1982 Clark et al. Meyer, 1983 Harris et al., 1984	Cross-sectional 1978	49 residents at high exposure and 33 at intermediate exposure Referent: 57 unexposed local residents	Carbon tetrachloride in well water >150 µg/l (high exposure) <45 µg/l (intermediate exposure)	Liver functions	Transient abnormalities of liver functions in exposed

Source: Expanded and adapted from Upton et al., 1989, with permission.

department reports on this subject, emerging international reports, and case studies of legal decisions that have evaluated epidemiologic evidence not otherwise available in the published literature. On the basis of this review, we will recommend research opportunities and developments for the field of environmental epidemiology.

REFERENCES

Ahlbom, A., O. Axelson, E.S. Hansen, C. Hogstedt, U.J. Jensen, and J. Olsen. 1990. Interpretation of "negative" studies in occupational epidemiology. Scand. J. Work Environ. Health:153-157.

Baker, D.B., S. Greenland, J. Mendlein, and P. Harmon. 1988. A health study of two communities near the Stringfellow Waste Disposal site. Arch. Environ. Health 43:325-334.

Black, B. 1990. Matching evidence about clustered health events with tort law requirements. Am. J. Epidemiol. 132:S79-S86.

Brady, J., F. Liberatore, P. Harper, P. Greenwald, W. Burnett, J.N. Davies, M. Bishop, A. Polan, and N. Vianna. 1977. Angiosarcoma of the liver: An epidemiologic survey. J. Natl. Cancer Inst. 59:1383-1385.

Buck, C. 1975. Popper's philosophy for epidemiologists. Int. J. Epidemiol. 4:159-168.

Budnick, L.D., D.C. Sokal, H. Falk, J.N. Logue, and J.M. Fox. 1984. Cancer and birth defects near the Drake Superfund site, Pennsylvania. Arch. Environ. Health 39:409-413.

Bullard, R.D. 1990. Dumping in Dixie: Race, Class, and Environmental Quality. Boulder, Colo.: Westview Press.

Bunge, M.A. 1963. Causality: The Place of the Causal Principle in Modern Science. Cleveland: World.

Burke, T.A., S. Gray, C.M. Krawiec, R.J. Katz, P.W. Preuss, and G. Paulson. 1980. An environmental investigation of clusters of leukemia and Hodgkin's disease in Rutherford, New Jersey. J. Med. Soc. N.J. 77:259-264.

California Department of Health Services. 1985. Pregnancy Outcomes in Santa Clara County 1980-1982: Reports of Two Epidemiological Studies. Berkeley: California Department of Health Services.

Chalmers, T.C., H. Levin, H.S. Sacks, D. Reitman, J. Berrier, and R. Nagalingam. 1987. Meta-analysis of clinical trials as a scientific discipline. I. Control of bias and comparison with large co-operative trials. Stat. Med. 6:315-328.

Clark, C.S., C.R. Meyer, P.S. Gartside, V.A. Majeti, B. Specker, W.F. Balisteri, and V.J. Elia. 1982. An environmental health survey of drinking water contamination by leachate from a pesticide waste dump in Hardeman County, Tennessee. Arch. Environ. Health 37:9-18.

CMA (Chemical Manufacturers Association). 1991. Guidelines for Good Epidemiology Practices for Occupational and Environmental Epidemiology Research. Washington, D.C.: Chemical Manufacturers Association.

Commission for Racial Justice, United Church of Christ. 1987. Toxic Wastes and Race in the United States: A National Report on the Racial and Socio-Economic Characteristics of Communities with Hazardous Waste Sites. [New York]: Public Data Access.

CRS (Congressional Research Service). 1980. Six Case Studies of Compensation for

Toxic Substances Pollution: Alabama, California, Michigan, Missouri, New Jersey, and Texas. Committee Print, 96th Congress, 2d Session, Serial No. 96-13. Washington, D.C.: U.S. Government Printing Office.

Davis, D.L. 1985. The "shotgun wedding" of science and law: Risk assessment and judicial review. Columbia J. Environ. Law 10:67-109.

Davis, D.L. 1988. Changing policy roles of environmental epidemiology. Stat. Sci. 3:281-285.

Doll, R., and R. Peto. 1978. Cigarette smoking and bronchial carcinoma: Dose and time relationships among regular smokers and lifelong non-smokers. J. Epidemiol. Community Health 32:303-313.

Environment and Health in Developing Countries. 1991. A newsletter published by Program on Environment and Health at Management Sciences for Health, Boston, Mass.

Feldman, R.G., J. Chirico-Post, and S.P. Proctor. 1988. Blink reflex latency after exposure to trichloroethylene in well water. Arch. Environ. Health 43:143-148.

Goldberg, S.J., M.D. Lebowitz, E.J. Graver, and S. Hicks. 1990. An association of human congenital cardiac malformations and drinking water contaminants. J. Am. Coll. Cardiol. 16:155-164.

Goldman, L.R., B. Paigen, M.M. Magnant, and J.H. Highland. 1985. Low birth weight, prematurity and birth defects in children living near the hazardous waste site, Love Canal. Haz. Waste Haz. Materials 2:209-223.

Goldsmith, J.R., ed. 1986. Environmental Epidemiology: Epidemiological Investigation of Community Environmental Health Problems. Boca Raton: CRC Press.

Greenland, S. 1988. Probability versus Popper: An elaboration of the insufficiency of current Popperian approaches for epidemiologic analysis. Pp. 95-104 in Causal Inference, K.J. Rothman, ed. Chestnut Hill, Mass.: Epidemiology Resources.

Greenland, S. 1990. Divergent Biases in Ecologic and Individual-Level Studies. Paper presented at the Second Annual Meeting of the International Society for Environmental Epidemiology, August 12-15, 1990, Berkeley, Calif.

Grisham, J.W., ed. 1986. Health Aspects of the Disposal of Waste Chemicals. New York: Pergamon.

Halperin, W., R. Altman, A. Stemhagen, A.W. Iaci, G. Caldwell, T. Mason, J. Bill, T. Abe, and J.F. Clark. 1980. Epidemiologic investigations of cluster of leukemia and Hodgkin's disease in Rutherford, New Jersey. J. Med. Soc. N.J. 77:267-273.

Harris, R.H., J.H. Highland, J.V. Rodricks, and S.S. Papadopulos. 1984. Adverse effects at a Tennessee hazardous waste disposal site. Hazardous Waste 1:183-204.

Heath, C.W., Jr., M.A. Nadel, M.M. Zack, Jr., A.T.L. Chen, M.A. Bender, and J. Preston. 1984. Cytogenic findings in persons living near the Love Canal. J. Am. Med. Assoc. 251:1437-1440.

Henderson, T.W. 1990. Toxic tort litigation: Medical and scientific principles in causation. Am. J. Epidemiol. 132(Suppl. 1):S69-S78.

Hertzman, C., M. Hayes, J. Singer, and J. Highland. 1987. Upper Ottawa Street Landfill Site health study. Environ. Health Perspect. 75:173-195.

Hill, A.B. 1953. Observation and experiment. N. Engl. J. Med. 248:995-1001.

Janerich, D.T., W.S. Burnett, G. Feck, M. Hoff, P. Nasca, A.P. Polednak, P. Greenwald, and N. Vianna. 1981. Cancer incidence in the Love Canal area. Science 212:1404-1407.

Johnson, B.L. 1988. Health effects of hazardous waste: The expanding functions of the Agency for Toxic Substances and Disease Registry. Environ. Law Reporter 18:10132-10138.

Johnson, B.L. 1990. Implementation of Superfund's health-related provisions by the

Agency for Toxic Substances and Disease Registry. Environ. Law Reporter 20:10277-10282.

Kopfler, F.C., and G.F. Craun. 1986. Environmental Epidemiology. Chelsea, Mich.: Lewis.

Lagakos, S.W., B.J. Wessen, and M. Zelen. 1986. An analysis of contaminated well water and health effects in Woburn, Massachusetts. J. Am. Statist. Assoc. 81:583-596.

Lilienfeld, A.M., and D.E. Lilienfeld. 1980. Foundations of Epidemiology, 2nd ed. New York: Oxford University Press.

Lilienfeld, D.E., E. Chan, J. Ehland, J. Godbold, P.J. Landrigan, G. Marsh, and D.P. Perl. 1989. Rising mortality from motoneuron disease in the USA, 1962-84 [see Comment in: Lancet 1989 Apr. 29; 1(8644):958]. Lancet 1(8640):710-713.

Logue, J.N., and J.M. Fox. 1986. Residential health study of families living near the Drake Chemical Superfund site in Lock Haven, Pennsylvania. Arch. Environ. Health 41:222-228.

Logue, J.N., R.M. Stroman, D. Reid, C.W. Hayes, and K. Sivarajah. 1985. Investigation of potential health effects associated with well water chemical contamination in Londonderry township, Pennsylvania. Arch. Environ. Health 40:155-160.

McKeown, T. 1976. The Modern Rise of Population. New York: Academic Press. 168 pp.

Meyer, C.R. 1983. Liver dysfunction in residents exposed to leachate from a toxic waste dump. Environ. Health Perspect. 48:9-13.

Miettinen, O.S. 1985. Theoretical Epidemiology: Principles of Occurrence Research in Medicine. New York: John Wiley & Sons.

Mill, J.S. 1865. An Examination of Sir William Hamilton's Philosophy. London: Longman.

NCI (National Cancer Institute). 1990. Cancer Statistics Review, 1973-1987. NIH Publ. No. 90-2789. Bethesda, Md.: U.S. Department of Health and Human Services.

Neuberger, J.S., M. Mulhall, M.C. Pomatto, J. Sheverbush, and R.S. Hassanein. 1990. Health problems in Galena, Kansas (USA): A heavy metal mining Superfund site. Sci. Total Environ. 94:261-272.

Neutra, R.R. 1990. Counterpoint from a cluster buster. Am. J. Epidemiol. 132:1-8.

NJDOH (New Jersey Department of Health) 1989. A Report on the Health Study of Residents Living Near the Lipari Landfill. Environmental Health Service. 120 pp.

NRC (National Research Council). 1983. Risk Assessment in the Federal Government. Managing the Process. Washington, D.C.: National Academy Press.

NRC (National Research Council). 1984. Assigned Share for Radiation as a Cause of Cancer. Review of Radioepidemiologic Tables Assigning Probabilities of Causation. Washington, D.C.: National Academy Press.

NRC (National Research Council). 1986a. Environmental Tobacco Smoke: Measuring Exposures and Assessing Health Effects. Washington, D.C.: National Academy Press.

NRC (National Research Council). 1986b. Drinking Water and Health, Vol. 6. Washington, D.C.: National Academy Press.

NRC (National Research Council). 1989. Biologic Markers in Reproductive Toxicology. Washington, D.C.: National Academy Press.

OTA (U.S. Congress, Office of Technology Assessment). 1989. Coming Clean: Superfund Problems Can Be Solved. OTA-ITE-433. Washington, D.C.: U.S. Government Printing Office. 223 pp.

Ozonoff, D., and L.I. Boden. 1987. Truth and consequences: Health agency responses to environmental health problems. Sci. Technol. Human Values 12:70-77.

Ozonoff, D., M.E. Colten, A. Cupples, T. Heeren, A. Schatzkin, T. Mangione, M. Dresner, and T. Colton. 1987. Health problems reported by residents of a neighborhood contaminated by a hazardous waste facility. Am. J. Ind. Med. 11:581-597.

Paigen, B., L.R. Goldman, J.H. Highland, M.M. Magnant, and A.T. Steegman, Jr. 1985. Prevalence of health problems in children living near Love Canal. Haz. Waste Haz. Materials 2:23-43.

Paigen, B. L.R. Goldman, M.M. Magnant, J.H. Highland, and A.T. Steegman, Jr. 1987. Growth of children living near the hazardous waste site, Love Canal. Hum. Biol. 59:489-508.

Rall, D.P. 1991. Carcinogens and human health: Part 2 [letter]. Science 251(4989):10-13.

Robbins, J. 1988. Alternative approaches to cluster investigations. Unabstracted presentation at the 21st Annual Meeting of the Society for Epidemiologic Research, Vancouver, British Columbia, Canada, June 1988.

Rosenman, K.D., J.E. Rizzo, M.G. Conomos, and G.J. Halpin. 1989. Central nervous system malformations in relation to two polyvinyl chloride production facilities. Arch. Environ. Health 44:279-282.

Rothenberg, R. 1981. Morbidity study at a chemical dump — New York. Morbid. Mortal. Week. Rep. 30:293-294.

Rothenberg, R.B., K.K. Steinberg, and S.B. Thacker. 1990. The public health importance of clusters: A note from the Centers for Disease Control. Am. J. Epidemiol. 132:S3-S5.

Rothman, K. 1986. Modern Epidemiology. Boston: Little, Brown.

Schuck, P.H. 1991. Two causation conundrums: Mass exposure and social causes. Courts Health Sci. Law 1:305-319.

Siegel, M.R. 1990. Integrating public health into Superfund: What has been the impact of the Agency for Toxic Substances and Disease Registry? Environ. Law Reporter 20:10013-10020.

Susser, M. 1973. Causal Thinking in the Health Sciences: Concepts and Strategies of Epidemiology. New York: Oxford University Press.

Swan, S.H., G. Shaw, J.A. Harris, and R.R. Neutra. 1989. Congenital cardiac anomalies in relation to water contamination, Santa Clara County, California, 1981-1983. Am. J. Epidemiol. 129:885-893.

Upton, A.C., T. Kneip, and P. Toniolo. 1989. Public health aspects of toxic chemical disposal sites. Annu. Rev. Public Health 10:1-25.

USDHHS (U.S. Department of Health and Human Services). 1976. The Health Consequences of Smoking. Report of the Surgeon General. Publ. No. CDC 78-8357. Washington, D.C.: Office of Smoking and Health, U.S. Department of Health and Human Services.

USDHHS (U.S. Department of Health and Human Services). 1986. The Health Consequences of Involuntary Smoking: A Report of the Surgeon General. DHHS Publication No. (CDC) 87-8398. Washington, D.C.: U.S. Department of Health and Human Services.

Utidjian, H.M.D. 1988. The interaction between epidemiology and animal studies in industrial toxicology. Pp. 309-329 in Perspectives in Basic and Applied Toxicology, B. Ballantyne, ed. London: Wright.

Vesselinovitch, S.D. 1969. Significance of the stage of perinatal development in the induction of tumors by a radiomimetic multicarcinogen. Pp. 511-515 in Radiation Biology of the Fetal and Juvenile Mammal. Oak Ridge, Tennessee: U.S. Atomic Energy Commission.

Vianna, N.J., and A.K. Polan. 1984. Incidence of low birth weight among Love Canal residents. Science 226(4679):1217-1219.

WHO (World Health Organization). 1983. Guidelines on Studies in Environmental Epidemiology. Environmental Health Criteria 27. Geneva: World Health Organization.

Wong, O., M.D. Whorton, N. Gordon, and R.W. Morgan. 1988. An epidemiologic investigation of the relationship between DBCP contamination in drinking water and birth rates in Fresno County, California. Am. J. Public Health 78:43-46.

2

State and Federal Context for Environmental Epidemiology of Hazardous Wastes

EDERAL AND STATE ENVIRONMENTAL policies have largely shaped the development of environmental epidemiology as it pertains to the study of hazardous-waste sites in the U.S. First, scientists working for state and federal agencies perform most of such studies. Second, federal and state regulations determine the nature and limitations of available data on environmental contamination related to hazardous-waste sites. Third, federal and state agencies are continuously involved in the process of defining which chemicals found in the environment are of concern for human health and the levels at which action should be taken to protect human health.

The environmental legislation that produced these government programs was clearly intended to protect human health. Congress and the states enacted strengthened legislation in the early 1980s in response to public concern about the impact of hazardous-waste sites on the health of nearby communities—concerns that persisted and escalated through the decade as the dimensions of the problem continued to expand. The U.S. Environmental Protection Agency (EPA) estimated that in 1981, 264 million metric tons of hazardous waste were produced (NRC, 1985). (One million metric tons equal approximately 1.1 million English [short] tons.) By 1988 the figure had risen: 5.5 billion metric tons of hazardous waste is produced each year in the U.S. (EPA, 1989a). Public opinion polls consistently rank hazardous-waste sites among the most serious environmental risks and the environment as the greatest public concern (Roberts, 1990). Hazardous-waste sites are a major public health management issue in every state. Half of the entire U.S. population and 95 percent of the rural population rely on groundwater as the main source of drinking water, and each year thousands of wells are closed because of hazardous-waste contamination (Wells, 1990). The public fears hazardous waste, wants it cleaned up, and is willing to pay the enormous sums currently spent on Superfund because of the belief that this program will protect public health.

Whether Superfund and other environmental programs are actually protecting human health is a critical question for environmental epidemiology with respect to federal and state efforts in environmental protection. To answer it would require information on the scope of potential and actual human exposures to hazardous wastes and on the health effects that could be associated with these exposures. Yet during the past 10 years, of the estimated $4.2 billion spent each year on hazardous-waste sites in the U.S. (OTA, 1989), less than 1 percent has been devoted to the evaluation of health risks at these sites. As a result, existing data on exposures and health effects are inadequate not only for decisions on the management of hazardous-waste sites, but for epidemiologic investigations of the health impact of the sites as well.

The purpose of this chapter is to describe how so much effort and money could have been spent with such a moderate yield in knowledge. This chapter will describe federal and state legislation, policies, and programs that determine how hazardous-waste sites are evaluated; what information on exposure and health effects is collected; how the data are analyzed and used in setting priorities and planning remediation programs; what proportion of hazardous-waste-control budgets is spent on assessing population exposures and risks; and what are the nature and extent of environmental epidemiology carried out by these agencies.

The intent of Congress in enacting legislation on hazardous-waste sites was clear. As set forth in the legislative history of the Comprehensive Environmental Response, Compensation, and Liability Act (CERCLA), passed in 1980 and generally known as Superfund, the goals of the bill included

> an inventory of inactive hazardous-waste sites in a systematic manner, establishment of priorities among the sites based on relative danger, a response program to contain dangerous releases from inactive hazardous-waste sites, acceleration of the elimination of unsafe hazardous-waste sites, and a systematic program of fund-

ing to identify, evaluate and take responsive actions at inactive hazardous-waste sites to assure protection of public health and the environment in a cost-effective manner. (Legislative History, P.L. 96-510, p. 25)

In essence, Congress wanted to know how widespread the problem of environmental contamination due to hazardous-waste sites is, and how serious a threat this is to human health; that the sites which present the worst problems would be dealt with first; what the actual health risks to communities living around specific hazardous-waste sites are, so that information could be used in making decisions about remediation; and that the remediation programs would do the most possible with limited resources to protect the health of the public.

These objectives are in fact the traditional elements of a public health strategy: The discovery and preliminary assessment of as many sites as possible, to describe the universe of potential exposures; the priority ranking of sites by a defined protocol, to identify and act on those most urgently requiring attention; the collection and use of data on current human exposures and health effects early in the triage and evaluation processes; and the development of remediation programs with direct and continuous attention to the public health effects of releases from the sites. As this review of the federal and state regulatory context for environmental epidemiology will reveal, however, the intent of Congress in creating Superfund has not been realized. Some 10 years after the program began, we are still unable to assess the impact of hazardous wastes on public health.

FEDERAL LEGISLATION, POLICIES, AND PROGRAMS

In 1980, CERCLA established the Superfund program as part of the Environmental Protection Agency. Under CERCLA, more than 31,000 sites have been reported to the CERCLA Information System (CERCLIS) inventory of sites that potentially require cleanup. EPA has completed more than 27,000 preliminary assessments and has conducted detailed investigations of more than 9000 sites (EPA, 1989a). As of March 1991, 1,189 sites were on EPA's final National Priorities List (NPL) (EPA, 1991). CERCLA was amended in 1986 in the Superfund Amendments and Reauthorization Act (SARA), and in 1990 it was reauthorized without amendment.

The Superfund program is responsible for the greatest part of hazardous-waste site evaluation and control at the federal level. It should be noted that CERCLA excludes the following from Superfund/EPA jurisdiction: petroleum and natural gas releases of nuclear materials or by-products; normal field application of fertilizers; engine exhausts;

certain workplace releases; and releases allowed by permits under other federal pollution control statutes (Wolf, 1988). Data on environmental releases of toxic substances, and more recently on health effects, are collected and analyzed at several stages of the evaluation and remediation processes. For readers not familiar with the organization and terminology of Superfund evaluations, the following is a brief description of activities proceeding from site identification to cleanup.

HAZARDOUS-WASTE SITE EVALUATION AND REMEDIATION

Identification: Sites are reported by states to Superfund; EPA decides whether to enter a site in the CERCLIS inventory.

Removal Action: This action starts any time after a site is identified because of emergency conditions that require fast action or to prevent deteriorating conditions that would make cleanup more difficult.

Preremedial Process

Preliminary Assessment (PA): Review of existing information on chemicals present at the site and on potential releases.

Site Inspection (SI): On-site inspection of some sites, as suggested by PA, and review of data.

Hazard Ranking System (HRS): Calculation of the HRS score: if the score is high enough, the site will be proposed for the NPL and will go on to the remedial process.

Remedial Process

Remedial Investigation/Feasibility Study (RI/FS): Evaluation of contamination, associated risks, and cleanup options.

Project Scoping: Review of SI data and sampling plans; formulation of preliminary remediation goals.

Site Characterization: Baseline risk assessment.

Remedial Action Objectives: Remedial goals refined, based on risk assessment and applicable or relevant and appropriate requirements (existing standards and guidelines).

Development and Screening of Alternatives

Detailed Analysis of Alternatives: Risk evaluation of alternative remedial strategies.

Record of Decision (ROD): Selected remedial strategies identified, federal government committed to actions that will reduce contamination to the level specified by the remedial objectives.
Remedial Design (RD): Plan for engineering and construction of the chosen remedy.
Remedial Action (RA): Implementation of remedial strategies. (based on OTA, 1989; EPA, 1989b)

The time required from the entry of a site into CERCLIS to the beginning of the remedial investigation and feasibility study (RI/FS) is usually four to five years. The entire process, through remediation, can take more than a decade under the best of circumstances. EPA Administrator Reilly has estimated that it will be 30 years before all of the sites currently on the NPL are fully remediated. Less than 10 percent of all sites in the CERCLIS inventory make it to the NPL, however; the rest are either referred to other federal or state authorities or determined not to require Superfund action (OTA, 1989). Complex sites are frequently divided into several parts for evaluation and cleanup, and the same site can have a number of distinct RI/FSs and RODs proceeding at different paces.

The preliminary assessment (PA) is usually a paper review of available information on the history and current contamination at the site. The site inspection (SI) involves at least a walk-around inspection of the site. Information gathered in the PA and SI are used to calculate a projected numerical site score using a standard formula, the hazard ranking system (HRS). This score is used to determine whether the site will merit further investigation, including placement on the NPL and progression to a full RI/FS. In general, only existing data on hazardous-waste releases, environmental contamination, and off-site migration are used in the preremedial process; extensive new sampling can be undertaken later, as part of the RI/FS.

The purpose of the remedial investigation (RI) is to develop a risk assessment for the site, representing the likely current and future risk associated with human exposures to releases from the site. The risk assessment includes hazard identification, a dose-response assessment, an exposure assessment, and risk characterization. The product of the risk assessment is "a numerical estimate of the public health consequences of exposure to an agent," used to establish cleanup goals; to set permit levels for discharge, storage, or transport of hazardous wastes, and to determine allowable levels of contamination (ATSDR, 1990a, pp. 2-5).

The exposure assessment developed as part of the RI/FS depends heavily on modeling rather than on actual measurement of exposure for people living near the site (EPA, 1989b). Sampling data are used to model the potential exposures of nearby residents, although the models employed in these assessments have not been adequately validated. The lack of sound exposure data for populations living near hazardous-waste sites not only undermines the capacity of federal agencies and other investigators to conduct epidemiologic studies, but it impedes the ability of Superfund managers to assess the public health impact of hazardous-waste-site exposures.

The original CERCLA legislation also created a new public health agency to deal with the human health effects of hazardous wastes: the Agency for Toxic Substances and Disease Registry (ATSDR), within the U.S. Public Health Service. Under CERCLA, EPA is the regulatory agency that administers Superfund, while ATSDR is the non-regulatory public health agency. ATSDR depends on EPA to endorse its funding requests, and EPA has initial approval over ATSDR's annual appropriation (Siegel, 1990). Although ATSDR was authorized by CERCLA in 1980, it was not until 1983 that it was formally established by the U.S. Public Health Service, following a lawsuit by the Environmental Defense Fund, the Chemical Manufacturers Association, and the American Petroleum Institute (Siegel, 1990). By the time Superfund was due for reauthorization in 1985, ATSDR—crippled by this late start, low budgets, and a lack of staff positions—still did not have a clear agenda and work plan and had not produced any significant work on the health aspects of hazardous-waste sites.

Although Congress was sharply critical of the early failure of the Superfund program to address the health effects of hazardous wastes, Congress in fact may have contributed to this problem by creating ATSDR (without authorization of staff and fiscal support adequate to influence the remediation process), thereby achieving the unintended effect of appearing to absolve EPA of the need to directly incorporate public health considerations into site assessments. Nevertheless, Congress attempted to resolve this problem with SARA. EPA was directed to revise its site evaluation process, and Congress gave new prominence and responsibility to ATSDR, which was directed to produce public health assessments of all Superfund sites proposed for the NPL, and for other sites in response to public petition. In addition, ATSDR was required to establish a priority list of hazardous substances found at CERCLA sites, to produce toxicologic profiles for each substance on this list, and to conduct research on the health effects of hazardous substances and hazardous-waste sites (P.L. 99-499).

SARA defined ATSDR's health assessments to include:

> preliminary assessments of the potential risk to human health posed by individual sites and facilities, based on such factors as

the nature and extent of contamination, the existence of potential
pathways of human exposure...the size and potential susceptibility of the community within the likely pathways of exposure, the
comparison of expected human exposure levels to the short-term
and long-term health effects associated with identified hazardous
substances and any available recommended exposure or toler-
ance limits for such hazardous substances, and the comparison of
existing morbidity and mortality data on diseases that may be
associated with the observed levels of exposure. (ATSDR, 1990a,
pp. 2-3, 4)

Although many aspects of EPA's risk assessment process and ATSDR's
health assessment process overlap, the distinction between them is
based primarily on the intended purpose of each type of assessment.
The EPA risk assessment is intended to serve as the quantitative basis for the selection of remedial objectives and strategies for the site;
the ATSDR health assessment is intended to provide the community
with qualitative information on the public health implications of the
site and to identify the need for further action to protect the health of
the community or to research the health effects associated with current or past releases from the site.

In response to ATSDR's slow start-up, Congress also set deadlines
for many of these mandated activities. Health assessments were to
be completed by the end of 1988 for all 951 Superfund sites listed on
the NPL before Oct. 17, 1986, and subsequent health assessments
were due within one year of proposal for NPL status. Significantly,
this meant that ATSDR's health assessment would normally be completed well before each RI/FS began. Because the RI/FS is the stage
at which the most extensive exposure and risk assessment information is produced, ATSDR has divided its health assessments into two
stages: the preliminary health assessment (PHA), prepared in the
first year after a site is proposed for listing, and the full health assessment, prepared when the RI/FS is complete. The full assessment
is used in determining the remediation objectives and the final record
of decision. As of Dec. 12, 1990, ATSDR had completed 600 preliminary assessments and 469 full assessments (J. Andrews, ATSDR, personal communication, 1991). With the backlog of unevaluated sites
now essentially eliminated, ATSDR can begin to evaluate sites as
soon as they are proposed for NPL listing, and it can begin to play a
more active role in the development of the RI/FS work plan.

Of the 951 NPL sites evaluated in the first round, ATSDR found
that 109 (11.5 percent) constituted a risk to human health because of
actual exposures (11 sites) or probable exposures (98 sites) to hazardous chemical agents that could have adverse health consequences.

These sites were listed in the categories of "urgent public health concern" or "public health concern." It is estimated that 725,000 persons live within a one-mile radius of the 109 sites (ATSDR, 1989a). In 1151 health assessments at NPL sites completed by mid-1990, ATSDR determined that 85 percent of the sites involved releases of hazardous substances and that about 15 percent of these merited further public health investigation (Johnson, 1990). More intensive analyses of 76 sites identified 32 percent (24) as needing some kind of health action (ATSDR, 1991). In characterizing the distribution of hazardous exposures at NPL sites, ATSDR reported frequent detection of a substantial number of hazardous substances, including lead at 43 percent of the sites and trichloroethylene at 42 percent of the sites (ATSDR, 1989a). These summary data indicate the breadth of the potential exposures associated with hazardous-waste sites. Figures 2-1, 2-2, and 2-3 indicate the types of exposure and sources of contamination at Superfund sites.

ATSDR found that the data available were adequate for evaluating environmental contamination and public health risks in only 31 percent of the 951 NPL sites assessed. Evaluation of the adequacy of

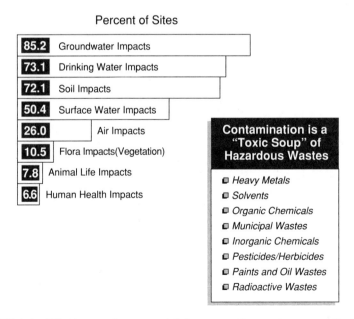

FIGURE 2-1   What were the potential threats to the environment that led to listing on the NPL? Source: Environmental Protection Agency, National Priorities List, Characterization Report, 1990.

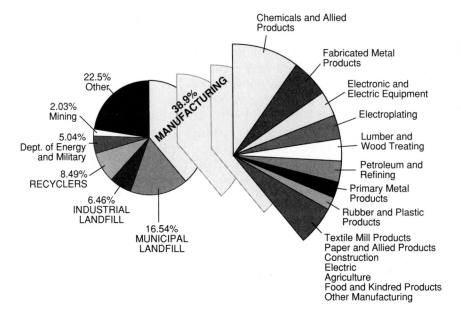

FIGURE 2-2 Wastes at NPL sites come from many sources. Source: Environmental Protection Agency, National Priorities List, Characterization Report, 1990.

data was conducted by ATSDR staff (ATSDR, 1989a). In all, there were adequate data for only 39 sites that could be eliminated as sources of public health concern either because remedial action had already mitigated earlier concerns or because there was no feasible pathway for human exposure (ATSDR, 1989a). Moreover, the population potentially exposed to these uncertain risks is quite large: ATSDR estimates that 4.1 million people live within one mile of 725 of the NPL sites for which population data exist, and 1.9 million of these persons are women of childbearing age, young children, or elderly persons—all of whom can be considered at particular risk from toxic chemical exposure.

Under CERCLA, ATSDR also was directed to issue public health advisories in cases of urgent public health concern. These notify the EPA administrator, state agencies, and the immediate community of recommendations for interim remediate actions, such as containment or the provision of alternative drinking-water supplies, required to protect the health of the public. In response to these advisories, the EPA administrator can direct an immediate removal action, place a

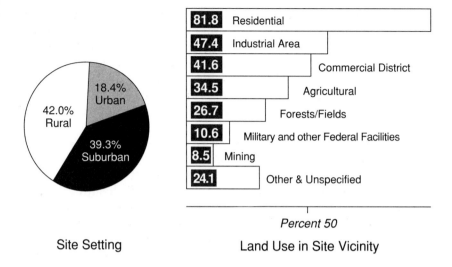

Site Setting   Land Use in Site Vicinity

FIGURE 2-3 NPL sites are located in all settings and areas. Source: Environmental Protection Agency, National Priorities List, Characterization Report, 1990.

site on the NPL or, if it is already listed, give it a higher priority (ATSDR, 1990a).

The Forest Glen site in Niagara Falls, New York, is illustrative of many of the limitations of these processes for site discovery, assessment, and the protection of public health. Previously used as an industrial landfill, Forest Glen had been developed as a mobile home park during the late 1970s. By 1989, a total of 150 people lived in 51 mobile homes atop the site. Hazardous wastes in the surface and subsurface soils included extraordinarily high concentrations of aniline, phenothiazine, benzothiazole, 2-mercaptobenzothiazole, and polyaromatic hydrocarbons, with dermal, ingestion, and inhalation exposures that carried associated risks of dermatitis, phytotoxic skin reactions, and cancer. The corrosion of drinking-water pipes by the chemicals raised the further possibility that drinking-water supplies could be, or had been, contaminated.

Although the Niagara County Health Department reportedly excavated some soil from the area in 1980 and EPA conducted an initial site inspection in 1987, no action had been taken to further assess the site, remediate the hazards, or relocate the residents until New York State and EPA invited ATSDR to conduct a public health assessment in 1989. ATSDR's assessment noted the potentially serious exposures for the families at the site and recommended the immediate relocation of the residents. By issuing the report as a public health advisory, ATSDR enabled EPA to immediately place Forest Glen on the NPL and allowed the Federal Emergency Management Agency to provide temporary relocation assistance for the residents. Within one month of the initial ATSDR site visit, all residents were notified of the health risks and offered the opportunity to relocate (J. Melius, New York State Department of Health, personal communication, 1991; ATSDR, 1989b).

Of the dozen public health advisories released by ATSDR to date, only two have been for sites that were already listed on the NPL but that required further immediate action to protect the health of the public. The other ten also represented urgent public health concerns, but they had not been reported to the Superfund program, had been rejected by CERCLIS, or were inventoried in CERCLIS but had not been proposed for the NPL. As listed in Table 2-1, these sites included a variety of hazardous substances, contaminated media, and routes of exposure.

Congress also directed ATSDR to undertake a further set of responsibilities, beyond the assessment of NPL sites, that were intended to build a science base for the health evaluation of hazardous-waste sites and exposures. With EPA, ATSDR has developed a priority list of 225 hazardous substances found at Superfund sites (see Table 3-2, and Appendixes 3-A and 3-B). These substances were chosen for their toxicity, their frequency of occurrence at NPL sites, and the potential for human contact. Toxicology profiles have been prepared for almost half of them. ATSDR has established criteria for determining the data gaps and research needs for each chemical, and is attempting to fill the gaps in collaboration with the National Institute for Environmental Health Sciences (NIEHS) and private industry. The lack of a specific congressional mandate and funding mechanism for this research has made it difficult for ATSDR to organize a logical and timely sequence of investigations in many cases.

In addition, ATSDR conducts pilot studies of human exposure to hazardous-waste-site releases, usually through biological monitoring or evaluations of symptom prevalence in surrounding populations (28 studies are in progress or complete); epidemiological studies (28 studies are in progress or complete); and a disease surveillance program, using health outcome data bases in 10 states. It also establishes registries of persons environmentally exposed to hazardous substances (trichloroethylene and dioxin, so far; a registry is proposed for benzene) and, in response to additional legislation, it prepares special reports for Congress (childhood lead poisoning, the health impact of medical waste) (Johnson, 1990).

TABLE 2-1 ATSDR Public Health Advisories

Site and Date	NPL Status When Advisory Released	Exposures of Concern	Population Exposed	Immediate Action Recommended
Times Beach, MO 12/23/82	No	dioxin (TCDD) in soil	residential areas contaminated by industrial oil applied on roadways, spread from flooding	1. intensive sampling 2. limit residents contact with soil, use protective clothing including dust filter masks 3. encourage residents who have moved away to remain off site
Glen Ridge, NJ 12/00/83	No	radium in soil, with indoor radon and gamma radiation	residential neighborhoods contaminated by waste from processed radium ore	1. requested EPA inform residents of high gamma rate areas, and of need to lower exposure by limiting time in those areas while awaiting remediation
Kelly-Koett Cincinnati, OH 8/13/87	No	radium in floors, walls and plumbing of buildings, with indoor radon	neighborhood access to abandoned industrial buildings contaminated by spill and cleanup, and removal of contaminated materials by intruders	1. prevent access to site
Ottowa, IL 4/04/88	No	radium in soil, indoor radon and gamma radiation	residential areas contaminated by industrial waste	1. intensive sampling 2. advise residents in exposed areas to (a) reduce indoor radon exposure, (b) reduce external gamma and internal radiation exposure, (c) not to smoke

72

TABLE 2-1 *Continued*

Site and Date	NPL Status When Advisory Released	Exposures of Concern	Population Exposed	Immediate Action Recommended
Radium Chemical Co. Queens, NY 2/10/89	No	radium, indoor radon and gamma radiation	radioactive waste stored at abandoned industrial site next to current industrial operations; neighborhood access to and removal of radioactive materials; fire/explosion risk at site	1. removal of radium sources 2. remediation and decontamination of building
Forest Glen Mobile Home Park Niagara Falls, NY 7/31/89	No	polyaromatic hydrocoarbons, analine, phenothiazine, benzothiazole, mercaptobenzothiazole	mobile home residents on top of hazardous waste site; possible contamination of water supplies	1. relocation of residents 2. place site on NPL
Newstead Site, Erie County, NY 8/22/89	No	lead and cadmium in soil; methylene chloride and benzene in drinking water well; physical injury	residents living on hazardous waste site	1. remove residents from site 2. measure blood lead and cadmium in residents on site 3. sample dusts within houses on site
Bunker Hill Kellogg, ID 10/5/89	No	arsenic in copper flue dust piles; lead, cadmium, arsenic in soil	active mining and ore concentrating; inactive smelter, sulfuric acid	1. restrict access to site 2. suspend all remediation activities and salvaging until safety plans approved

Site	NPL listing	Contaminants	Exposure/Population	Recommendations
		and asbestos on grounds; physical injury	plant and phosphate/fertilizer plant; unrestricted access to and recreational use of site; soils carried by wind into nearby residential areas	1. identify and follow former employees and surrounding population in health survey 2. protect current on-site workers and family members from exposures 3. intensive sampling
Caldwell Systems, Inc. Lenoir, NC 7/25/90	No (RCRA closure pending)	incineration products of furniture manufacturing and waste torpedo fuel	employees and family members at former incinerator and adjacent landfill and lands where waste was dumped; inhalation exposure to incinerator emissions among nearby residents; potential groundwater contamination	
Navajo-Brown Vanderver Navajo-Desiderio Uranium Mining Areas Bluewater, NM 11/21/90	No	uranium in soil, radon and gamma radiation; heavy metals in soil; physical hazards	residents living on mining areas contaminated with radioactive mine wastes; adjacent residential properties	1. place on NPL 2. restrict access to site 3. advise residents of risks and steps to reduce exposures 4. follow population in health surveillance 5. further sampling
White Chemical Co. Newark, NJ 11/21/90	No	materials and wastes from manufacture of acid chlorides and flame retardants	ongoing release of fumes and liquids from containers on-site; threat of catastrophic release of hazardous substances in heavily populated former industrial area	1. take actions to stabilize site 2. restrict access to site 3. further sampling 4. develop emergency response and notification procedures 5. train local emergency response personnel

TABLE 2-1 *Continued*

Site and Date	NPL Status When Advisory Released	Exposures of Concern	Population Exposed	Immediate Action Recommended
Asbestos Disposal Sites Passaic, NJ 12/20/90	No	chrysotile asbestos in soil	residents living on and nearby hazardous waste site; employees in small firms on site	1. relocate residents from contaminated homes 2. further sampling in homes of residents on or near site 3. restrict access to site 4. restrict cleanup activities likely to generate airborne dusts 5. sample homes of cleanup employees

Finally, as its name—the Agency for Toxic Substances and Disease Registry—implies, Congress intended that the Public Health Service establish registries of populations exposed to hazardous wastes and follow these populations over time to observe associated health effects. Because of the uncertain end points and utility and great expense of starting and maintaining site-specific, open-ended registries, ATSDR has resisted congressional and community pressures to establish them. Instead, the agency has developed specialized registries to study the long-term health effects of exposure to specific chemicals at hazardous-waste sites, with the intention of combining data from several sites where similar exposures have occurred to achieve populations large enough that the associated health effects can be detected.

Other federal statutes have established programs that are much more limited in their capacity to evaluate and control exposures at active and abandoned sites. Although Resource Conservation and Recovery Act (RCRA) amendments authorized ATSDR to conduct health assessments at the request of EPA at landfills and surface impoundments, many of these sites are still held by EPA from entry into the CERCLIS system and will not reach ATSDR's attention for some time. The Safe Drinking Water Act and the Clean Air Act mandate monitoring of a limited set of priority chemicals, but they are not intended to identify or track specific sources of pollution, such as hazardous-waste sites, and are therefore of limited use in characterizing the releases from such sites. In particular, the Safe Drinking Water Act does not include domestic wells, which are frequently the pathway of exposure of greatest concern at NPL sites. Although routine monitoring of drinking water and air quality are state responsibilities, state direction of this monitoring to assess potential emissions from hazardous-waste sites is made even less likely by the fact that EPA's regional offices do not notify the relevant state agencies when off-site migration is suspected or confirmed.

DISTRIBUTION OF EXPOSURE

How well does this system characterize the distribution of human exposures to chemicals released from hazardous-waste sites? For the purposes of environmental epidemiology, this question has two parts: For each site, how well are the potential human exposures characterized in terms of the contamination of media; the identification of on-site human contact, environmental pathways, and off-site migration; of off-site human contact with contaminated media; of populations at risk; and of indicators of human exposure? For hazardous-waste sites as a whole—including non-NPL sites—how well known is the range and distribution of human exposure to hazardous substances? The importance of the latter is often poorly understood. While epidemiology may fruitfully investigate the physiologic changes and disease end points associated with one or more exposures at a particular site, the tasks of epidemiology include the characterization of the extent and nature of such outcomes resulting from hazardous-waste sites (and other environmental sources) in the entire population.

UNIVERSE OF POTENTIAL EXPOSURES

A substantial number of hazardous-waste sites are not reported to CERCLIS. Sites also are reported to or known to the Emergency Response Notification System, the Federal Facilities Hazardous Waste Compliance Docket, RCRA, the Department of Defense, the Department of the Interior's Abandoned Mine Lands Remediation Program, and the Leaking Underground Storage Tank (LUST) program. Not all of these agencies or programs maintain inventories or data bases of sites reported to them. The congressional Office of Technology Assessment (OTA) recently concluded that the maximum number of potential sites from which CERCLIS and NPL sites are drawn is approximately 439,000. These sites include RCRA Subtitle C and D facilities, mining waste sites, nonpetroleum leaking underground storage tanks, pesticide-contaminated sites, federal facilities, radioactive releases, underground injection wells, municipal gas facilities, and wood-preserving plants, among others, but not sites assigned to the other remediation programs listed above. If even 10 percent of the CERCLIS-eligible sites ultimately require cleanup, the result would be a total NPL of 43,900 sites (OTA, 1989).

State programs also track and record hazardous-waste sites. A 1986 survey found 32,910 sites on state lists, in comparison with 24,544 sites then in CERCLIS (OTA, 1989). No guidance exists on the criteria and processes for reporting sites to CERCLIS, and many states screen sites and report to EPA only those sites for which they regard EPA management as potentially helpful. OTA reports that EPA itself holds thousands of hazardous-waste sites outside the CERCLIS inventory, to control the resource and management problems posed by congressional deadlines for preliminary assessments on CERCLIS sites. As a result, there is no single, common inventory of hazardous-waste sites in the U.S. (OTA, 1989).

There also is no national program of hazardous-waste-site discovery. As the 1989 OTA report on Superfund states, "EPA has never requested funds from Congress for site discovery. EPA has no site discovery program, has no budget for site discovery, and does not allow States to spend Superfund monies for site discovery" (OTA, 1989, p. 88). EPA had initiated a comprehensive site discovery program in 1980, known as the 200 Cities Hazardous-waste Site Discovery Plan, but canceled it a year later when the agency's comptroller informed the contracting laboratory that EPA already had more sites than there was money for, and did not need more (OTA, 1989). EPA's Office of Research and Development later produced guidelines for an expanded program to finish the 200-city search and to analyze 150 sites. OTA estimated the total costs through fiscal year (FY) 1986 at $6.4 million for discovery and site analysis; these funds were never requested by the agency.

In FY90, the total EPA budget request for PAs, SIs, and HRS scoring work was $47 million. This annual cost of preremedial site evaluation is comparable to the cost of cleaning up one large site, and it represents only about 3 percent of the annual Superfund budget (OTA, 1989). OTA has estimated that a revised 200 cities plan would cost about $100 million over a five-year period, including assessment of an estimated 7500 sites found as a result of the program. As OTA points out, this would be well within the current Superfund expenditures for site characterization and remediation. OTA further estimates all current expenditures on site characterization and remediation, public and private, at $242-612 million annually (OTA, 1989).

The lack of a site discovery system—and of a common site inventory—are the result of the federal policy of controlling CERCLIS to manage EPA's work load. EPA's resources are already strained by the need to meet congressional deadlines for assessing CERCLIS and NPL sites. By far the greatest share of this burden occurs in the remedial phase after a site is listed on the NPL, during the lengthy and expensive processes of the RI/FS and in the ultimate cleanup. In comparison, the preremedial evaluation of sites is relatively inexpensive. Relevant cost estimates are summarized in Table 2-2. It is important to note that only a relatively small portion of the cost estimates for EPA's PA and SI evaluations presented here are devoted to assessments of potential or actual human exposures. The bulk of the costs are incurred in engineering studies of the need for and feasibility of remediation.

The lack of a site discovery program and a comprehensive inventory presents a particular problem from a public health perspective. The range and distribution of human exposure to releases from hazardous-waste sites is both unknown and unknowable. EPA now acknowledges that undiscovered sites could well represent significant health risks (OTA, 1989). This is a reversal of previous statements

TABLE 2-2   Cost Estimates: Preremedial Assessments of
Hazardous-Waste Sites

Agency	Stage	Cost ($ Million)
EPA (FY91)	Preliminary Assessment	7
	Site Inspection	25
	Listing Site Inspection	75
	NPL Listing	88
	Subtotal	195
ATSDR (FY89)	Preliminary Health Assessment	25

that most sites with serious potential for harm had been detected
(OTA, 1989).   The assumption that potential health risks are missed
in the current nonsystem of reporting to CERCLIS is supported by
several state reviews of the subject.   The California State Department
of Health, in reviewing the 93 sites on the state's Superfund list in
1984, found that 19 of the sites were also on the federal NPL.   Yet 46
of the sites showed evidence of waste release into groundwater, and
in 34 of these cases the groundwater was known to be used for drinking.   Extensive or systematic sampling existed for only 22 of the sites,
despite the evidence of potential human exposure.   In all 19 of the
California sites with known contamination of groundwater, moreover, more than 10,000 persons were potentially exposed (Layefsky
et al., 1988).

The discovery and preliminary assessment of hazardous-waste sites
represent, in epidemiologic terms, case-finding: identifying potentially serious exposures that require both further assessment and intervention to protect the health of the community.   For environmental epidemiology to be of help to us in understanding the overall
health risks associated with hazardous-waste releases, the ability to
know the universe of potential risk is critical (Marsh and Caplan,
1986).   Because exposures vary so greatly from one site to the next,
the incomplete descriptions of the sites and the failure to fully assess
the exposures that result from releases at many identified sites put
the epidemiologist at risk of missing health effects associated with
high levels of exposure at undetected sites, of incorrectly estimating
the frequency or amount of population exposures to specific releases,
and of missing opportunities to combine data from several populations to achieve greater power in studies of specific chemicals.

CHARACTERIZATION OF EXPOSURE

PREREMEDIATION PHASE

Because less than 10 percent of CERCLIS sites are ever placed on the NPL by EPA, it is important to examine both the nature of the preremedial assessment itself and the criteria used to select sites for the NPL. For most of the sites reported to Superfund, the only environmental contamination and health assessment data available are those assembled during preremedial assessment: the preliminary assessment (PA), the site inspection (SI), and the hazard ranking system (HRS) score.

In most cases, the PA is simply a review of existing data about the site. As a part of the PA, a probable HRS score is calculated; if it is below the cut-off for proposal for the NPL, the site will be designated "no further remedial action planned" (NFRAP). NFRAP sites also include those that never received CERCLA hazardous substances, those that have no potential to release CERCLA hazardous substances into the environment, and those that do not fall under EPA jurisdiction (such as uranium mill tailings that fall under a Department of Energy program). According to OTA and EPA documents, the PA was originally applied as a screen to identify sites that required immediate removal actions (OTA, 1989). All other sites were automatically forwarded to SI unless the information was sufficient to conclude that no threat existed. Now, however, sites that could represent a threat to public health but that lie beyond Superfund jurisdiction or that do not score high enough on the projected HRS are eliminated before the SI stage. In other words, sites with clearly present or potential hazards can be rejected after a paper review and deferred to the states or simply held on CERCLIS with no further action. EPA has revised its management of the site evaluation process to limit the number of sites going through the system at each stage. Although limiting the number of sites evaluated because of resource constraints makes good sense for the purposes of program management, this approach has had an unfortunate effect as well. It has artificially constrained the number of sites recognized as needing further evaluation. Congressional deadlines for the evaluation of sites are clocked from the date of listing on CERCLIS or of proposal for the NPL and do not permit EPA to maintain lists of sites that need evaluation but cannot be processed because funds are limited.

As a result, there is a growing body of "rejects" from the preremedial Superfund process. A substantial proportion of these sites could present serious threats to the health of the public and thereby merit both immediate public health assessment and, in some cases, environmental epidemiology investigations. EPA's Region 5 compared HRS scores projected during the preremedial process with actual HRS scores assigned after an SI, and found both false positives and false negatives: Only 30 percent of sites with high projected scores actually ended up with scores above the Superfund threshold, and 10 percent of the sites with low priority projections ultimately received HRS scores above the Superfund threshold for NPL ranking. OTA estimates that as many as 2000 of the 17,000 CERCLIS sites rejected for the NPL could be "false negatives"—sites not listed on the NPL because of incorrect decisions or errors (OTA, 1989, pp. 112-114).

EPA is now re-evaluating a subset of sites rejected for NPL listing during the preremedial process, although the criteria for review and the quality of the data available could limit the validity of this review. A 1989 EPA report on the congressionally mandated revision of the hazard ranking system stated that the legislative intent in SARA "makes clear that this mandate does not require detailed risk assessments, but directs EPA to rank sites as accurately as feasible based simply on information available from preliminary assessments and site inspections consistent with the goal of 'expeditiously' identifying candidates for response actions" (EPA, 1990a, p. i).

This implies that the only consequence of the preremedial assessment is to prioritize sites for more detailed assessment. For most sites, in fact, no attempt is made to characterize the potential public health impact or the need for action to protect the health of the public in this preremedial phase. Because the vast majority of sites never receive more than a preremedial assessment, moreover, the implications for accurate evaluation of health hazards at these sites and for environmental epidemiology are critical. The problem is particularly serious because of the growing number of sites in the CERCLIS inventory, as seen in Figure 2-4.

REMEDIATION PHASE

As noted earlier, less than 10 percent of CERCLIS sites assessed in the preremedial phase are proposed for NPL listing. Sites listed on the NPL enter what is known as the remedial phase, and are subjected to a full remedial investigation and feasibility study (RI/FS) for the purposes of selecting and implementing a remediation strategy. It is in this stage that extensive sampling is conducted at the direction of Superfund managers and contractors.

Over the past decade, the Superfund RI/FS has relied almost exclusively on measurements of on-site releases and contamination of

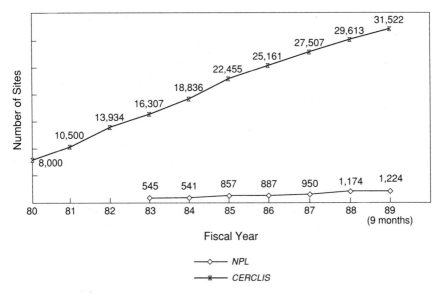

FIGURE 2-4   CERCLIS inventory and NPL sites.   Source: OTA, 1989.

media. Off-site contamination and human exposure have been modeled rather than measured directly in off-site sampling of groundwater, drinking water, soil, and air. The estimates of off-site contamination of media derived from these models are then used as surrogates for actual exposure measurements in the calculation of risk assessments for each contaminant. The lack of validation studies for many of these modeling approaches may introduce errors in exposure estimates, which in turn introduce further uncertainty in the risk-assessment process. In ATSDR's review of 951 NPL sites, 75-80 percent were found to have reached the NPL without adequate off-site sampling, such as sampling of nearby homeowners' wells for drinking-water contamination suggested by migration models or sampling of soil in near off-site locations where lead contamination was likely (H. Emmett, ATSDR, personal communication, 1990). Groundwater was most likely to be monitored off-site; surface water, air, and soil releases were even more rarely sampled, although citizen reports of odors and concerns about airborne chemicals frequently are the complaints that lead to site evaluations (Layefsky et al., 1988). Recently, EPA has begun to direct more resources to off-site sampling, and the agency has incorporated more direct measures of population exposure in the revised HRS (EPA, 1990b).

Minimum data requirements for sampling pathways of exposure

and points of human contact have not been established, although extensive requirements exist for on-site exposures. The EPA manual for risk assessment prepared in 1989 gives substantial attention to on-site monitoring and to modeling of off-site migration, but it offers little guidance for off-site sampling of current human exposure points or for the use of such data in the calculation of risk (EPA, 1989b). If the earlier emphasis on environmental monitoring to evaluate the feasibility of remediation strategies is to be balanced by monitoring to address human health concerns, the development of a minimum data set and of usable, standard measurements of exposure will be increasingly important. As Buffler (Buffler et al., 1985) and others have underscored, moreover, obtaining accurate information on routes of exposure and doses received will be particularly critical to selecting appropriate target organs and health end points for epidemiologic study.

An internal review of Superfund management in 1988 discussed the need to strengthen the public health aspects of site evaluations (EPA, 1989a). Nevertheless, EPA documents and operations reflect a continuing ambivalence about the agency's capacity for, and interest in, integrating health considerations into this process, which has been driven almost exclusively by risk assessment. The EPA risk assessment manual reports that the agency's staff "considers the information in a health assessment along with the results of the baseline risk assessment to give a complete picture of health threats" (EPA, 1989b, pp. 3-2, 3-3). But EPA has no public health professionals or other staff members trained in the public health aspects of site evaluation to rely upon in this regard; it is ATSDR, in fact, that incorporates the EPA risk assessments generated in the RI/FS process into EPA's full health assessment (EPA, 1989b).

The EPA remedial project manager (RPM) is responsible for "scoping" at each site, that is, for determining the appropriate level of effort and the level of detail necessary for the RI/FS, including the evaluation of potential and actual human exposures and health effects. Without public health training or input, the RPM "must make up-front decisions about, for example, the scope of the baseline risk assessment, the appropriate level of detail and documentation, trade-offs between depth and breadth in the analysis and the staff and monetary resources to commit" (EPA, 1989b, p. 2). Detailed instructions are given in the EPA manual for planning data needs for the RI/FS, without reference either to ATSDR's preliminary health assessment or to the need for consultation with ATSDR staff (EPA, 1989b).

EPA and ATSDR are beginning to experiment with the coordination of agency efforts in the initial stages of the RI/FS. ATSDR participation with EPA regional staff in the scoping phase of Superfund remedial investigations—during which both the sampling plans and the preliminary remedial goals are established—will be tested at six sites during FY91 (H. Emmett, ATSDR, personal communication, 1991). As ATSDR has cleared the backlog of health assessments on pre-existing NPL sites, moreover, an important role has emerged for ATSDR's health assessments in the selection of remediation strategies by EPA. The preliminary health assessment is initiated by ATSDR when EPA proposes a site for NPL listing in the *Federal Register*, that is, after the EPA preremedial evaluation has been completed but well before the RI/FS begins (the RI/FS frequently does not begin for another four to five years). Under these conditions the health assessment becomes the main evaluation of the public health impact of a site proposed for NPL listing, and this information is directly available to the community, to policy makers, and to research scientists, including environmental epidemiologists.

Although the full ATSDR health assessment is not completed until the RI/FS has been concluded, the preliminary health assessment attempts to cover much of the same ground with the data at hand. ATSDR's deputy administrator has argued that the agency's assessments need to draw on more information about the health concerns of the community and local health care providers (Johnson, 1990). This is particularly important because ATSDR increasingly functions as a "communication" arm of the Superfund program with concerned communities. Finally, ATSDR is now compiling the results of the more than 1000 health assessments completed to date at NPL sites to create a data base of health-related information. This data base will be used to identify patterns of hazardous-chemical releases from particular types of sites and to identify those releases most frequently found among all sites (ATSDR, 1989a).

DEFERRAL OF SITES AND NFRAP DESIGNATION

Sites submitted to the Superfund program for initial entry in the CERCLIS inventory can be rejected and deferred to the responsibility of other federal or state agencies that have jurisdiction. A site that enters the CERCLIS inventory can subsequently be designated "no further remedial action planned" (NFRAP) if it is determined to be outside Superfund jurisdiction or if its projected HRS score is too low for proposal for NPL status. Superfund responsibility for the site is then terminated. In most cases responsibility for these sites reverts to the states, although it can revert to another federal agency, such as the Department of Defense or the Department of Energy. Because most sites designated NFRAP have at best had a preliminary assessment, the quality and quantity of information available usually is inadequate to support a clear conclusion about the potential hazard of the site. Thus, an undetermined number of sites with potentially significant public health hazards are dropped from the CERCLIS inventory each year. Because there is no federal system for tracking sites after they are deferred, no information is available about the subsequent evaluation or remediation of these sites or of changes in their use and associated human exposures.

FEDERAL POLICIES AND ENVIRONMENTAL EPIDEMIOLOGY

The result of the federal programs and policies described here has been to create multiple and overlapping, but incomplete, inventories of hazardous-waste sites. On-site sampling of environmental contamination to estimate off-site human exposure is in some cases inadequate for the assessment of potential human exposure; these cases should be identified and off-site samples obtained. There is no routine review of early site assessments to determine the need for public health interventions or epidemiologic studies. The information used in decisions about subsequent site listing and remediation is inadequate as well. The attendant cost has been a great deal of confusion about the actual risks that hazardous-waste sites pose to human health and the loss of multiple opportunities for epidemiologic research. Clues to the potential scale of human exposure to toxic chemicals released from hazardous-waste sites are emerging, however.

As one of the federal agencies with responsibility for environmental epidemiology, ATSDR has assembled a small professional staff in epidemiology and the related fields of toxicology, environmental medicine, and risk communication. Because the agency has only limited authority and a narrow mandate, and because of its equally limited budget, ATSDR's current programs can do little more than establish a framework for evaluating health effects and for developing research that will be needed to address the issue of hazardous-waste sites adequately in the future. The agency conducts or supports epidemiologic investigations in cases where human exposure to hazardous substances has occurred or is occurring, where a potentially exposed population can be identified, where the exposure can be measured, and where the possible health effects are known or biologically plausible (ATSDR, 1989a).

The broader plan for ATSDR health surveillance activities prepared for FY90 includes site-specific studies at sites that contain compounds of public health importance and for which there are significant data gaps; studies that combine data from multiple sites; long-term surveillance of populations that have been permanently relocated because of exposure to hazardous-waste releases in their original communities; state-based surveillance, usually conducted as ecologic studies that link existing data bases such as birth weight, birth defects, and cancer incidence to geographic distributions of environmental contamination; surveillance of workers employed in the cleanup of hazardous waste; and development of a public health reporting and surveillance system for hazardous-waste material emergencies (ATSDR, 1990b).

ATSDR also is investigating the use of "sentinel health events" as additional indicators of environmental contamination. The concept was first developed for public health surveillance of morbidity and mortality that results from preventable causes, such as deaths from infectious diseases that are preventable by immunization or chronic obstructive pulmonary disease that results from cigarette smoking (Rutstein et al., 1983). Such indicators are most useful when they identify causes of morbidity and mortality that are uniquely or predominantly associated with specific and preventable exposures. For example, mesothelioma is almost exclusively associated with exposure to asbestos fibers, and hepatic angiosarcoma is predominantly associated with exposure to vinyl chloride.

Environmental sentinel health events are designed to serve as warning signals of particular environmental exposures, using existing data systems such as vital records, hospital discharge data, and tumor registries. Some illnesses, such as methemoglobinemia that results from excessive amounts of nitrate in water, indicate hazardous environmental exposure even when they occur as single cases. Other diseases indicate potential environmental exposures when they occur at elevated rates among larger populations, such as bladder cancer among nonsmokers or chronic respiratory disease among children. The further development and application of this approach to environmental surveillance holds particular promise for the epidemiologic investigation of populations exposed to hazardous wastes.

Although ATSDR is vigorously pursuing the development of an intramural research program in environmental epidemiology and has extended this to include a number of states through cooperative agreements, in FY90 ATSDR's total budget for programs that assess hazardous-waste sites was $15.8 million (J. Andrews, ATSDR, personal communication, 1990). The National Institute of Environmental Health Sciences (NIEHS), a sister agency within the U.S. Public Health Service, also receives Superfund monies to support a basic research program in ecology, engineering, and hydrogeology integrated with biomedical research to improve the sensitivity and specificity of techniques for detecting adverse effects in humans or in ecologic systems. In FY91, NIEHS received $21.9 million for the program, which it distributed in 11 grants to academic institutions. In addition, NIEHS sponsors research in environmental epidemiology, using $13.7 million for the support of 39 epidemiologic studies by the end of calendar year 1990, although most of these studies do not assess populations exposed to hazardous-waste sites (A.P. Sassaman, NIEHS, personal communication, 1991). Table 2-3 shows funding sources and the kinds of affiliations of the principal investigators reporting environmental epidemiologic studies in the published literature.

STATE PROGRAMS

The public concerns that led to the enactment of CERCLA also led to the development of similar laws in state legislatures. In many states, new departments for handling hazardous-waste sites were founded, or existing environmental protection agencies were expanded. The formal organization of these agencies varied greatly among the states, as did their statutory and programmatic mandates. The development of separate environmental agencies exacerbated the previous separation and lack of coordination between environmental and other public health programs (Institute of Medicine, 1988).

State hazardous-waste-site programs were largely modeled after the Superfund program. Site evaluation depended mainly on exposure modeling and risk assessment. Program staff were drawn primarily from engineering and law. With little training in risk communication and with little capacity for assessing actual health effects, state programs initially faced public concerns similar to those faced by the federal programs, but with much greater pressure from local constituents. A common result was the emergence of large departments devoted to environmental management that became entangled in the processes of risk assessment and prolonged legal battles, and remediation that, from the public point of view, seemed to do little either to reassure or to protect it.

Exceptions to this general pattern occurred, primarily when public health professionals were more involved in evaluating the sites and in working with the affected communities. For example, New York State has developed a program in which Department of Health staff work closely with Department of Environmental Conservation staff at every stage of the site assessment and remediation process. This integration helps to ensure that public health concerns (off-site exposures, drinking water) are appropriately evaluated and controlled

TABLE 2-3 Environmental Epidemiology: Investigators and Funding Sources

Study Location and Year of Publication	Study Design and Period of Observation	Exposure Measure	Reported Outcome	Principal Investigator Affiliation	Funding Source
Tucson, AZ 1990 Goldberg et al.	Case-control 1969-1987	Child conceived and first trimester spent in Tucson Valley	Significant association between parental exposure to CWA and increased proportion of congenital heart disease among live births	University of Arizona	State of Arizona
Fresno County, CA 1988 Wong et al.	Retrospective follow-up 1978-1982	Surrogate: residence in Fresno county	No decrease in birth rate	Environmental Health Associates, Inc.	Not available
Stringfellow Site Glen Avon, CA 1988 Baker et al.	Cross-sectional 1983	Proximity to site	Weak to moderate positive associations: ear infection, bronchitis, asthma, angina pectoris, and skin rash	Mount Sinai School of Medicine	State of California
Santa Clara County, CA 1985 CA Dept. of Health Services	Retrospective follow-up 1980-1981 1981-1982	Surrogate: residence in households served by contaminated water at the time of chemical leak	1980-1982: significant excess of spontaneous abortions and congential malformations	CA Dept. of Health	State of California

TABLE 2-3 *Continued*

Study Location and Year of Publication	Study Design and Period of Observation	Exposure Measure	Reported Outcome	Principal Investigator Affiliation	Funding Source
			1981-1982: excess incidence of cardiac defects within and outside the study area. No support for an association with the chemical leak		
Santa Clara County, CA 1989 Swan et al.	Retrospective follow-up 1981-1983	Surrogate: residence in households served by contaminated water	Increased prevalence of cardiac anomalies but temporal distribution suggests solvent leak not responsible	CA Dept. of Health Services	State of California
Galena, KS 1990 Neuberger et al.	Retrospective follow-up 1980-1985	Residence in towns for at least 5 years prior to 1980	Significant associations of stroke, anemia, hypertension, heart disease, skin cancer with exposure	University of Kansas	University
Lowell, MA 1987 Ozonoff et al.	Cross-sectional 1983	Surrogate: residence in households within a given distance from site	Increased prevalence of minor symptoms, irregular heart beat, fatigue, bowel complaints	Boston University	Commonwealth of Massachusetts

Location/Study	Design/Dates	Exposure Measure	Findings	Institution	Funding
Woburn, MA 1986 Lagakos et al.	Case-control 1964-1983	Surrogate: residence in households served by contaminated wells	Significant association of childhood leukemia with estimated exposure	Harvard School of Public Health	Private and Federal
Woburn, MA 1986 Lagakos et al.	Retrospective follow-up 1960-1982	Surrogate: residence in households served by contaminated wells	Association with perinatal deaths, eye/ear anomalies, CNS anomalies; association with kidney/urinary tract infection	Harvard School of Public Health	Private and Federal
Woburn, MA 1988 Feldman et al.	Clinical case-control 1987(?)	Surrogate: residence in households served by contaminated wells	Significant differences in blink reflex function when means were compared	Boston University	University
Rutherford, NJ 1980 Burke et al., Halperin et al.	Case-control 1973-1978	Surrogate: residence in the area	Reduced prevalence of rubella vaccination in leukemia cases. Excess of prior vaccinations and tonsellectomies in Hodgkin's cases	NJ Depts. Health, Environmental Protection	State of New Jersey
Hyde Park, NY 1981 Rothenberg	Cross-sectional 1979	Surrogate: employment in plants near site	Increased prevalence of hiatus hernia and other minor gastrointestinal problems	NY State Dept. of Health; National Institute for Occupational Safety and Health	Federal

TABLE 2-3 *Continued*

Study Location and Year of Publication	Study Design and Period of Observation	Exposure Measure	Reported Outcome	Principal Investigator Affiliation	Funding Source
Love Canal, NY 1981 Janerich et al.	Retrospective follow-up (census tract) 1955–1977	Surrogate: proximity to dump site	Incidence: no increase in cancer	NY Dept. of Health	State of New York
Love Canal, NY 1984 Health et al.	Cross-sectional 1982	Surrogate: testing of chemicals (two years before) in the house of exposed	No difference in SCE or chromosal aberrations	Centers for Disease Control	Federal
Love Canal, NY 1984 Vianna and Polan	Retrospective follow-up 1941–1978	Surrogate: proximity to dump site and at least 5 months residence	Elevated incidence of low birthweight among exposed	NY Dept. of Health	State of New York
Love Canal, NY 1985 Paigen et al.	Cross-sectional 1980	Surrogate: proximity to dump site	Increased prevalence of health problems: seizures, learning problems, hyperactivity, eye irritation, skin rash, abdominal pain, incontinence	Children's Hospital Medical Center	Private foundation
Love Canal, NY 1987 Paigen et al	Cross-sectional 1980	Surrogate: proximity to dump site	Increased prevalence of shorter stature	Children's Hospital Medical Center	Private foundation

Location, Year, Author	Study design and period	Exposure	Findings	Institution	Sponsor
1987 Hertzman et al.	follow-up Workers: 1965-1980; Residents: 1976-1980	employment on or adjacent to site; Residents: long/short-term residence in area during 1976-1980	of respiratory, skin, narcotic, and mood disorders; Residents: confirmed association between landfill site exposure and mood, narcotic, skin, and respiratory conditions	University of British Columbia	Province of Ontario
Clinton County, PA 1984 Budnick et al.	Mortality 1950-1979	Surrogate: residence in the area	Increased bladder cancer mortality in male resident population after 1970	Chronic Disease Division, Center for Health Services, U.S. Dept. of Health and Human Services	Federal
Clinton County, PA 1985 Logue et al.	Cross-sectional 1983	Surrogate: residence in the area	Increased prevalence of skin problems and sleepiness	Division of Environmental Health, PA Dept. of Health	State of Pennsylvania
Dauphin County, PA 1986 Logue and Fox	Cross-sectional 1983	Surrogate: residence in households with past contamination of water with TCE	Increased prevalence of eye irritation, diarrhea, and sleepiness	Division of Environmental Health, PA Dept. of Health	State of Pennsylvania
Hardeman County, TN 1982 Clark et al. Meyer, 1983 Harris et al., 1984	Cross-sectional 1978	Carbon tetrachloride in well water >150 µg/l (high exposure <45 µg/l (intermediate exposure)	Transient abnormalities of liver functions in exposed	Dept. of Environmental Health, University of Cincinnati Medical Center	Federal

Source: Expanded and adapted from Upton et al., 1989, with permission.

early in the assessment process. State health departments have been assisted by ATSDR funding through cooperative agreements, representing $5.2 million of the total $15.8 million ATSDR budget for health assessments in FY90 (J. Andrews, ATSDR, personal communication, 1990). ATSDR also has provided support for private sector organizations, such as the Association of State and Territorial Health Officers, the Association of State and Territorial Risk Assessors, and the National Governors' Association, to establish programs within state health departments and to provide policy leadership within professional organizations.

States have taken independent action to close or restrict access to more than 1705 sites because of contamination with toxic substances, as reported in a 1989 survey conducted by the National Governors' Association with ATSDR support. The most common reason for site restrictions is groundwater contamination (69 percent of sites), because this affects drinking-water supplies (7479 groundwater wells were closed at these sites) (Wells, 1990). In the same survey, state environmental (and combined environmental and health) agencies reported having the most extensive authority to identify, restrict, and remediate contaminated sites. Mirroring the distinction between EPA and ATSDR, most state health agencies have primary responsibility for assessing human exposures and for epidemiologic studies of associated health effects (Wells, 1990).

The major source of funding for state programs for the evaluation and cleanup of hazardous-waste sites is that provided by the Superfund program under cooperative agreements. EPA does not allow states to use cooperative agreement funds for site discovery. Some states have invested additional funds in site discovery, in more complete initial assessments, and in outreach programs to work with groups of citizens who are concerned about waste sites in their communities. The most recent survey of state expenditures estimates that about $500 million is spent on hazardous-waste-site cleanups each year; no similar information is available for the health assessment aspect of these activities alone (OTA, 1989).

Most environmental epidemiology studies of health effects associated with hazardous wastes are conducted by state health departments, even in states that have separate departments for environmental management. State capacity in environmental epidemiology varies greatly. Some have several doctoral-level epidemiologists who conduct environmental epidemiology studies full time; in others, communicable disease or chronic disease epidemiologists also respond to environmental concerns when necessary; other states simply refer these issues to ATSDR or the Centers for Disease Control.

Although ATSDR funding for state health departments has provided impetus for studies of exposed populations, the most compelling pressure has been the continuous public demand for health studies of specific sites. Politically, such studies are an appealing way to cope with frightened and outraged communities, particularly when cleanup is far in the future. In many states, these demands for health studies are focused on reported clusters of cancer or other illnesses. The states with the largest programs, California, New York, New Jersey, and Minnesota, have developed triage systems that sort out the scientific plausibility and methodologic feasibility of responding to the increasing stream of requests (R.R. Neutra, California State Department of Health Services, personal communication, 1990). These programs also have led to extensive discussions within the field of epidemiology about the methodologic issues associated with the study of reported clusters (American Journal of Epidemiology, 1990). Relatively few of the environmental epidemiology studies conducted by the states make their way into the published literature. Directly published state reports often serve the agencies better, and many investigations are not designed or completed in a form that is appropriate for publication in the regular scientific literature.

A REVISED FORM OF INITIAL SITE ASSESSMENT

Congress has charged the federal government—EPA, along with ATSDR and NIEHS—with the job of protecting the health of the public from hazardous-waste sites. Three components of this responsibility are also among the critical tasks of environmental epidemiology: characterizing current and potential human exposures; evaluating the potential harm to human health of these exposures; and investigating the actual health effects associated with the exposures.

As our review of federal programs concludes, there is no comprehensive national inventory of hazardous-waste sites, no site discovery program, no minimum data set on potential human exposures, no adequate system for the early identification of sites for which immediate action to protect public health or continued surveillance of health effects could be necessary, and no validation or evaluation of the component parts of the site assessment process. EPA and ATSDR are instituting some improvements in each of these areas, but these improvements are largely limited to sites that are proposed for or already listed on the NPL.

During the past 10 years, of the estimated $4.2 billion spent each year on hazardous-waste sites in the U.S. (OTA, 1989), less than 1 percent has been devoted to the study of health risks at these sites.

As a result, existing data on exposures and health effects are inadequate not only for decisions on the management of hazardous-waste sites, but for epidemiologic investigations of the health impact of the sites as well.

Some states have mounted systematic discovery programs, have comprehensive inventories, and routinely undertake off-site sampling to identify potential human exposures. The California State Department of Health, in reviewing the 93 sites on the state's Superfund list in 1984, found that 19 of the sites were also on the federal NPL. Yet 46 of the sites showed evidence of waste release into groundwater, and in 34 of these cases the groundwater was known to be used for drinking. Extensive or systematic sampling existed for only 22 of the sites, despite the evidence of potential human exposure. In all 19 of the California sites with known contamination of groundwater, moreover, more than 10,000 persons were potentially exposed (Layefsky et al., 1988). Their experiences could serve as a model for the development of an effective discovery and initial assessment program. Such a program might rapidly establish public confidence that the "worst" sites are aggressively sought and dealt with, and that Superfund resources are effectively applied to remove the most serious risks. Data collected by such a national program would also provide a comprehensive data base containing preliminary (and later, more refined) information on the substances known to be present at hazardous-waste sites, on the media contaminated, on the routes of exposure, and on the human populations potentially at risk.

Even without the establishment of a site discovery program, the development and validation of an adequate initial assessment methodology for hazardous-waste sites is an urgent recommendation of this committee. Epidemiology is not merely a passive science, cataloguing exposures and effects. It is an active tool for identifying potentially hazardous exposures and directing interventions to prevent further exposures. Because the evaluation of human exposures and health effects associated with hazardous-waste sites is not integrated into early site evaluation and interim remediation decisions, the real contributions of public health and epidemiology are lost.

This is of grave concern, because some hazardous wastes do constitute a significant public health hazard to specific populations at specific sites, as discussed in Chapters 4, 5, and 6. As ATSDR has documented, and other reports confirm, human exposure to hazardous-chemical releases are common at some of these sites. The health of the public has remained in jeopardy at many sites long after the risks could have—and should have—been identified (Hazardous Waste Treatment Council, 1990).

To explore the feasibility of a revised approach to the preliminary assessment of hazardous-waste sites, we provide an estimate (Table 2-4) of the cost of EPA's preremedial engineering and exposure assessments (the preliminary assessment and site inspection) in combination with ATSDR's preremedial health assessment (the preliminary health assessment).

This revised preliminary assessment includes both the preliminary engineering studies (physical characteristics of the site, estimates of contamination, and feasibility of remediation strategies) and the preliminary health assessment. Nevertheless, applying the full revised preliminary assessment (PA, SI + PHA) at all currently listed CERCLIS sites would cost $1.824 billion. Spread over a five-year period, this would come to approximately $365 million per year, or one-third of the total FY91 Superfund budget. Because many sites will require only the EPA PA and the ATSDR PHA, this in fact is an overestimate of the actual costs of applying such an approach. If the EPA and ATSDR functions are maintained separately, $165 million per year would be allocated to the ATSDR budget for health assessments, a substantial increase from the ATSDR FY89 budget of $15.8 million. Savings could be realized by reorganizing the assessment process to directly incorporate health assessments—and staff with health expertise—into the management and implementation of preliminary assessments.

CONCLUSION

We know enough about some exposures at some sites—chiefly from ATSDR's assessments of those sites on the NPL—to suggest the potential benefit of further epidemiologic studies at these and other sites. A site discovery program and a revised preliminary site assessment would identify sites for such studies, as well as for the purposes of public health protection, and would provide the basis for a significantly expanded national program of environmental epidemiology. Some of the necessary support and related components for an

TABLE 2-4 Revised Prelimary Assessment: Estimated Costs

EPA	Preliminary Assessment (PA) and	
	Site Inspection (SI)	$32,000
ATSDR	Preliminary Health Assessment (PHA)	$25,000
TOTAL		$57,000

32,000 CERCLIS sites × $57,000/site = $1824 billion

environmental epidemiology program are now under development at ATSDR, including toxicologic profiles, screening values as benchmarks for hazardous levels of exposure to priority substances (ATSDR, 1990a), pilot studies of human exposure, standardized protocols for the collection of data, and the identification of data gaps and the development of a research agenda.

An expanded and strengthened program of environmental epidemiology must be developed as an integral part of federal environmental programs.

• Establish an active and coordinated system of site discovery for hazardous-waste sites, based in the EPA and providing technical assistance to other federal and state programs. An aggressive site discovery program, in combination with improved assessments and triage of sites for interim and final remediation, will restore the original congressional intent to protect the health of the public from hazardous-waste-site exposures.

• Define a revised approach to site assessments that integrates public health determinations of population exposures, health effects, and the necessity of interim and final remediation or other actions into a continuum of site evaluation. Establish protocols and criteria for the revised preliminary assessment of all sites, with triggers for interim remediation or other action, such as relocation, and require that all sites undergo a revised preliminary assessment within one year of discovery.

• Establish a comprehensive national inventory of hazardous-waste sites that will track the status of all sites through assessment and remediation or closure. Use the inventory to ensure that sites are not deferred or placed in closure status without a revised preliminary assessment as described above.

• Rigorously evaluate the data and methodologies used in site assessment, including the characterization of potential and actual releases to groundwater, surface water, air, and soil that result in human exposure; methodologies for the estimation of populations exposed to hazardous-waste-site emissions; the use of this information in the preliminary assessment and in determining actions to protect the public health; and compliance with public health recommendations for the protection of exposed populations and site remediation. In fact, the entire process from the preliminary assessment (PA) through the site inspection (SI) and the RI/FS is largely conducted by contractors working for EPA or by "potentially responsible parties"—those responsible for the original deposition or management of the waste. The process as a whole is directed at remediation rather than at the assessment of public health risks.

• Improve and expand research in environmental epidemiology to illuminate the distribution and severity of exposures, risks, and health effects associated with hazardous-waste sites. Authorize ATSDR to direct responsible parties to conduct research to fill prioritized data gaps on critical substances. Expand the ATSDR mandate to establish an extensive program of applied research, including exposure registries linked to priority substances, and further the development of surveillance methods such as community health data bases, biologic monitoring, and sentinel events. Regularly monitor the literature on health effects of toxic-waste sites and publish reviews when indicated. As appropriate, meta-analyses can be conducted of these studies, provided that the studies meet the criteria required for such aggregate analysis.

• Direct ATSDR to expand cooperative agreements with states and to develop a comprehensive program of technical assistance for state and local agencies. Provide increased funding for competitive grants in environmental epidemiology through ATSDR and NIEHS.

A decade after implementation of Superfund, and despite congressional efforts to redirect the program, substantial public health concerns remain, and critical information on the distribution of exposures and health effects associated with hazardous-waste sites is still lacking. Whether for the purposes of environmental epidemiology or for the protection of public health, the nation is failing to adequately identify, assess, or prioritize hazardous-waste-site exposures.

The legislative mandates, policies, and programs of the federal and state agencies that currently manage hazardous-waste sites are inadequate to the task of protecting the health of the public. Although extensive evidence suggests that specific populations near specific sites are exposed to substantial risks, the distribution and frequency of these exposures are impossible to ascertain. At sites where potentially critical exposures are detected, there is no regular application of an adequate system of early assessment of the health risks involved or of the need for interim action to protect the health of exposed populations. As a result of the failure to construct a system for managing hazardous-waste sites that incorporates these essential components, we find that the health of some members of the public is in danger, and that the conditions for development of environmental epidemiology are so adverse as to impede the development of useful scientific investigations of many important questions.

REFERENCES

American Journal of Epidemiology. 1990. National Conference on Clustering of Health Events (entire issue) 132(Suppl. 1).

ATSDR (U.S. Public Health Service, Agency for Toxic Substances and Disease Registry). 1989a. ATSDR Biennial Report to Congress: October 17, 1986-September 30, 1988. Atlanta: Agency for Toxic Substances and Disease Registry. 2 vols.

ATSDR (U.S. Public Health Service, Agency for Toxic Substances and Disease Registry). 1989b. Preliminary Health Assessment for Forest Glen Mobile Home Park, Niagara Falls, Niagara County, New York. July 21. Atlanta: Agency for Toxic Substances and Disease Registry.

ATSDR (U.S. Public Health Service, Agency for Toxic Substances and Disease Registry). 1990a. Health Assessment Guidance Manual (Draft). Atlanta: Agency for Toxic Substances and Disease Registry.

ATSDR (U.S. Public Health Service, Agency for Toxic Substances and Disease Registry). 1990b. Summary of the Division of Health Studies Surveillance Plan. October 5. Atlanta: Agency for Toxic Substances and Disease Registry.

ATSDR (U.S. Public Health Service, Agency for Toxic Substances and Disease Registry). 1991. ATSDR Biennial Report to Congress: 1989 and 1990. Atlanta: Agency for Toxic Substances and Disease Registry.

Baker, D.B., S. Greenland, J. Mendlein, and P. Harmon. 1988. A health study of two communities near the Stringfellow Waste Disposal site. Arch. Environ. Health 43:325-334.

Budnick, L.D., D.C. Sokal, H. Falk, J.N. Logue, and J.M. Fox. 1984. Cancer and birth defects near the Drake Superfund site, Pennsylvania. Arch. Environ. Health 39:409-413.

Buffler, P.A., M. Crane, and M.M. Key. 1985. Possibilities of detecting health effects by studies of populations exposed to chemicals from waste disposal sites. Environ. Health Perspect. 62:423-456.

Burke, T.A., S. Gray, C.M. Krawiec, R.J. Katz, P.W. Preuss, and G. Paulson. 1980. An environmental investigation of clusters of leukemia and Hodgkin's disease in Rutherford, New Jersey. J. Med. Soc. N.J. 77:259-264.

California Department of Health Services. 1985. Pregnancy Outcomes in Santa Clara County 1980-1982: Reports of Two Epidemiological Studies. Berkeley: California Department of Health Services.

Clark, C.S., C.R. Meyer, P.S. Gartside, V.A. Majeti, B. Specker, W.F. Balisteri, and V.J. Elia. 1982. An environmental health survey of drinking water contamination by leachate from a pesticide waste dump in Hardeman County, Tennessee. Arch. Environ. Health 37:9-18.

EPA (U.S. Environmental Protection Agency). 1989a. A Management Review of the Superfund Program. Washington, D.C.: U.S. Environmental Protection Agency.

EPA (U.S. Environmental Protection Agency). 1989b. Risk Assessment Guidance for Superfund, Volume I: Human Health Evaluation Manual. Interim Final. EPA/540/1-89/002. Washington, D.C.: U.S. Environmental Protection Agency.

EPA (U.S. Environmental Protection Agency). 1990a. Field Test of the Proposed Revised Hazard Ranking System (HRS). EPA/540/P-90/001. Washington, D.C.: U.S. Environmental Protection Agency.

EPA (U.S. Environmental Protection Agency). 1990b. Hazard Ranking System. Final Rule. December 14. Fed. Regis. 55 (241):51532.

EPA (U.S. Environmental Protection Agency). 1991. National Priorities List for uncontrolled hazardous waste sites. Final Rule. February 11. Fed. Regis. 56(28):5598-5631.

Feldman, R.G., J. Chirico-Post, and S.P. Proctor. 1988. Blink reflex latency after exposure to trichloroethylene in well water. Arch. Environ. Health 43:143-148.

Goldberg, S.J., M.D. Lebowitz, E.J. Graver, and S. Hicks. 1990. An association of human congenital cardiac malformations and drinking water contaminants. J. Am. Coll. Cardiol. 16:155-164.

Halperin, W., R. Altman, A. Stemhagen, A.W. Iaci, G. Caldwell, T. Mason, J. Bill, T. Abe, and J.F. Clark. 1980. Epidemiologic investigations of cluster of leukemia and Hodgkin's disease in Rutherford, New Jersey. J. Med. Soc. N.J. 77:267-273.

Harris, R.H., J.H. Highland, J.V. Rodricks, and S.S. Papadopulos. 1984. Adverse effects at a Tennessee hazardous waste disposal site. Hazardous Waste 1:183-204.

Heath, C.W., Jr., M.A. Nadel, M.M. Zack Jr., A.T.L. Chen, M.A. Bender, and J. Preston. 1984. Cytogenic findings in persons living near the Love Canal. J. Am. Med. Assoc. 251:1437-1440.

Hazardous Waste Treatment Council. 1990. Tracking Superfund: Where the Program Stands: A Comprehensive Environmental-Industry Report on Recent EPA Cleanup Decisions. Washington, D.C.: Hazardous Waste Treatment Council.

Hertzman, C., M. Hayes, J. Singer, and J. Highland. 1987. Upper Ottawa Street Landfill Site health study. Environ. Health Perspect. 75:173-195.

Institute of Medicine. 1988. The Future of Public Health. Washington, D.C.: National Academy Press.

Janerich, D.T., W.S. Burnett, G. Feck, M. Hoff, P. Nasca, A.P. Polednak, P. Greenwald, and N. Vianna. 1981. Cancer incidence in the Love Canal area. Science 212:1404-1407.

Johnson, B.L. 1990. Implementation of Superfund's health-related provisions by the Agency for Toxic Substances and Disease Registry. Environ. Law Reporter 20:10277-10282.

Lagakos, S.W., B.J. Wessen, and M. Zelen. 1986. An analysis of contaminated well water and health effects in Woburn, Massachusetts. J. Am. Stat. Assoc. 81:583-596.

Layefsky, M.E., D.F. Smith, M.J. Mendell, R.D. Schlag, and R.R. Neutra. 1988. California Superfund sites: Insights from a computerized database. Haz. Waste Haz. Materials 5:313-320.

Logue, J.N., and J.M. Fox. 1986. Residential health study of families living near the Drake Chemical Superfund site in Lock Haven, Pennsylvania. Arch. Environ. Health 41:222-228.

Logue, J.N., R.M. Stroman, D. Reid, C.W. Hayes, and K. Sivarajah. 1985. Investigation of potential health effects associated with well water chemical contamination in Londonderry township, Pennsylvania. Arch. Environ. Health 40:155-160.

Marsh, G.M., and R.J. Caplan. 1986. The feasibility of conducting epidemiologic studies of populations residing near hazardous waste disposal sites. Pp. 67-88 in Environmental Epidemiology, F.C. Kopfler and G.F. Craun, eds. Chelsea, Mich.: Lewis.

Meyer, C.R. 1983. Liver dysfunction in residents exposed to leachate from a toxic waste dump. Environ. Health Perspect. 48:9-13.

Neuberger, J.S., M. Mulhall, M.C. Pomatto, J. Sheverbush, and R.S. Hassanein. 1990. Health problems in Galena, Kansas (USA): A heavy metal mining Superfund site. Sci. Total Environ. 94:261-272.

NRC (National Research Council). 1985. Reducing Hazardous Waste Generation: An Evaluation and a Call for Action. Washington, D.C.: National Academy Press.

OTA (U.S. Congress, Office of Technology Assessment). 1989. Coming Clean: Superfund's Problems Can be Solved. OTA-ITE-433. Washington, D.C.: U.S. Government Printing Office.

Ozonoff, D., M.E. Colten, A. Cupples, T. Heeren, A. Schatzkin, T. Mangione, M. Dresner, and T. Colton. 1987. Health problems reported by residents of a neighborhood contaminated by a hazardous waste facility. Am. J. Ind. Med. 11:581-597.

Paigen, B., L.R. Goldman, J.H. Highland, M.M. Magnant, and A.T. Steegman, Jr. 1985. Prevalence of health problems in children living near Love Canal. Haz. Waste Haz. Materials 2:23-43.

Paigen, B. L.R. Goldman, M.M. Magnant, J.H. Highland, and A.T. Steegman, Jr. 1987. Growth of children living near the hazardous waste site, Love Canal. Hum. Biol. 59:489-508.

Roberts, L. 1990. Counting on science at EPA. Science 249:616-618.

Rothenberg, R. 1981. Morbidity study at a chemical dump — New York. Morbid. Mortal. Week. Rep. 30:293-294.

Rutstein, D.D., R.J. Mullan, T.M. Frazier, W.E. Halperin, J.M. Melius, and J.P. Sestito. 1983. Sentinel Health Events (occupational): A basis for physician recognition and public health surveillance. Am. J. Public Health 73:1054-1062.

Siegel, M.R. 1990. Integrating public health into Superfund: What has been the impact of the Agency for Toxic Substances and Disease Registry? Environ. Law Reporter 20:10013-10020.

Swan, S.H., G. Shaw, J.A. Harris, and R.R. Neutra. 1989. Congenital cardiac anomalies in relation to water contamination, Santa Clara County, California, 1981-1983. Am. J. Epidemiol. 129:885-893.

Upton, A.C., T. Kneip, and P. Toniolo. 1989. Public health aspects of toxic chemical disposal sites. Annu. Rev. Public Health 10:1-25.

Vianna, N.J., and A.K. Polan. 1984. Incidence of low birth weight among Love Canal residents. Science 226(4679):1217-1219.

Wells, B. 1990. Restrictions Imposed on Contaminated Sites: A Status of State Actions. Washington, D.C.: National Governors' Association, Center for Policy Research, Natural Resources Policy Studies Unit, Environment, Health and Safety Program.

Wolf, S.M. 1988. Pollution Law Handbook. Westport, Conn.: Greenwood Press.

Wong, O., M.D. Whorton, N. Gordon, and R.W. Morgan. 1988. An epidemiologic investigation of the relationship between DBCP contamination in drinking water and birth rates in Fresno County, California. Am. J. Public Health 78:43-46.

3

Dimensions of the Problem: Exposure Assessment

E XPOSURE ASSESSMENT IS A crucial component of environmental epidemiology studies that seek to establish causal relationships between exposure to chemical and physical agents from hazardous-waste sites and adverse consequences to human health. The discipline of exposure assessment encompasses numerous techniques to measure or estimate the contaminant, its source, the environmental media of exposure, avenues of transport through each medium, chemical and physical transformations, routes of entry to the body, intensity and frequency of contact, and spatial and temporal concentration patterns. Exposure to a contaminant is defined as "an event that occurs when there is contact at a boundary between a human and the environment at a specific contaminant concentration for a specified period of time; the units to express exposure are concentration multiplied by time" (NRC, 1991, p. 3).

In environmental epidemiology, exposure assessment has proved difficult. Epidemiologic research typically involves retrospective studies. When data are gathered retrospectively, there is an enormous opportunity for exposure assessment to be influenced by apparent disease occurrence, and vice versa. Records of environmental pollution can sometimes provide a surrogate for exposure, but these surrogates are not always available, and direct measures of past exposures have not usually been recorded.

Rothman (1990) noted estimates of exposure are very often heterogenious, poorly described, and involve low concentrations of toxicants. Although essential to well-designed epidemiologic investigations, exposure assessment has been and continues to be an inadequately developed component of environmental epidemiology, because

• the temporal characteristics of site discovery and investigation make it difficult;
• the conceptual framework and techniques for evaluation have only recently been established;
• epidemiologists often have not understood or given sufficient attention to exposure evaluation.

This chapter has three sections. The first describes the potential for human exposure by identifying toxic chemicals found at hazardous-waste sites. This includes direct site contamination, contamination by unidentified or uncharacterized pollutants, and groundwater contamination from other sources. The second section discusses approaches to exposure assessment and their attendant problems. The third section examines reported exposure assessments associated with hazardous-waste sites and reviews the strengths and weaknesses of the reports.

TOXIC-CHEMICAL EXPOSURE AT WASTE SITES

Although much of the waste produced annually in the U.S. is not listed as hazardous, the U.S. Environmental Protection Agency (EPA) estimated in 1988 that the amount of hazardous waste managed by approximately 3000 licensed facilities was 275 million metric tons (EPA, 1988). In addition, there are a substantial number of uncontrolled disposal sites that contain hazardous wastes and that could present serious environmental or public health problems. For example, municipal waste sludge and incinerator ash can contain toxic materials such as lead, cadmium, mercury, and other toxic materials.

In the late 1970s there was widespread publicity about the indiscriminate dumping of waste that was resulting in release of toxic agents into the environment. The national failure to address the many known and suspected hazards from uncontrolled hazardous waste sites led Congress to pass the Comprehensive Environmental Response, Compensation, and Liability Act of 1980 (CERCLA), generally known as the Superfund law. Under CERCLA's terms, more than 31,000 sites have been reported to EPA's CERCLA Information System (CERCLIS) inventory of sites that could require cleanup. EPA has completed more than 27,000 preliminary assessments, and more than 9000 sites have been investigated in detail (EPA, 1988). As of June 1988, EPA's National Priorities List (NPL), included 1236 sites, about 30 percent of which have had initial actions to reduce immediate threats. The number of identified sites represents a small proportion of the sites that are expected to be identified in the future (OTA, 1989).

HAZARDOUS-WASTE SITES

Within the past decade, estimates of the number of potential NPL sites have shifted dramatically. The Office of Technology Assessment (OTA, 1989) concludes that there could be as many as 439,000 candidate sites. This is more than 10 times that estimated earlier by EPA. These sites include Resource Conservation and Recovery Act (RCRA) Subtitle C and D facilities, mining waste sites, underground leaking storage tanks (nonpetroleum), pesticide-contaminated sites, federal facilities, radioactive release sites, underground injection wells, municipal gas facilities, and wood-preserving plants, among others.

One recent EPA survey found that more than 40 million people live within four miles and about 4 million reside within one mile of a Superfund site. Residential proximity does not per se mean that exposures and health risks are occurring, but the potential for exposure is increased. As of December 1988, the Agency for Toxic Substances and Disease Registry (ATSDR) concluded that 109 NPL sites (11.5 percent) were associated with a risk to human health because of actual exposures (11 sites) or probable exposure (98 sites) to hazardous chemical agents that could cause harm to human health. These NPL sites were listed in the categories of "urgent public health concern" or "public health concern."

The states with the largest number of NPL sites are New Jersey, Pennsylvania, California, Michigan, and New York. They accounted for 464 of 1236 (37.5 percent) sites as of 1991 (Figure 3-1). The activities associated with these sites are shown in Table 3-1. Figure 3-2 depicts the observed contamination of various media as a percentage of 1189 final sites on the NPL as of February 1991. Note that a site can have more than one type of contamination.

Data derived from the 951 ATSDR health assessments at hazardous-waste sites indicate the existence of more than 600 different chemical substances. Some of them are listed in Table 3-2. The documented migration of substances into water, soil, air, and food also is listed in Table 3-2. Most of the identified agents are toxic and represent potential threats to the public health, depending on the degree of expo-

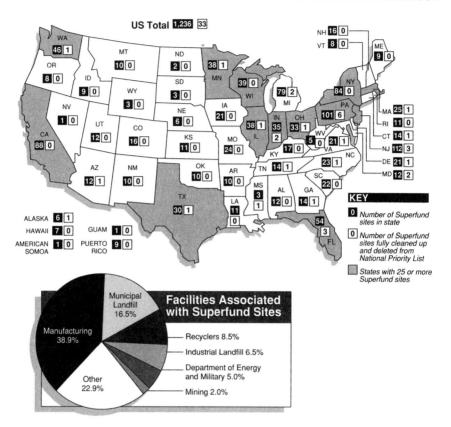

FIGURE 3-1 Few Superfund sites completely cleaned up. Source: Adapted from Viviano, 1991, with permission.

sure. Of the compounds identified at more than 100 sites, lead, chromium, arsenic, cadmium, nickel, trichloroethylene (TCE), perchloroethylene (PCE), vinyl chloride, methylene chloride, chloroform, benzene, ethylene dichloride (EDC), and polychlorinated biphenyls (PCB) have been identified as either human or animal carcinogens and are classified in group 1 of the ATSDR-EPA list of the 100 most hazardous substances. A list of agents identified at more than 10 proposed and final NPL sites is listed in Appendix 3-A to this chapter, and the original ATSDR list of priority substances can be found in Appendix 3-B.

Buffler et al. (1985) have reviewed the adverse health effects associated with specific toxicants identified at hazardous-waste sites. While discussing the types of chemicals found, the review addresses whether health effects could be detected in studies of populations exposed to these chemicals at waste-disposal sites. Skin and central nervous

TABLE 3-1 Types of Activities at Hazardous-Waste Sites in the United States (Includes 1177 Final and Proposed Sites Placed on the National Priorities List as of June 1988)

Activity	Final	Proposed	Total
Surface impoundments	295	137	432
Landfills, commercial/ industrial	299	113	412
Containers/drums	229	64	293
Other manufacturing/ industrial	102	137	239
Landfills, municipal	157	56	213
Spills	111	73	184
Chemical processing/ manufacturing	82	78	160
Waste piles	73	46	119
Leaking containers	80	36	116
Tanks, above-ground	80	28	108
Tanks, below-ground	46	42	88
Groundwater plumes	63	12	75
Electroplating	36	27	63
Wood preserving	39	16	55
Waste oil processing	34	16	50
Ore processing/refining smelting	27	9	36
Open burning	24	12	36
Solvent recovery	24	11	35
Outfall, surface water	20	15	35
Military ordnance production/storage/ disposal	19	14	33
Military testing & maintenance	16	10	26
Landfarm, land treatment/ spreading	18	7	25
Battery recycling	17	6	23
Incinerators	17	1	18
Mining sites, surface	11	4	15
Underground injection	11	2	13
Drum recycling	8	4	12
Sand and gravel pits	7	3	10
Mining sites, subsurface	6	3	9
Road oiling	7	1	8
Laundries/dry cleaners	2	5	7
Sinkholes	6	1	7
Explosive disposal/ detonation	2	1	3
Tire storage/recycling	2	0	2
Total sites[a]:	799	378	1177

[a]Since each site may have more than one activity, the number of activities is greater than the number of sites.

Source: U.S. Environmental Protection Agency, Office of Emergency Response, Washington, D.C. 20460.

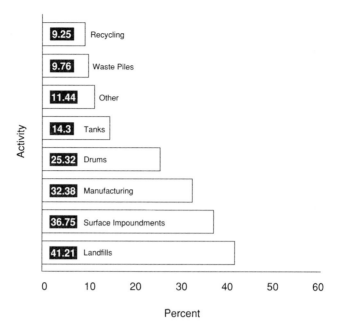

FIGURE 3-2   NPL: Types of activities at 1189 final sites. Source: Environmental Protection Agency, Office of Solid Waste and Emergency Response, 1991.

system (CNS) effects were the most likely effects to occur from direct contact with waste site chemicals. Hepatic, hematopoietic, renal, reproductive, and CNS effects were the most likely indicators of chronic, low-dose exposure through ingestion.

UNIDENTIFIED OR UNCHARACTERIZED CONTAMINANTS

To date, attention has focused on a relatively small number of chemical contaminants identified at hazardous-waste sites. Many identified or unidentified potential contaminants have received little scrutiny. These uncharacterized pollutants include substances that are not on the ATSDR-EPA list of 100 most hazardous substances, compounds that cannot be identified by standardized or accepted analytical methods, previously unidentified substances that result from in situ transformation processes, and by-products of treatment techniques. MacKay et al. (1989) suggest that large quantities of these potentially toxic compounds may be relatively mobile in the subsurface environment, and a potential exists for these compounds to contaminate groundwater.

One EPA evaluation (Bramlett et al., 1987) of the composition of leachates from hazardous-waste sites documents the potential problem. The chemical composition of leachates from 13 sites located throughout the U.S. was analyzed. Only 4 percent of the total organic carbon (TOC) in the leachate was characterized by gas chromatography/mass spectroscopy according to their chemical structure. More than 200 separate compounds were identified in the 4 percent fraction. This included 42 organic acids, 43 oxygenated and heteroaromatic hydrocarbons, 39 halogenated hydrocarbons, 26 organic bases, 32 aromatic hydrocarbons, 8 alkanes, and 13 metals. The unidentified 96 percent of organic carbon is of unknown toxicity. Overall, the number of chemical agents found in the 4 percent of the leachate studied is large, and yet this represents only a fraction of the overall organic contribution. In addition to the toxicity of these chemical agents, whether the mobile compounds promote transport of chemical toxicants is an important subject for research.

Research in California by MacKay et al. (1989) has documented the examples of uncharacterized compounds that could have important toxicologic properties or significance for transport. Chlorobenzenesulfonic acids have been identified at the Stringfellow Acid Pits in Glen Avon and at the BKK landfill in West Covina; arsenicals were found at a site in Rancho Cordova; and brominated alkanes were found at the Casmalia hazardous-waste disposal site, along with high melting explosive (HMX) (cyclotetramethylene tetramintriamine), research department explosive (RDX) (cyclonite), and mutagenic explosive byproducts from the Lawrence Livermore National Laboratory, to name just a few.

NONPOINT SOURCES

As important as the NPL sites are, focusing attention solely on the chemicals identified at these sites understates the potential scope of the problem of groundwater contamination. Toxic contaminants in groundwater can be considered as "hazardous waste" in a public health or toxicologic context, in contrast to the regulatory framework for defining hazardous waste. Secondly, contaminated groundwater close to defined hazardous-waste sites may act as a confounder in environmental epidemiologic investigation. In California, for example, 70 percent of public drinking water comes from groundwater (Leeden et al., 1990). Moreover, recent surveys show that problems with groundwater are not unique to California. In 1986, EPA reported to Congress that groundwater contamination from organic chemicals had occurred or was occurring in 70 percent of the states; 65 percent and

TABLE 3-2 Selected Hazardous Substances at 951 National Priorities List Sites: Number and Percentage of Sites and Documented Migration of Substances into Specific Media

Substance	ATSDR Priority Group	No.	%	Sites with Migration	Ground-water	Surface Water	Soil	Air	Food	Sediment
Metallic Elements										
Lead	1	564	59	327	234	138	122	37	50	114
Chromium	1	404	43	224	159	84	88	28	39	84
Arsenic	1	329	35	142	93	55	48	12	15	46
Cadmium	1	262	28	36	92	46	54	16	19	50
Mercury	2	232	24	112	72	49	45	18	21	44
Nickel	1	129	14	58	29	24	20	6	10	19
		126	13	55	30	24	15	3	8	21
Beryllium	1	21	2	9	2	3	1	0	0	3
Volatile Organic Compounds (VOCs)										
Trichloroethylene	1	518	54	268	236	88	81	71	31	58
Benzene	1	402	42	231	204	63	41	44	19	27
Tetrachloroethylene	1	323	34	139	115	41	27	29	9	24
Toluene	2	267	28	125	116	28	22	34	11	17
Vinyl Chloride	1	256	27	101	78	26	29	26	6	20
Methylene Chloride	1	187	20	87	80	16	14	18	7	9
Chloroform	1	183	19	81	61	21	16	17	4	9
		142	15	74	61	20	8	7	3	9
1,4-Dichlorobenzene	1	31	3	7	6	0	1	1	1	1
Polychlorinated Biphenyls (PCBs)	1	162	17	86	43	25	40	11	25	39

Polycyclic Aromatic Hydrocarbons (PAH)		187	20	75	32	22	31	4	6	38
Benzo(a)pyrene	1	56	6	18	6	6	9	0	2	8
Benzo(a)anthracene	1	32	3	10	3	4	8	0	1	6
Benzo(a)fluoroanthene	1	25	3	10	1	3	5	0	0	4
Chrysene	1	23	2	6	2	1	3	0	1	4
Dibenzo(a,h)anthracene	1	4	<1	1	0	0	1	0	0	0
Phthalates		106	11	35	22	13	17	5	5	16
Bis(2-ethylhexyl)phthalate	1	88	9	35	22	13	16	3	5	16
Pesticides		82	9	25	13	8	17	6	7	12
Dieldrin/aldrin	1	29	3	13	8	2	6	3	2	3
Heptachlor/heptachlor epoxide	1	15	2	4	2	0	1	0	0	1
Dioxins		47	5	21	8	7	16	2	7	11
2,3,7,8-Tetrachlorodibenzo-p-dioxin	1	19	2	15	5	3	8	3	7	10
Other										
Cyanide	1	74	8	23	13	9	7	3	2	8
N-Nitrosodiphenylamine	1	8	1	4	2	1	2	0	1	2

Source: Adapted from ATSDR, 1989.

60 percent had groundwater contamination from metals and pesticides, respectively (EPA, 1987a). Contamination from nonpoint sources, such as agricultural runoff, may not derive from a specific hazardous-waste site, but is toxic waste and could pose significant health hazards unless recognized and controlled. For example, according to EPA (Appendix 3-A), the reproductive toxicant and carcinogen dibromochloropropane (DBCP) has been identified at only one NPL site. Although DBCP use was suspended in California in 1979, it persists in the environment and has been detected in more than one-fifth of drinking water wells in California not related to NPL sites. MacKay and Smith (1990) have reviewed the status of groundwater monitoring in California for "active" ingredients from pesticides, based on samplings from 1975 to 1988 of 10,929 wells. DBCP was detected in 2353 wells; in more than 1000 wells, it exceeded the state maximum contaminant level (MCL) of 0.2 parts per billion (ppb). About 100 of the wells that exceeded the limit were in public supply systems that serve large numbers of customers. One hundred were in smaller public supply systems, and others were private supply wells. It is estimated that approximately 500,000 Californians have DBCP in their drinking water supply.

In addition to the active ingredients in pesticides, so-called "inert" ingredients also contaminate groundwater in California and elsewhere. Cohen and Bowes (1984) have estimated that 200 million pounds of inert ingredients were released to the land in pesticide use between 1971 and 1981. These are rough estimates because the composition of inert ingredients in a commercial pesticide formulation is proprietary. In some cases, materials that have been banned as active ingredients continued to be used as inert ingredients. Reports published by MacKay and co-workers (MacKay et al., 1987; Smith et al., 1990) note that inert ingredients can include TCE, PCE, formaldehyde, pentachlorophenol, ethylene dichloride, and 1,4-dichlorobenzene, all of which are known to be toxic. In 1987, EPA confirmed that these and other inert ingredients can have toxicologic significance (EPA, 1987b). Of the approximately 1200 substances used as inert ingredients in pesticide products, EPA (1987b) has determined that about 50 are of "significant toxicological concern" on the basis of their carcinogenicity, adverse reproductive effects, neurotoxicity, or other chronic effects. An additional 60 compounds were considered "potentially toxic." These pollutants are not derived from hazardous-waste sites, but they illustrate the potential for groundwater contamination from agricultural chemical waste. They constitute a hazardous-waste hazard in themselves, whereas their impact on epidemiologic investigation of hazardous-waste sites would be that of a confounder.

Since 1984, public drinking water supplies in California have been investigated by the California Department of Health Services (DHS) to determine the extent of groundwater contamination in the state (Smith et al., 1990). During the period 1984-1988, approximately 7000 large and small supply systems were evaluated, and about 1500 wells were found to be contaminated with organic chemicals. The chemicals identified in this monitoring included pesticides and solvents such as PCE, TCE, chloroform, EDC, TCA, and carbon tetrachloride. A total of 409 (5.6 percent) wells had one or more chemicals exceeding the state's action level or the Maximum Contaminant Level (MCL), and 18.3 percent of the wells had some contamination. Since early 1986, the state has sought to identify the sources of organic chemical pollution of contaminated supply wells identified by the monitoring program, but there is no comprehensive effort to identify new sources of groundwater contamination, and the evaluation of existing sources is slow. The MacKay and Smith study (1990) also documents groundwater contamination from a variety of solvents and toxic active ingredients in pesticides. These include 1,2-dichloropropane and ethylene dibromide (EDB), atrazine, simazine, bentazon, aldicarb, diuron, prometon, and bromacil, all of which have been linked with adverse human health effects. These data indicate the need for periodic screening of groundwater supplies in areas of high chemical use.

Table 3-3 lists the major causes of groundwater contamination reported by states. NPL sites are included, but other sources of contamination are also important. The groundwater contamination from sources other than hazardous-waste sites is relevant to the conduct of exposure assessment in environmental epidemiology. For example, in the city of Santa Maria, California, which is adjacent to the operating Casmalia hazardous-waste site, numerous wells were closed because of contamination by organic solvents (Breslow et al., 1989). Possible sources of well water contamination include leaching from the Casmalia hazardous-waste disposal site (unlikely), use of such solvents as TCE and PCE to clean septic tanks (likely), and runoff of agricultural chemicals (likely). Groundwater contamination of this type from unrecognized nonpoint sources poses a twofold problem. Such contamination may provide important additional exposures that increase the overall health risk and can reduce the likelihood of finding effects in studies that fail to take these exposures into account.

ASSESSMENT OF THE NATURE AND EXTENT OF EXPOSURE

There is no question that large quantities of highly toxic chemicals are found at hazardous-waste sites. Even though it is not always

TABLE 3-3　Activities Contributing to Groundwater Contamination in the United States

Activity	States Citing	Estimated Sites	Contaminants Frequently Cited as Result of Activity
Waste disposal:			
Septic systems	41	22 million	Bacteria, viruses, nitrate, phosphate, chloride, and organic compounds such as trichloroethylene.
Landfills (active)	51	16,400	Dissolved solids, iron, manganese, trace metals, acids, organic compounds, and pesticides.
Surface impoundments	32	191,800	Brines, acidic mine wastes, feedlot wastes, trace metals, and organic compounds.
Injection wells	10	280,800	Dissolved solids, bacteria, sodium, chloride, nitrate, phosphate, organic compounds, pesticides, and acids.
Land application of wastes	12	19,000 land application units	Bacteria, nitrate, phosphate, trace metals, and organic compounds.
Storage and handling of materials:			
Underground storage tanks	39	2.4-4.8 million	Benzene, toluene, xylene, and petroleum products.
Above-ground storage tanks	16	Unknown	Organic compounds, acids, metals, and petroleum products.
Material handling and transfers	29	10,000-16,000 spills per year	Petroleum products, aluminum, iron, sulfate, and trace metals.
Mining activities:			
Mining and spoil disposal-coal mines	23	15,000 active; 67,000 inactive	Acids, iron, manganese, sulfate, uranium, thorium, radium, molybdenum, selenium, and trace metals.
Oil and gas activities:			
Wells	20	550,000 production; 1.2 million abandoned	Brines.

TABLE 3-3 *Continued*

Activity	States Citing	Estimated Sites	Contaminants Frequently Cited as Result of Activity
Agricultural activities:			
Fertilizer and pesticide applications	44	363 million acres	Nitrate, phosphate, and pesticides.
Irrigation practices	22	376,000 wells; 49 million acres irrigated	Dissolved solids, nitrate, phosphate, and pesticides
Animal feedlots	17	1900	Nitrate, phosphate, and bacteria.
Urban activities:			
Runoff	15	47.3 million acres urban land	Bacteria, hydrocarbons, dissolved solids, lead, cadmium, and trace metals.
Deicing chemical storage and use	14	Not reported	Sodium chloride, ferric ferrocyanide, sodium ferrocyanide, phosphate, and chromate.
Other:			
Saline intrusion or upconing	29	Not reported	Dissolved solids and brines.

Source: Adapted from U.S. Geological Survey, 1988.

feasible to identify them completely, there is little doubt that the sites are large repositories of potentially dangerous substances. That information notwithstanding, the issue in an epidemiologic and public health context is whether there are pathways from a hazardous-waste site to nearby residents that will allow exposures that can damage human health (see Figure 3-3). The issue of whether off-site migration results in public exposure is a matter of concern in exposure assessment associated with epidemiologic studies of waste-chemical facilities.

The purpose of exposure assessment in environmental epidemiology is to facilitate investigation of and to establish cause-effect relationships between environmental exposure and adverse health outcomes. Causation may be implied in descriptive studies in which no direct determination of exposure is carried out, but well-conducted studies of population exposure enhance confidence in the interpretation of a causal relationship between exposure and health outcome.

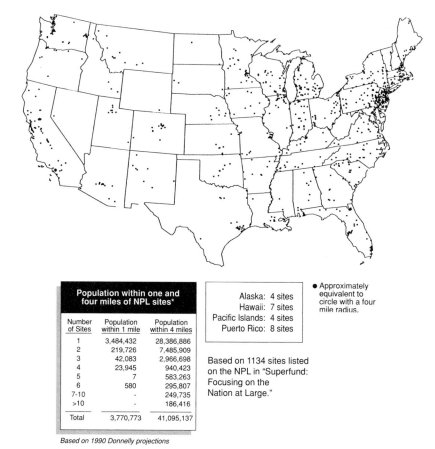

Population within one and four miles of NPL sites*		
Number of Sites	Population within 1 mile	Population within 4 miles
1	3,484,432	28,386,886
2	219,726	7,485,909
3	42,083	2,966,698
4	23,945	940,423
5	7	583,263
6	580	295,807
7-10	-	249,735
>10	-	186,416
Total	3,770,773	41,095,137

Based on 1990 Donnelly projections

Alaska: 4 sites
Hawaii: 7 sites
Pacific Islands: 4 sites
Puerto Rico: 8 sites

Based on 1134 sites listed on the NPL in "Superfund: Focusing on the Nation at Large."

● Approximately equivalent to circle with a four mile radius.

FIGURE 3-3a NPL sites and population resident within 1 and 4 miles. Source: Environmental Protection Agency, Office of Solid Waste and Emergency Response, 1991.

Within this overall context, exposure assessment strategies have several secondary objectives:

1. To facilitate identification of persons at risk for adverse health consequences from exposure to toxic chemical agents—i.e., to identify with reasonable accuracy persons who are being or have been exposed to materials considered hazardous waste.

2. To define the nature of the exposure—e.g., whether exposure is derived from a single source, such as inhalation of materials, or from multiple sources, such as air and water. This objective requires identification of specific toxic chemicals. Assessment of potential interactive effects (such as potentiation or synergy) of simultaneous chemical exposures is advantageous.

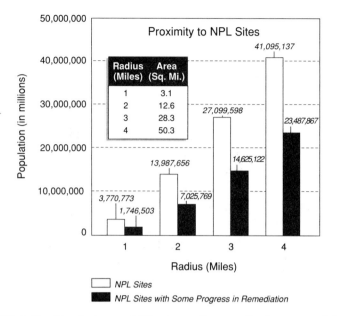

FIGURE 3-3b Proximity to NPL sites. Source: Environmental Protection Agency, Office of Solid Waste and Emergency Response, 1991.

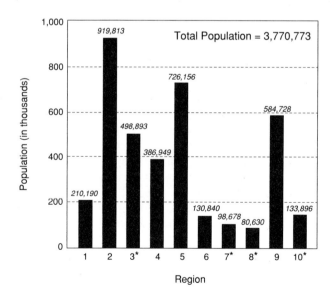

FIGURE 3-3c Population living within 1 mile of a Superfund site(s). *Regions likely to be undercounted because of missing location data. Source: Environmental Protection Agency, Office of Solid Waste and Emergency Response, 1991.

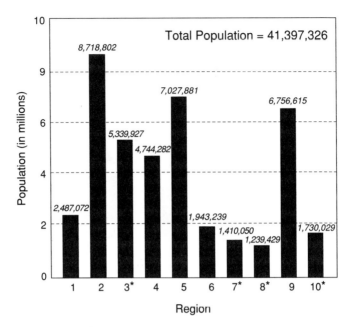

FIGURE 3-3d Population living within 4 miles of a Superfund site(s).
*Regions likely to be undercounted because of missing location data. Source:
Environmental Protection Agency, Office of Solid Waste and Emergency Response, 1991.

3. To assess the nature of potentially confounding exposures, including groundwater contamination that may occur from numerous sources, such as agricultural runoff, and may increase the health risk of a study population or inhibit population identification and characterization and identification of causal factors in epidemiologic investigations.

4. To determine the temporal characteristics of exposure—to identify the period over which exposure has occurred and the duration of exposure. Exposure within a given geographic area may change as a result of contamination migration, so surrogate measures of exposure based on distance from a point source (fixed site) have the disadvantage of not taking the movement of chemicals into consideration.

5. To quantify the degree of exposure of individuals or defined populations. This may be accomplished by direct measurement of exposure (including personal sampling, and use of biologic biomarkers) or indirect measurement (e.g., measurement of contaminant concentrations in water or air, that is, microenvironmental monitoring).

The NRC report (1991) on human exposure assessment for airborne pollutants, which reviews progress in addressing total human exposure, is particularly valuable for pursuing those objectives. The report describes the framework and specific methods for exposure assessment. It recommends that scientists and regulators consistently use its definitions of exposure and exposure assessment to ensure standardization across disciplines. This approach has special significance for studies of possible adverse health outcomes associated with hazardous-waste sites because of the potential for multiple chemical exposure, the wide range of pathways for transport of contaminants, and the complex temporal characteristics of exposure.

The NRC report (1991) summarized the requisite entities to be determined in exposure assessment:

• concentration distributions in time and space for different environmental media;
  • populations or groups at high and low risk;
  • chemical and physical contributions of various sources;
  • factors that control contaminant release into environmental media, routes of environmental transport, and routes of entry into humans.

ROUTES OF EXPOSURE

In general, all routes of exposure and all environmental media should be assessed to determine their relative contribution to the overall exposure associated with a waste site. Such work has been done, but generally not in the context of epidemiologic investigation. Likely media of exposure from hazardous-waste sites include air, water, food, and soil (Figure 3-4). Exposure to toxic chemicals would most likely occur through contaminated groundwater that has leached or run off from waste sites to enter the drinking water supply. Other sources of exposure include direct contact with contaminated sediment; accidental ingestion of contaminated soil or surface water; release of volatile agents into the air; and ingestion of contaminated vegetables, fruit, meat, poultry, or fish.

Exposure to contaminated water can derive from showering or bathing, from drinking water, and from using water in food preparation. Those routes of exposure have received considerable attention as a result of EPA's Total Exposure Assessment Methodology (TEAM) studies (Wallace et al., 1986, 1987, 1988), the work of Andelman et al. (1986, 1990), and the work of Lioy and co-workers (Jo et al., 1990a,b). The results of the investigations illustrate the importance of indoor

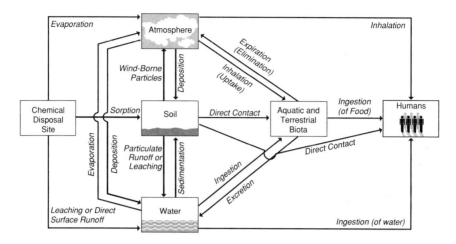

FIGURE 3-4 Physical and biological routes of transport of hazardous substances, their release from disposal sites, and potential for human exposure. Source: Adapted from Grisham, 1986, with permission.

environment exposure to volatile organic compounds (VOCs). For example, Andelman (1990) has developed an indoor air model validated by air measurements of TCE from residential bathrooms. He found that TCE inhalation exposures from a six-minute shower are comparable to ingestion of TCE in drinking water. Jo et al. (1990a,b) found that breath concentration after showering was approximately twice as high as that after inhalation-only exposure; thus dermal absorption was equivalent to inhalation absorption.

Percolation of VOCs into the home from contaminated soil under or around houses is another pathway for exposure. For example, at Love Canal, New York, migration of chemical leachates through the soil and evaporation through porous basement walls resulted in the presence of benzene, toluene, chloroform, TCE, PCE, and hexane in the air inside homes (Paigen et al., 1987).

Lioy (1990) has pointed out that contaminant exposure through ingestion of soil and inhalation of dust from soil has begun to receive attention (Pierce, 1985; Travis and Hattemer-Frey, 1987; Severn, 1987). Estimates of the quantity of soil ingested by children and adults have been made (Lioy, 1990). Daily ingestion rates range from milligrams per kilogram of body weight per day to grams per kilogram per day and are important for estimating exposure. Exposure to soil dust through inhalation has received little attention.

The relevance of the total environmental exposure model in assessing exposure to risk from hazardous-waste sites has been illustrated by Lioy et al. (1988) as these authors sought to define total exposure to benzopyrene (BAP). The study was carried out in Phillipsburg, New Jersey, where there is a metal pipe foundry. The foundry was the point source for BAP emissions and could represent a surrogate for a hazardous-waste site. In this study indoor and outdoor air, food, and water exposure analyses were conducted. Additional multimedia studies of this type will be useful in defining protocols for exposure assessment at hazardous-waste sites.

MEASUREMENT OF EXPOSURE

This section addresses what constitutes appropriate approaches to the measurement of exposure in order to identify and characterize an exposed population and then considers potential problems in the estimation of exposure to the public associated with hazardous-waste sites.

ATSDR health assessments could be important sources of information about the possible routes of human exposure and the types and amounts of hazardous materials present at NPL sites. The conceptual model ATSDR has adopted for conducting its health assessments seeks to emphasize early identification of potential public health problems and interventions that would ameliorate problems at a site. The health assessments have generally not been published in the peer-reviewed literature and are therefore not within the scope of this report. The committee has reviewed the abstracts for the 951 health assessments and evaluated some assessments in detail.

The assessments provide information about the specific toxic chemicals found at NPL sites, the degree of contamination, and potential routes of off-site exposure of the public. There is little information about the degree of off-site contamination. Virtually no information about actual exposure to the public is derived from personal sampling, direct measurement of exposure of individuals, or total exposure assessment modeling. The ATSDR health assessments are in reality hazard assessments with limited information about potential human health effects from off-site migration of chemical wastes. They do not constitute epidemiologic investigations nor were they intended to be used for those purposes. They provide a starting point for epidemiologic investigations, insofar as they contain information about some of the chemicals identified at hazardous-waste sites. Their lack of information on the fate and transport of contaminants and on exposures of persons near the sites makes them of limited use for identification of a potentially exposed population in environmental epidemiologic investigations.

Site-specific investigations have also not proceeded to the steps of defining the populations at risk and quantitatively evaluating exposure to toxic contaminants. The characterizations of the sites more often reflect requirements of environmental engineering and site remediation than assessment of public health considerations. Whether the toxic contaminants pose a risk to the exposed population cannot be determined in the absence of more detailed information about human exposures. Instead of focusing on the toxic chemicals that have been identified at a site itself, it is necessary to develop estimates of exposure to define and assess the population at risk, including estimation of the size and exposure-related characteristics.

In development of estimates of human exposure and estimating population exposure in connection with waste sites, a hierarchy of exposure or surrogate exposure data can be useful in establishing a sampling strategy (Table 3-4). Direct measurement of exposure assessment includes personal monitoring and use of biologic markers (see Chapter 7) (NRC, 1991). Personal monitoring is advantageous insofar as it enables direct measurement of the concentration of air contaminants in the breathing zone of a subject. Biologic markers are potentially indicative of total dose, in that they integrate the dose from multiple routes of exposure. For environmental epidemiologic investigations, these types of data provide a basis for analysis of exposure as a continuous variable and are potentially valuable for identifying the etiologic basis of an adverse outcome as a function of dose. Other types of data (categories 2-7 on Table 3-4) are generally

TABLE 3-4 Hierarchy of Exposure Data or Surrogates

Types of Data	Approximation to actual exposure
1. Quantified personal measurements	Best
2. Quantified area or ambient measurements in the vicinity of the residence or other sites of activity	
3. Quantified surrogates of exposure (e.g., estimates of drinking water use)	
4. Distance from site and duration of residence	
5. Distance or duration of residence	
6. Residence or employment in geographic area in reasonable proximity to site where exposure can be assumed.	
7. Residence or employment in defined geographical area (e.g., a county) of the site	Poorest

considered indirect measurements of dose and can be subdivided into information derived from quantification of the concentration of toxic contaminants in a particular microenvironment and information that does not use quantitative estimates of exposure but rather surrogates of exposure, such as proximity to a site or county of residence.

Quantification of microenvironment concentrations implies monitoring of contaminant concentrations in the location where exposures occur—for example, monitoring of contaminants in drinking water, measurement of the concentration of air contaminants in the general location of the subjects in the study, and determination of the degree of contamination of food and soil. Monitoring of this nature provides a realistic basis for assessment of individual exposure. But it is often not possible to obtain either personal or microenvironmental data in a timely fashion. The studies reviewed to date make limited use of these approaches and instead use surrogates of exposure (types 4-7) including proximity to a site, duration of residence, or residence in a specific geographic region, such as a county. Data derived from studies of this type are easier to obtain and may provide useful inferences about causative factors for adverse health effects associated with hazardous-waste sites, but they are clearly limited in scope and prone to misclassification (see below).

Gann (1986) has asked what kind of exposure data epidemiologists need. The answer should depend on the research question before the investigator and will depend, in part, on the biologic model of the exposure-response relationship. Marsh and Caplan (1987) define three levels of a health effects investigation: Level I includes ecologic studies and is based on existing, routine, and easily accessible records of exposure. Exposure assessment in ecologic studies has generally made use of the type of information found in categories 4-7 (Table 3-4) of the exposure information hierarchy. Many of the studies to be reviewed here fall into this category. Level II studies as defined by Marsh and Caplan (1987) include cross-sectional, case-control, or short-term cohort studies. Level III consists of prospective studies. Quantitative assessment of personal exposure and microenvironment monitoring to determine the concentrations of chemical toxicants in a variety of media are especially appropriate for Level II and III studies. Improved quantitative exposure data could enhance study population identification and improve ecologic studies, but that information has not been pursued, because ecologic studies have relied on surrogates of exposure. Ecologic studies are often considered hypothesis-generating, and in-depth exposure evaluations would not necessarily be considered appropriate to a design of this type. However, failure to identify the population at risk accurately may limit study findings, and more careful attention to the exposure question is probably warranted.

There are three relevant approaches to estimating personal exposure: measurement of potential dose, measurement of internal dose, and measurement of the dose at the biologic target (Figure 3-5). The dose at the target site, or the biologically effective dose, is the fraction of the contaminant or its metabolite identified at the site of action in the body from which the ensuing health effect derives. Investigators would prefer to have information on the biologically effective dose for each exposed individual over time (see Chapter 7).

Absent such information, internal dose measures the contribution of exposure to a contaminant from all media. Internal dose is generally assessed by means of biologic monitoring when biological monitoring techniques are available. But biologic monitoring is difficult if the investigator must assess exposure to multiple chemicals. The difficulty derives in part from paucity of validated biologic monitoring assays and the sparseness of development of toxicokinetic models to describe toxicant metabolism. Method development for biologic monitoring is a priority for assessment of exposure to chemical mixtures. Biologic monitoring is useful if the object of a study is to find or characterize an association between specific chemicals and various health end points, because it enables an investigator to determine dose from inhalation, ingestion, and dermal contact. Evalua-

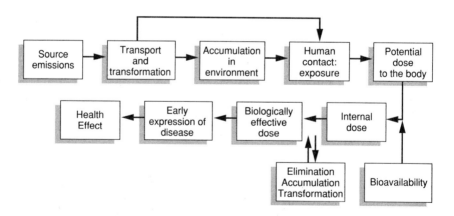

FIGURE 3-5 Continuum from emission of a contaminant to a health effect. Source: Lioy et al., 1990. Reprinted with permission from *Environ. Sci. Technol.* **1990**, *24*, 940[942]. Copyright 1990 American Chemical Society.

tion of exposure based on determination of concentrations of contaminants in various media requires multiple measurements, each with its own limitations, such as the accuracy of monitoring systems, whereas biologic monitoring integrates an exposure dose.

Biologic monitoring has additional limitations as a measure of internal dose in exposure assessment of hazardous waste sites. How to address complex mixtures is one issue, whereas a second concerns the question of how to address variability in biological monitoring (Droz and Wu, 1991). Third, biologic monitoring generally addresses current exposure although there are notable exceptions such as x-ray fluorescence of lead in bone, which serves as a basis to estimate long term absorption of lead (EHP, 1991).

Toxicokinetic models that quantitatively describe rates of absorption, distribution, biotransformation, and excretion of toxicants are necessary for the development and validation of biologic monitoring techniques that address assessment of both short- and long-term exposures. Toxicokinetic modeling has been particularly valuable in describing the overall dynamics of lead metabolism (Landrigan, et al., 1985), nonlinearities in the biotransformation of methylene chloride (Hattis, 1990), the relationship between sperm count and ethylene oxide exposure (Smith 1988) and the neurotoxicity of acrylamide (Hattis and Shapiro, 1990); for better estimation of target-tissue dose for purposes of risk assessment for butadiene (Hattis and Wasson, 1987) and ethylene oxide (Hattis, 1987); and for risk assessment of drinking water with particular reference to the quantitative estimation of uncertainty (NRC, 1987; Hattis and Froines, in press). Advancing the development and use of toxicokinetic modeling should have high priority.

The problem of using biologic monitoring or contaminant concentration to assess exposure where there are complex mixtures can be addressed in part by using a marker which serves as a surrogate for the complex mixture. Hammond (1991) has suggested that within a population exposed to a mixture which is qualitatively similar to a known toxicant, a marker of exposure can make possible a quantitative estimate of exposure level. This approach does assume that given a situation in which exposure to a complex mixture is related to some adverse health consequences, that there will be a relationship between the marker of exposure and the disease outcome. The use of pack years as a surrogate for exposure estimation in the investigation of health risk from smoking is a good example of the utility of estimates of exposure where the specific etiologic agents have not been identified.

Personal monitoring of exposure to airborne toxicants provides a direct measurement of their concentrations in the breathing zone of an individual. However, exposure derived from hazardous waste sites may be derived primarily from ingestion, e.g., drinking water and food, or dermal exposure, e.g., soil contamination, and inhalation may not represent the most significant exposure route. In this context microenvironmental monitoring in the locations where exposure occurs in the particular media of concern will represent the approach of choice. Lioy (1990) and the National Research Council (NRC, 1991) have described the parameters required to calculate the potential and internal dose (Figure 3-6). These parameters derive from the need to link environmental source, transport, and receptor models to estimate exposure.

Limited attention has been given to date to the development of models to estimate exposure. A model in this context would make use of both measured and modeled microenvironmental concentrations and would address the temporal characteristics of the exposures. The NRC report on estimation of human exposure described the principal advantage of models as their ability to estimate concentrations in different microenvironments or exposures on which there is little direct information.

Where personal or biologic monitoring, microenvironment characterization, and modeling cannot be readily accomplished, surrogate measures of exposures are the last resort; they were the method of choice in the earlier ecologic investigations reviewed here. With one exception (Clark et al., 1982), virtually no studies have attempted to quantify personal exposure to contaminants that have migrated off site from waste sites. There have been no estimates of exposure from microenvironment monitoring, such as the EPA TEAM studies (Wallace et al., 1986, 1987, 1988). These are excellent examples of the type of microenvironmental monitoring that would usefully be models for assessment of exposure associated with waste sites.

Surrogates of exposure may provide evidence that adverse health outcomes are related to a hazardous-waste site exposure. They have some utility for initial screening, although a negative result could result in no follow-up studies and a false-negative finding. In this regard, Baker and colleagues (1988) have strongly warned against the presumption of no adverse effects of exposure to toxic agents from Stringfellow Acid Pits in Glen Avon, California. They caution investigators that lack of good exposure estimates may have biased their results. Use of surrogate exposures should generally be viewed in this context.

Airborne contaminant

I. Concentrations ($\mu g/m^3$, ppb)
   A. Microenvironments
   B. Personal
II. Patterns of exposure
   A. Intensity "episode" concentrations versus normal levels (average)
   B. Frequency and duration of contact
III. Transport
   A. Dispersion and advection
   B. Other meteorology-related removal rates (washout, fallout)
   C. Indoor ventilation and removal rates
IV. Chemistry
   A. Formation rates
   B. Transformation rates
V. Deposition rate ($\mu g/cm^2$)
   A. Environmental
   B. Lung
VI. Contact
   A. Inhalation (dependent on exercise regimen) ($m^3/time$)
   B. Dermal deposition and permeability ($\mu g/cm^2/time$)
   C. Ingestion (food, soil) ($\mu g/g/time$)
VII. Absorption
   A. Within tissue
   B. Into the blood and other fluids

Water contaminant

I. Concentration ($\mu g/L$, ppm)
   A. Tap water
   B. Water uses
   C. Effluent
      1. Industrial
      2. Commercial
      3. Residential
      4. Uncontrolled dumps
II. Patterns of exposure
   A. Drinking
   B. Swimming
   C. Cooking
   D. Bathing
   E. Laundry
   F. Showering

III. Solubility of contaminant
IV. Volatility of contaminant
V. Transport
   A. Groundwater
   B. Surface water
   C. Domestic supply
VI. Chemistry
   A. Formation rates
   B. Transformation rates
   C. Degradation
VII. Contact rate ($\mu g/L/time$) via exposure route
   A. Ingestion
   B. Skin
   C. Inhalation (volatilized)
VIII. Absorption
   A. Dermal deposition and permeability
   B. Gastrointestinal tract

Soil and sediment

I. Concentrations ($\mu g/g$)
   A. Dusts
      1. Outdoor
      2. Indoor
   B. Contaminated soil
      1. Uncontrolled dumps
      2. Airborne deposition
      3. Landfills
      4. Resuspension
II. Patterns of exposure
   A. Frequency and duration
   B. Intensity of contact
III. Percolation rate
   A. Soil composition
   B. Water table
   C. Solubility
   D. Transport
IV. Volatilization
   A. Contaminant
   B. Soil composition
   C. Top soil and cover
V. Contact rate via exposure route
   A. Dermal deposition and permeability
   B. Lung
   C. Gastrointestinal tract (pica)
      1. Normal population
      2. Abnormal ingestion behavior
Vi. Body parameter
   A. Lung volume

   B. Exposed skin surface (condition of skin)
VII. Absorption
   A. Soil composition
   B. Contact and absorption rates

All media: Can be supplemented by measuring a biological marker of accumulated single-medium or multi-media exposures in blood, urine, feces, and so forth. Many of these usually are nonmedia specific.

Body weight: Used for lifetime exposure and dose calculation.

Food (commercial and home-grown produce)

I. Concentrations ($\mu g/g$)
   A. Plants
   B. Vegetables and fruit
   C. Milk
   D. Animals and fish
   E. Cooked foods
   F. Beverages and water-based foods ($\mu g/L$)
II. Patterns of exposure
   A. Rate ($\mu g/L/time$) ($\mu g/g/time$)
   B. Frequency
   C. Origin of food
      1. Home grown
      2. Commercial distribution
      3. Local farms
      4. Processed foods
III. Source of contamination
   A. Naturally occurring contaminants
   B. Airborne deposition
   C. Fertilization
   D. Pest control
   E. Waste dumps
   F. Water supply
   G. Preparation and cooking techniques
IV. Contact rate
   A. Gastrointestinal (GI)
   B. Inhalation (cooking only)
V. Absorption through GI tract

FIGURE 3-6 Parameters required to calculate the potential and internal dose. Source: Lioy, 1990, with permission.

LIMITATIONS OF DATA ON EXPOSURE

All too often, the data on exposure available to the epidemiologic investigator are limited, especially if the study was triggered by public concern about a disease or illness cluster or by perceived rather than documented exposures to toxicants at a hazardous-waste site. In some cases no quantitative information on exposure is available and investigators are forced to use a dichotomous approach rather than having estimates of continuous variables. They are required to divide the study population into groups of exposed and unexposed persons (ever/never) or even into groups of those who are likely to have been exposed and those who are not likely to have been exposed. This approach may represent the only alternative where exposure occurred in the past, but in many cases some estimate of exposure could be made by monitoring the concentration of contaminants. The fact that monitoring may not have occurred may be more a matter of resources, especially where the investigations are carried out by state health departments.

Lioy (1990) has suggested that scientific techniques and tools to measure exposure have advanced more quickly than have the strategies currently used to assess exposure in environmental epidemiologic studies. As Rothman (1990) points out, exposure assessment receives a low level of attention in study after study of chronic disease clusters. Upton et al. (1989) have suggested that a major weakness of environmental epidemiologic studies is their lack of exposure assessment. They report that the vast majority of the studies use surrogate measures of exposure based on the location of the at-risk population in relation to the hazardous-waste site or source of contamination. Buffler et al. (1985) have reviewed exposure assessment associated with environmental episodes at waste sites and other point sources. Their review cites 24 investigations that used indirect exposure estimates; 4 used surrogate indicators, although 15 had used some form of biological monitoring assessment. They concluded that direct measures of exposure were rarely available.

The specific aim of an environmental epidemiologic study of hazardous waste sites is to identify and establish a relationship between exposures derived from a site and adverse health outcomes. Identification and subsequent characterization of the study population represents the challenge before the investigator. The selection of sampling site is then crucial and the sampling site chosen should be relevant to potential human exposure (NRC, 1988). Table 3-5 is a summary of designs that can be used in the choice of sampling sites (NRC, 1988 and discussions therein).

TABLE 3-5 Spatial Considerations: Summary of Sampling Designs and When They Are Most Useful

Sampling Design	Condition for Most Useful Application
Haphazard sampling	Only valid when target population is homogeneous in space and time; hence, not generally recommended
Purposive sampling	Target population well defined and homogeneous, so sample-selection bias is not a problem; or specific environmental samples selected for unique value and interest, rather than for making inferences to wider population
Probability sampling	
Simple random sampling	Homogeneous population
Stratified random sampling	Homogeneous population within strata (subregions); might consider strata as domains of study
Systematic sampling	Frequently most useful; trends over time and space must be quantified
Multistage sampling	Target population large and homogeneous; simple random sampling used to select contiguous groups of population units
Cluster sampling	Economical when population units cluster (e.g., schools of fish); ideally, cluster means are similar in value, but concentrations within clusters should vary widely
Double sampling	Must be strong linear relation between variable of interest and less expensive or more easily measured variable

Source: NRC, 1988, 1991.

How exposures are characterized across individuals, locations, and time is a crucial issue in the design of an exposure assessment strategy. The precision of derived risk estimates is proportional to the population size under study, and validity is improved by reducing measurement error in the actual exposure data (Checkoway et al., 1989). Therefore, an exposure assessment strategy that gathers in-depth, quantitative exposure data on individuals might reduce measurement error, but it will probably do so at the expense of study size because of resource limitations. The loss in number of subjects needs to be juxtaposed against the possible gain in quantitative information about exposure.

For purposes of epidemiologic investigation, the larger the study population, the greater the ability to detect an effect when present. However, the conduct of extensive personal and microenvironmental monitoring is both time consuming and resource intensive. For example, the TEAM study in New Jersey evaluated exposure to volatile organic compounds (VOCs) of 355 residents. This in-depth evaluation involved giving each resident a diary and a specially designed, miniaturized pump connected to a 6-inch Tenax cartridge which was carried throughout the day. The TEAM New Jersey study concluded that the levels of 11 important organic compounds were significantly higher indoors than outdoors. These data appeared to reject the hypothesis that personal exposures to VOCs were directly related to releases from point sources. The study may have had sufficient sample size and probability sampling to permit extrapolation to the general population. However, whether a study of this size would meet the requirements of an epidemiologic investigation of hazardous-waste-site consequences is questionable. Studies which focus on low prevalence diseases such as cancer are particularly difficult because of low statistical power associated with small sample sizes (Ozonoff et al., 1987). Thus, there is a potential conflict between an in-depth exposure study in a small population versus the requirements of an epidemiologic investigation which must be addressed. Case-control approaches such as the two radon exposure studies being conducted by the New Jersey Health Department and the Argonne National Laboratories are useful examples of approaches to the in-depth estimation of exposure in a defined study population (NRC, 1991).

One useful approach for resolving the apparent contradiction between the requirements for in-depth exposure assessment and study population size is through the use of nested exposure-assessment designs in which a small number of the overall study population is subject to extensive direct and indirect measurements of exposure including personal and microenvironmental monitoring, biomarkers, and modeling. This population will serve as a surrogate to the larger study population and may be linked via indirect measures such as questionnaires or by modeling (NRC, 1991).

A second approach to resolving the apparent contradiction between population size and exposure assessment involves modeling exposure in which the results of microenvironmental monitoring are combined with individual activity patterns (NRC, 1991). This indirect approach seeks to develop exposure profiles by combining activity patterns with the expected concentrations of contaminants. Mathematical modeling is of particular value here. (A larger discussion of these issues will be addressed in Volume II.)

Bailar (1989) lists a number of common problems with all types of human exposure data (Table 3-6). The NRC reports on Human Exposure Assessment for Airborne Pollutants (1991) and Complex Mixtures (1988) have discussed these issues in detail and they will be addressed in our second report. This section will only highlight certain issues for purposes of illustration. For example, Bailar raises the important question of what to measure: Are we interested in peak exposure or cumulative exposure? Gillette (1987) expands the question to ask whether the incidence and magnitude of the biological response are most closely related to maximum concentration, average concentration, minimum concentration, or the total dose of the biologically active form of the toxicant. Our theoretical and practical understanding of how to address dose rate, an analogue of exposure concentration that can vary over time, is a problem that has been given no attention in environmental epidemiologic studies. Effects of exposure pattern or dose rate on health or biologic end points are more readily assessed once the relationship between exposure and response has been ascertained. The exploratory nature of many environmental epidemiologic investigations precludes this level of analysis.

Buffler et al. (1985) suggest that estimating the extent of exposures

TABLE 3-6 Some Common Problems with All Types of Human Exposure Data

---

High variability of human exposure, past and present
    Time to time
    Person to person
Lead times of decades
Synergy
Questions of what to measure:
    Peak exposure vs. time-weighted average (short or long)
    Short-term vs. lifetime
    High correlations
Incomplete and inaccurate monitor systems
    Ambient vs. indoor vs. personal monitors
Sample-to-sample variation
High costs, and small samples

- -

Self-selection, and confounders
Nonresponse, and incomplete follow-up
Reporting errors
Investigator or interviewer bias

Source: Bailar, 1989, with permission.

from waste sites can be extremely difficult. Where contamination results in a study population exposed to low concentrations of contaminant, the probability of detecting adverse health outcomes is also low. This problem is made more difficult when many toxic substances are found at low levels, and multiple health outcomes need to be studied. Nonspecificity of many potential health effects associated with chemical exposure, especially those with high background sites, represent important study constraints.

As discussed in the first chapter of this monograph, to determine whether a coincident finding is likely to be causal, the finding should make sense biologically, that is, the results should reflect a plausible hypothesis of the relationship between the studied exposures and diseases. In studies of groundwater and public health, associations have sometimes been proposed between chemical exposures and adverse health outcomes that are not well rooted in biology, but chiefly derive from the analytic capability to detect pollutants. Failure to conduct adequate exposure assessments can result in false-positive associations because the true causative agent has not been identified.

In evaluating biological plausibility, sometimes acute effects associated with higher occupational exposures are studied to see whether such effects may be caused by much lower concentrations from environmental exposures. Caution must be evident in associating signs and symptoms to certain chemicals known to be toxic at levels that are orders of magnitude greater than those commonly encountered by populations in proximity to waste sites.

Another problem in exposure assessment stems from the misclassification of exposure, a failure to place subjects in correct categories according to their levels of exposure. Misclassification generally weakens the association between exposure and outcome, and thereby compromises a study's validity. Unfortunately, the availability of more accurate information on exposure solves only part of the problem of misclassification. Even where the specific exposures studied may be correctly classified, other relevant exposures are crucial, including such confounding factors as tobacco smoke, workplace exposures, or the effect of other chemicals found at a site. Accurate assessment for the important exposure covariates is important, especially where the other exposure classification includes a strong risk factor for the disease such as occurs with cigarette smoking and lung cancer. In general, low levels of risk are found in environmental epidemiology studies (Gann, 1986; NRC, 1991), making accurate exposure information even more critical.

Landrigan (1983) has illustrated the problem of grouped versus individual data in comments on a study of arsenic in drinking water conducted by the Centers for Disease Control and the Alaska Division of Public Health. The concentration of arsenic in well water was a poor indicator of individual exposure because some of the persons studied had supplemented their consumption or switched completely to drinking bottled water. When estimates of bottled drinking water consumption were incorporated, the correlation between arsenic exposure and well water consumption strengthened the dose-response relationship.

EXPOSURE ASSESSMENT IN SPECIFIC EPIDEMIOLOGIC INVESTIGATIONS

The committee reviewed epidemiologic studies of hazardous-waste sites or water contamination to evaluate the exposure assessment in each. Landrigan (1983), Heath (1983), Anderson (1985), Marsh and Caplan (1987), and Hertzmann et al. (1987) argue that it is difficult at best to establish etiologic associations in relation to hazardous-waste sites unless some conditions are met before a study is done. These include identification of the nature and quantity of pollutant emissions from the site under study, identification of probable routes of human exposure, assessment of individual exposure in contrast to population-based data, and identification of populations that had high exposures and so are high-risk groups, such as persons who are exposed in the workplace. To meet these criteria, high-quality exposure information would have to have been collected.

The studies reviewed here all used *surrogate measures* to gather population-based exposure data. These studies were noteworthy for their attempts to define surrogates to characterize exposure and, in particular, to use a continuous, cumulative metric of exposure, rather than the more common dichotomous (ever-never) approach.

WOBURN, MASSACHUSETTS

A study of the association between childhood leukemia and exposure to solvent-contaminated drinking water from two wells in Woburn, Massachusetts, by Lagakos et al. (1986) used both a dichotomous and a continuous approach. In this study there was concern regarding public exposure to water from two wells (G and H) contaminated with chlorinated organic solvents that operated during the 15 years from 1964 to 1979. Residents of Woburn received a blend of water from eight wells including wells G and H, and the specific blend depended on the location of the residence and time the water was received.

In developing the exposure estimates the authors made use of a report prepared by the state (Waldorf and Cleary, 1983), which estimated the regional and temporal distribution of water from wells G and H during the study period. The study was possible because the monthly amounts of water pumped by each of Woburn's wells was routinely recorded, and therefore, the proportion of water to each household from G and H could be identified. The state's report made possible an estimate of each household's annual water supply from wells G and H, and these data were merged with other data to determine an exposure history for each child in the study. The exposure determination also took into account changes in residence over each child's lifetime and the proportion of G and H water supplied to each child's home during each year of life.

Several problems with the exposure assessment for the Woburn study mitigate the success of the estimation of each household's exposure to the contaminated water. First, there are no qualitative or quantitative data on the nature and amount of chemicals in the wells before 1979, when the chlorinated solvents were first detected. Second, estimates of exposure could be made only on the household samples; there was no way to estimate additional exposure outside the home—for example, in schools.

The authors acknowledge that the entire leukemia excess could not be explained by exposure to water from wells G and H. MacMahon (1986) has criticized the Woburn study on a number of grounds and has suggested that the greater complexity of measurement of exposure has not been successful in illuminating the limited associations that have been identified. The levels of contaminants in G and H water are low and would not be expected to result in a doubling of leukemia risk. MacMahon (1986) argues that the data are inconsistent with an underlying linear relationship between cumulative exposure and rate of disease. These criticisms notwithstanding, the exposure assessment in this study is relevant insofar as it reaches beyond the traditional dichotomous approach to exposure and establishes limited estimates of individual dose.

FRESNO COUNTY, CALIFORNIA

Whorton and co-workers (Whorton et al., 1988; Wong et al., 1988, 1989) conducted an ecologic and case-control study of the relationship between drinking water contaminated with DBCP and birth rates, gastric cancer, and leukemia in Fresno County, California. The ecologic study required an exposure estimate for each census tract, and the case-control study required determination of the drinking water source and its quality for the residence of the individual.

First, drinking water systems and private wells were identified, mean contaminant levels of DBCP for individual wells were determined from state-derived data, and an evaluation was made of which water system supplied drinking water to each census tract. By using mapping techniques, the authors were able to estimate the geographic percentage of the census tract supplied by each water system. Based on these data, specific weighted averages of arsenic, nitrate, and DBCP by census tract were determined and used in the subsequent ecologic and case-control studies. Mean DBCP levels ranged from 0.0041 to 5.7543 ppb among census tracts. Fourteen (12.8 percent) census tracts had DBCP concentrations in excess of the state's MCL of 1.0 ppb.

There are limitations associated with the studies—for example, no estimate of individual exposure accounts for bottled-water use or other use patterns and whether there is sufficient latency, that is time from first exposure to the development of the disease. But the DBCP studies are serious attempts at defining the historical exposure in greater detail than is generally found in environmental studies, and they should serve as useful models for future investigations.

The findings of the studies are complex. No correlation was found between gastric cancer or leukemia and DBCP exposure in the ecologic analysis. The case-control study did not identify any relationship between gastric cancer and DBCP in drinking water. However, the variable "Hispanic surname" was a risk factor for gastric cancer; Hispanics had a relative risk of gastric cancer of 2.77, compared with non-Hispanics. Hispanics tended to live in areas where the drinking water was more contaminated than did other groups. In addition, farm workers seem to have an increased risk of leukemia, possibly because of occupational exposures—although this will require further study. Dietary factors have not been evaluated. Overall, the case-control study found no association between exposure to DBCP and risk of developing leukemia in persons who live in Fresno County.

SANTA CLARA COUNTY, CALIFORNIA

The California Department of Health Services (Deane et al., 1989; Swan et al., 1989; Wrensch et al., 1990a,b) has reported on a number of studies designed to assess the basis for an excess of adverse pregnancy outcomes, such as statistically significant spontaneous abortions and birth defects, in Santa Clara County. There were significant concerns in the community that adverse pregnancy outcomes might have occurred as a result of contamination of a single well with trichloroethane (TCA) that had leaked from an underground storage tank owned by a semiconductor manufacturer.

The exposure assessment was designed to investigate two census tracts, both of which were assumed to have comparable exposure to well water contaminated by the leaking tank. This assessment had two distinct components. The first component estimated the time of initiation of the leak, the rate at which the TCA plume migrated to the well in question, and the concentrations of TCA found in this and other wells. The second component estimated the water flow from the contaminated well to the two census tracts. The model developed to estimate water flow was validated through field testing. The water distribution analysis gave the probability that water from the contaminated well was delivered to each of 112 specific water pipe junctions within the water system. Quantitative modeling was restricted to 1981, but pumping logs were also reviewed for 1979 through 1980 and showed there were no major differences in water distribution to the study areas during that period as well. Both components of the exposure assessment were conducted by a consulting engineer who had no knowledge of the temporal and spatial distribution of pregnancy outcome in the study census tracts. The probabilities of exposure to contaminated water were multiplied by the estimated concentration of TCA to give an estimated exposure by month.

Estimated exposures to TCA could then be compared to the frequency of spontaneous abortions and congenital malformations. In comparing two census tracts, the tract with the highest spontaneous abortion and birth defects rates had a lower TCA exposure than a comparable tract. Women with adverse pregnancy outcomes did not appear to have been exposed to higher concentrations of TCA than women with live births (see Chapter 5 for further discussion of these investigations). Uncertainties in the modeling have resulted in criticism of the conclusions of this study although the hydrogeologic modeling was carefully constructed. The controversy surrounding this study illustrates the difficulties encountered in exposure assessment that seeks to recreate environmental exposures. Unfortunately, there is no obvious approach that would resolve these ambiguities. Toxicologic investigations that evaluate the potential of the chemicals in question to produce adverse reproductive effects might be valuable in providing indirect confirmation of the epidemiologic investigations.

MCCOLL SITE, FULLERTON, CALIFORNIA

An interesting surrogate of exposure was used by California researchers (Lipscomb et al., in press) to investigate community concerns about potential health problems from the McColl Waste Disposal Site in Fullerton Hills, California. Rather than measure chemical concentrations in ambient air, the researchers investigated the relative frequency of detecting odors from the site. This 20-acre site consists of 12 waste pits that were in use from the early 1940s to 1946. In 1978, residents complained of odors in the neighborhood surrounding the site and were concerned that there might be health problems associated with chemical exposure. Results of an early survey demonstrated higher than expected rates of complaints about noxious odors and of complaints of 22 symptoms such as nausea, skin irritation, wheezing, dizziness, chest pain, loss of appetite, fatigue, and earaches (Satin et al., 1983).

A study by Duffee and Errera (1982) was based on the use of an extensive odor survey in which the McColl study area was divided into five "odor zones." Exposure was then defined by surrogate measures, such as the relative frequency of detecting odors or the proximity to the waste site. The odor zones were used to classify exposure areas. In the most recent survey (Lipscomb et al., in press), the highest three odor zones (92 households), the lowest odor zone (217 households), and a comparison area (242 households) were selected to attempt to identify a dose-response relationship between areas. The study determined that prevalence odds ratios comparing symptom reporting between high exposed and comparison area residents were greater than they were for an earlier survey (Duffee and Errera, 1982) for 89 percent of the symptoms. The authors noted symptoms reported in excess did not represent a single organ system or suggest a mechanism of response. They suggest that living near a hazardous-waste site and being concerned about the environment can result in "recall bias" that could affect findings more than does the toxicity of the chemicals found in the site. Unfortunately, the report provides no environmental monitoring data. Although the exposures are presumably in the parts-per-billion range, considerably below the levels at which health effects have been identified, this site contains a large number of chemicals, combinations of which could be harmful. Even if the primary effects were derived from stress and concern, there might have been a contribution from chemical exposure. These issues are treated as dichotomous variables. The authors' conclusions would have been strengthened by a more detailed exposure evaluation.

STRINGFELLOW SITE, GLEN AVON, CALIFORNIA

A study by Baker et al. (1988) used surrogates of exposure to evaluate nonspecific symptoms. Baker and his co-workers investigated public concern over potential health problems among residents living near the Stringfellow Waste Disposal Site in Glen Avon, California. This site operated from 1956 to 1976, when approximately 33 million gallons of liquid industrial waste was discharged at the site. It is approximately 4000 feet from the nearest residential property in Glen Avon and is located in Pyrite Canyon. Heavy rainfall has resulted in the waste ponds at the site overflowing their containment berms, washing waste down the channel that runs through the town of Glen Avon. Baker and co-workers conducted a health survey to assess whether there were increased rates of mortality, adverse pregnancy outcomes, disease incidence, or symptom prevalence, such as blurred vision, pain in ears, daily cough for more than a month, nausea, frequent diarrhea, unsteadiness when walking, and frequent urination among individuals living near the waste site.

The exposure surrogate they chose was based on "relative exposure likelihood of residents to toxic waste from the Stringfellow site" (Baker et al., 1988, p. 326). The investigators assumed that the most likely routes of exposure were surface water runoff and airborne contamination, and their exposure classifications were determined primarily by proximity to the site and to the Pyrite channel. Three communities were chosen: residents with the highest likelihood of exposure, those with small potential for exposure, and a reference group of unexposed persons. The study revealed that mortality, cancer incidence, and pregnancy outcomes did not differ among the three study areas; there were differences among the study areas for reported diseases (ear infections, bronchitis, asthma, angina pectoris, and skin rashes) and symptoms. The authors conclude that the apparent broad-based elevation in reported diseases and symptoms derives from increased perception or recall of conditions by subjects living near the site. This is similar to the conclusions reached by Lipscomb et al. (in press). In the Baker study (1988), the lack of exposure assessment weakens the conclusions, and exposure misclassification could be an important issue. The authors do discuss the possible "toxicological mechanisms" associated with various end points and with the uniform increase in symptom prevalence. Because no toxicants were identified or quantified as part of an exposure evaluation, the discussion of toxicologic mechanism has no objective validity. Baker et al. acknowledge these weaknesses and conclude, "Our experience indicates the fundamental need for health studies of toxic waste disposal sites to be based on environmental monitoring and modeling of past exposures sufficient to identify potential exposure to specific chemicals at an individual or household level" (Baker et al., 1988, p. 333).

LOWELL, MASSACHUSETTS

Ozonoff et al. (1987) conducted a symptom prevalence survey in a neighborhood assumed to be exposed to airborne hazardous wastes. The study population included households within 400 meters of a hazardous-waste site in Lowell, Massachusetts; the unexposed controls were those households within a radius of 800 to 1200 meters from the site. Linear distance of each residence to the center of the site was determined, thereby providing a further breakdown of potential exposure. The exposure surrogate was distance from the hazardous-waste site. In contrast to the aforementioned studies by Baker et al. (1988) and Lipscomb et al. (in press), Ozonoff et al. concluded that the study "raised the possibility that exposure to relatively low levels of airborne chemicals may have increased the prevalence of respiratory and constitutional symptoms in adults in the affected neighborhood" (Ozonoff et al., 1987, p. 596). They noted that the most serious potential problem in the study was recall bias—special importance being given by respondents to particular symptoms. Careful evaluation of the potential for recall bias indicated that six symptoms exhibited a "biological gradient" (a dose-response relationship) and recall bias does not account for the study findings.

It is outside the scope of this chapter to review each of the last three studies described (Stringfellow, McColl, and Lowell) in more detail, but it is important to point out that their exposure assessments were very sparse. That limits the confidence in a positive association between the exposed populations and subjective health outcomes. Absence of an association is equally problematic, given the lack of individual exposure data, information derived from microenvironmental monitoring, or indirect methods based on modeling. The potential for misclassification in these studies seems to be particularly high.

The problem of chemical identification and false linkages is even more intractable when we consider findings based on subjective reporting. It will be difficult to resolve these differences entirely without an improved understanding of the nature and scope of exposure.

HAMILTON, ONTARIO

Like Ozonoff et al. (1987), who studied distance from the waste site, Hertzman et al. (1987) used distance as their surrogate for exposure in investigations of adverse health effects associated with the Upper Ottawa Street Landfill Site in Hamilton, Ontario. In addition, they carried out a prospective morbidity study of workers as a hypothesis-generating study. There was no individual exposure assessment of workers, and no specific chemical agents were suggested as being causative in the employee study. The resident study identified six groups for health survey interviews, combining distance and time of residence as a basis for selection. For example, Group A consisted of those living 250-500 meters from the dumpface at the time of interview and who had been residents there for three or more years between 1976 and 1980. Group D was made up of those who lived 500-750 meters from the landfill and who had been residents for fewer than three years during the same period—the period of highest volume of disposal of industrial waste.

The authors report an association between psychological, narcotic (headaches, dizziness, lethargy, and balance problems), skin, and respiratory conditions with landfill site exposure that was confirmed by the following criteria: strength of association, consistency with a simultaneous study of workers at the landfill, risk gradient by duration of residence and proximity to the landfill, absence of evidence that less healthy people had moved to the area, specificity, and lack of recall bias. These data resulted in a conclusion that the adverse effects were more likely the result of chemical exposure than of perception of risk. Unfortunately, it was difficult to evaluate the accuracy of the conclusions of this study because there were more than 100 substances found at the landfill and the health end points in the study population were common and nonspecific. Although no environmental measurements are reported in this study, the authors assume that exposures occurred from airborne contact or from direct skin exposure during recreational activities in and around the landfill. There was no discussion of the potential for groundwater contamination which could result in infiltration of homes from the cellar or through ingestion.

LOVE CANAL, NEW YORK

A number of studies have been published (Vianna and Polan, 1984; Goldman et al., 1985; Paigen et al., 1985, 1987) on the hazardous-waste site at Love Canal. These reports are discussed elsewhere in this monograph. The authors briefly review the potential exposures to citizens in the Love Canal area and correctly point out that exposure to residents of Love Canal is not well understood, especially given the fact that more than 200 chemicals have been found in the Love Canal dump site. Selection of the study population and the exposure surrogate were based on residence in the Love Canal neighborhoods.

COUNTY OF RESIDENCE AS SURROGATE

Studies by Day et al. (1990) and Budnick et al. (1984) used residence in a county known to have chemical contamination as the surrogate of exposure. These ecologic studies used other counties, the state in which the counties were located, and U.S. rates for comparison. Day and co-workers point out the difficulty in drawing inferences from ecologic studies where the study population could have been occupationally exposed and suggest that occupational histories will need to be taken in future studies, or surrogate indications of occupation entered into such analyses to increase their utility.

The study by Budnick et al. (1984) focuses on a particular Superfund site in Clinton County, Pennsylvania. These authors were careful to document that the Drake Chemical Company, the American Color Chemical Corporation, and their predecessor companies used, manufactured, or stored the known human carcinogens β-naphthylamine, benzidine, and benzene. Thus, their finding of an increased number of bladder cancer deaths among white males in the area has biologic plausibility, but the authors note that white females did not exhibit an increase in bladder cancer deaths. The excess of cancer-caused deaths in males could reflect occupational rather than environmental exposure. The authors suggest that more definitive studies will be needed to further assess health risks that could play a role in other excess cancers found. An in-depth case-control study of bladder cancers with exposure ascertainment would help address the question of the possible environmental sources of some cancer deaths. A subsequent community survey of health complaints (Logue and Fox, 1986) did not find evidence of any serious and chronic health conditions.

OTHER STUDIES OF CONTAMINATED DRINKING WATER

Drinking water contaminated by hazardous wastes has served as the basis for exposure assessment in a number of studies. The adverse health end points of concern included leukemia, liver dysfunction, congenital cardiac malformations, eye irritation, diarrhea, sleepiness, and an electrophysiologic measurement of the blink reflex.

With the exception of the leachate from a pesticide waste dump in Hardeman County, Tennessee (Clark et al., 1982), the principal toxicant identified in the other studies was trichloroethylene (TCE). Thus, one finds very low levels of TCE associated with leukemia, cardiac malformations, eye irritation, diarrhea, sleepiness, and neurologic changes. These results suggest the need to conduct more detailed studies of the toxicology of TCE. It is hoped that the ease of identification of TCE by analytic chemical methods—that is, the ability to detect low levels of TCE—is not the basis for the association.

Dawson et al. (1990) approached the problem of associating specific health end points to chemical exposure by developing an animal model to explain the cardiac malformations associated with exposure to drinking water contamination by TCE and dichloroethylene (DCE) in Tucson, Arizona (Goldberg et al., 1990). These authors conclude that both DCE and TCE could be potent cardiac teratogens. The epidemiologic findings of cardiac malformations associated with drinking water contaminated with TCE and DCE are strengthened by the toxicologic research of Dawson et al. (1990). The value of the toxicologic confirmation of the association is relevant insofar as one of the limitations of the epidemiologic study cited by its authors was the inability to estimate individual doses because of limited sampling data, variability in exposure, lack of precise information on the geographic area of contamination, and the temporal characteristics of the contamination and exposures.

There also is ample evidence that TCE can act as a chemical neurotoxicant, as Feldman et al. (1988) have cited. However, other findings of TCE-related illnesses where the exposure levels are very low must be confirmed by additional epidemiologic findings or by toxicologic study or both.

The paper by Feldman et al. (1988) on blink reflex latency after exposure to TCE in well water from Woburn, Massachusetts, used a control group that had no stated history of occupational or environmental exposure to neurotoxicants. The authors conclude that the study subjects may have suffered subclinical cranial nerve damage as a result of their chronic ingestion of TCE contaminated water.

In studies, such as Feldman's, that rely on subjects' and controls' self-reporting of other occupational or environmental exposures, it might be useful to use hazard surveillance data on industry and occupation versus chemical exposure to ensure that neither group has an unrecognized workplace exposure that could compromise the validity of the results. The four-digit Standard Industrial Classification (SIC) code can be used to identify potential exposures that can be confirmed in interviews if necessary (Froines et al., 1986, 1989).

The ecologic study by Fagliano et al. (1990) examined the relation of the incidence of leukemia and the presence of volatile organic compounds (VOCs) in public drinking water supplies in several cities in New Jersey. The authors conclude that the results appear to suggest an association between nontrihalomethane (non-THM) VOCs and an increased incidence of leukemia among women. The incidence was elevated only in towns in the category ranked highest for potential exposure to VOCs based on actual water-sampling data collected by the State of New Jersey during 1984-1985. However, the authors acknowledge that misclassification of exposure may exist at both the population and individual level, in that the actual sampling data were collected after exposure was known to have occurred. Occupational exposures and local toxic air emissions were not accounted for in this study. The authors do note that ecologic studies of this type with potential biases and multicolinearity are improved by using narrow exposure strata and regression to estimate effect. The study could not verify whether subjects actually drank tap water or purchased bottled water. Similarly, occupational exposures were not studied.

The research by Clark et al. (1982), of the Hardeman County, Tennessee, dump site, was rooted in a clear understanding of the toxicology of the contaminants, namely that carbon tetrachloride is a potent hepatotoxicant (a toxicant that destroys liver cells). Carbon tetrachloride was the most abundant contaminant detected in wells serving individuals living near the 200-acre pesticide waste dump site. The dump operated between 1964 and 1972, during which time approximately 300,000 barrels of liquid and solid waste were buried in shallow trenches. In 1977 residents became alarmed by unusual odors and tastes in their well water and reported a high number of symptoms (skin and eye irritation; weakness in the upper and lower extremities; upper respiratory infection; shortness of breath; and severe gastrointestinal symptoms including nausea, diarrhea, and abdominal cramping) which they associated with contaminated drinking water. The most common contaminant detected in private wells serving the exposed study population was carbon tetrachloride, which was identified in concentrations as high as 18,700 micrograms per liter. The study found that residents who drank contaminated water had elevated concentrations of the serum enzymes alkaline phosphatase and serum glutamic oxaloacetic transaminase. The finding of a relationship between ingestion of drinking water contaminated with carbon tetrachloride and liver abnormalities is an example of a finding with significant biologic plausibility, because of the numerous toxicologic data identifying carbon tetrachloride as a potent hepatotoxin. In addition, the study's authors made a significant effort to assess actual exposures to solvents. For example, water from selected homes was analyzed, air samples were collected from bathrooms while showers were running, and urine samples were analyzed for the presence of solvents. Measurements of indoor air concentrations of selected organic compounds in houses with contaminated groundwater demonstrated detectable levels of hexachlorocyclopentadiene, carbon tetrachloride, and tetrachloroethylene. As other evidence of the effect of exposure to contaminated water, abnormalities in the liver tests were significantly reduced when the investigators rescreened subjects two months after all use of contaminated water had ceased. This study stands in marked contrast to other investigations that used surrogates of exposure.

Harris et al. (1984) conducted a follow-up risk assessment of the Hardeman County population based on animal toxicity data and concluded that adults and children living near the landfill were at high risk of sustaining liver damage and thereby at increased risk of contracting cancer. This research suggests that the health risk assessments should play an important role in guiding epidemiologic investigation and that risk estimates that use animal toxicity data will also be of value.

Logue and Fox (1986) investigated potential health effects associated with contaminated well water from a dump site in Pennsylvania. They found that significantly more individuals in the exposed group than in the control group experienced eye irritation, diarrhea, and sleepiness during the 12-month period before the survey. Exposure was defined as the experience of residential well-water contamination from a dump site at the former Olmsted Air Force Base. A possible linkage with TCE exposure was made, but the authors hypothesize that the finding could derive from the limitations of the exposure assessment.

CONCLUSIONS

Repositories of potentially dangerous substances can be found at a number of hazardous-waste sites and have been generated by agricultural, mining, storage, and other activities. The available characterizations of these materials generally reflect data requirements of environmental engineering and site remediation, rather than public health considerations. Accordingly, whether these materials pose a future risk to public health cannot readily be determined, in the absence of more detailed information about potential human exposures. Also, their current impact on public health, while likely to be negligible in the majority of cases, may be substantial in a smaller number of cases, and cannot readily be estimated.

This chapter has detailed major difficulties in assessing the more than 600 chemical compounds identified at hazardous-waste sites, along with the hundreds or thousands of unidentified pollutants, in the context of environmental epidemiology. The potential for exposure is of such a magnitude that researchers who develop exposure assessment strategies will have to direct their attention to an analysis of contaminants at hazardous-waste sites, and to off-site migration and public exposure. In this context, methods for exposure assessment—including direct methods, such as personal exposure monitoring, and indirect methods, such as microenvironmental monitoring and mathematical models—although often difficult, must receive greater scientific attention, if appropriate associations are to be made between contaminants, exposures, and potential health effects. Evaluations of exposure associated with hazardous-waste sites must consider all possible media as potential sources of toxic contaminants.

Regarding the specific pollutants measured, evidence indicates that uncharacterized pollutants are a potentially important source of chemical exposures. In some cases, these compounds have recognized toxicity; in others, the toxicity is unknown. Moreover, some preliminary toxicologic studies suggest that these contaminants and so-called inert pesticide ingredients may have important biologic properties, environmental persistence, and mobility. Additional studies need to be conducted to characterize the mixture of materials deposited as hazardous wastes and to estimate better their potential transport and fate in the environment. Toxicologic evaluation of the concentration of leachate appears to represent an appropriate subject of investigation. Short-term in vitro assays and long-term animal studies to assess toxicity of the mixtures would be useful. In the broadest sense, these unidentified, unregulated substances represent a risk of unknown magnitude.

The focus of many studies has been on site-specific characterization, but pollutants do not respect such boundaries. Given the potential movement of materials in groundwater and the importance of multiple routes of exposure, efforts need to proceed to estimate plume characteristics and groundwater staging in order to improve the ability to anticipate movements of pollutants and ultimately to prevent greater exposures.

Similarly, exposure from domestic water is not limited to ingestion, but includes airborne exposures to materials that outgas during showering, bathing, cooking, or other uses. Therefore, estimates of exposure from domestic water need to be expanded to take into account the role of airborne and transdermal exposures.

Although direct ingestion of soil poses a risk chiefly to children, risks may also be incurred by adults who eat food grown in such soil or who otherwise come into regular contact through their work or personal habits. Sophisticated methods have recently been devised for improving the ability to assess soil exposures. These refined methods need to be applied in epidemiologic studies to improve the ability to estimate exposures in connection with soil, including studies of ingested plants and fish from contaminated water, characterization of chemical transformation, and better measurements of residues.

Weaknesses in data employed on exposure are common to most studies of hazardous-waste sites that the committee has reviewed. The flaws reflect historical tendencies to collect data to conform to environmental needs, rather than to meet the needs of public health assessment. Usually, exposure estimates are made with one medium—water—although others may be critical. Site assessments should use more realistic exposure measures, including direct studies of contaminants at the tap of incoming domestic water supplies, in order to improve their utility for epidemiologic research. In addition, where concerns have been raised, efforts should be made to include relevant soil and airborne measurements, so that integrated exposure assessment can be conducted.

APPENDIX 3-A

Frequency of Substances Reported at Final and Proposed NPL Sites* (3/91)

1,1,2-TRICHLOROETHYLENE (TCE)	401
LEAD (PB)	395
CHROMIUM AND COMPOUNDS, NOS (CR)	310
TOLUENE	281
BENZENE	249
TETRACHLOROETHENE	210
1,1,1-TRICHLOROETHANE	202
CHLOROFORM	196
ARSENIC	187
POLYCHLORINATED BIPHENYLS, NOS	185
CADMIUM (CD)	179
ZINC AND COMPOUNDS, NOS (ZN)	159
COPPER AND COMPOUNDS, NOS (CU)	150
XYLENE	136
1,2-TRANS-DICHLOROETHYLENE	134
ETHYLBENZENE	130
PHENOL	126
1,1-DICHLOROETHANE	124
METHYLENE CHLORIDE	107
1,1-DICHLOROETHENE	106
MERCURY	97
VINYL CHLORIDE	92
CYANIDES (SOLUBLE SALTS), NOS	90
NICKEL AND COMPOUNDS, NOS (NI)	83
CARBON TETRACHLORIDE	81
1,2-DICHLOROETHANE	77

APPENDIX 3-A *Continued*

CHLOROBENZENE	65
PENTACHLOROPHENOL (PCP)	62
NAPHTHALENE	60
DDT	50
METHYL ETHYL KETONE	56
TRICHLOROETHANE, NOS	49
MORE THAN 15 SUBSTANCES LISTED	48
BARIUM	47
MANGANESE AND COMPOUNDS, NOS (MN)	44
PHENANTHRENE	41
HEAVY METALS, NOS	40
ACETONE	40
BENZO(A)PYRENE	37
IRON AND COMPOUNDS, NOS (FE)	33
CHLORDANE	33
VOLATILE ORGANICS, NOS	33
BENZO(J,K)FLUORENE	30
CHROMIUM, HEXAVALENT	30
PYRENE	29
CIS-1,2-DICHLOROETHYLENE	29
LINDANE	28
1,1,2-TRICHLOROETHANE	28
ARSENIC AND COMPOUNDS, NOS (AS)	27
BIS(2-ETHYLHEXYL)PHTHALATE	27
DICHLOROETHYLENE, NOS	26
ANTHRACENE	26
1,1,2,2-TETRACHLOROETHANE	26
STYRENE	23
URANIUM AND COMPOUNDS, NOS (U)	22
DDE	22
TETRACHLOROETHANE, NOS	21
CREOSOTE	19
FLUORENE, NOS	19
DIOXIN	18
SELENIUM	19
ETHYL CHLORIDE	18
CHRYSENE	18
RADON AND COMPOUNDS, NOS (RN)	18
ASBESTOS	17
TRINITROTOLUENE (TNT)	17
DDD	17
DICHLOROETHANE, NOS	17
DIELDRIN	17
SULFURIC ACID	17
WASTE OILS/SLUDGES	17
ACENAPHTHENE	16
RADIUM AND COMPOUNDS, NOS (RA)	16
ALDRIN	16
AROCLOR 1260	16
ENDRIN	16

APPENDIX 3-A *Continued*

TRICHLOROFLUOROMETHANE	16
1,4-DICHLOROBENZENE	16
ACID, NOS	15
DI-N-BUTYL PHTHALATE	15
DICHLOROBENZENE, NOS	15
METHYL ISOBUTYL KETONE	15
M-XYLENE	14
1,2-DICHLOROBENZENE	14
ALUMINUM AND COMPOUNDS, NOS (AL)	14
CHLOROMETHANE	14
AMMONIA	13
TETRAHYDROFURAN	12
THORIUM AND COMPOUNDS, NOS (TH)	12
HEXACHLOROBENZENE	12
HEPTACHLOR	11
TOXAPHENE	11
TRIBROMOMETHANE	11
1,2-DICHLOROPROPANE	11
RDX (CYCLOTRIMETHYLENETRINITRAMINE)	10
ANTIMONY AND COMPOUNDS, NOS (SB)	10
BARIUM AND COMPOUNDS, NOS (BA)	10
BERYLLIUM AND COMPOUNDS, NOS (BE)	10

*This list is a frequency of substances documented during HRS score preparation, not a complete inventory of substances at all sites.

"NOS"—Not otherwise specified, e.g., not identified as to specific isomer or congener.

APPENDIX 3-B

ATSDR Priority List of Substances for Toxicological Profiles (Listed in Federal Register 52(74), Friday April 17, 1987, p. 12869)

CAS No.	Substance Name
Priority Group 1	
50328	Benzo(a)pyrene
53703	Dibenzo(a,h)anthracene
56553	Benzo(a)anthracene
57125	Cyanide
60571	Dieldrin/aldrin
67663	Chloroform
71432	Benzene
75014	Vinyl chloride
75092	Methylene chloride
76448	Heptachlor/heptachlor epoxide
79016	Trichloroethene

APPENDIX 3-B *Continued*

86306	N-Nitrosodiphenylamine
106467	1,4-Dichlorobenzene
117817	Bis(2-ethylhexyl)phthalate
127184	Tetrachloroethene
205992	Benzo(b)fluoranthene
218019	Chrysene
1745016	p-Dioxin
7439921	Lead
7440020	Nickel
7440382	Arsenic
7440417	Beryllium
7440439	Cadmium
7440473	Chromium
11196825	PCB-1260,54,48,42,32,21,1016

Priority Group 2

56235	Carbon tetrachloride
57749	Chlordane
62759	N-Nitrosodimethylamine
72559	4,4'DDE, DDT, DDD
75003	Chloroethane
75274	Bromodichloromethane
75354	1,1-Dichloroethene
78591	Isophorone
78875	1,2-Dichloropropane
79005	1,1,2,-Trichloroethane
79435	1,1,2,2-Tetrachloroethane
87865	Pentachlorophenol
91941	3,3'-Dichlorobenzidine
92875	Benzidine
107062	1,2-Dichloroethane
108883	Toluene
108952	Phenol
111444	Bis(2-chloroethyl)ether
121142	2,4,-Dinitrotoluene
319846	BHC-alpha, gamma, beta, delta
542881	Bis(chloromethyl)ether
621647	N-nitrosodi-n-propylamino
7439976	Mercury
7440666	Zinc
7782492	Selenium

Priority Group 3

71556	1,1,1-Trichloroethane
74873	Chloromethane
75218	Oxirane
75252	Bromoform
75343	1,1-Dichloroethane
84742	Di-N-butyl phthalate

APPENDIX 3-B *Continued*

88062	2,4,6-Trichlorophenol
91203	Naphthalene
98953	Nitrobenzene
100414	Ethylbenzene
107028	Acrolein
107131	Acrylonitrile
108907	Chlorobenzene
118741	Hexachlorobenzene
122667	1,2-Diphenylhydrazine
124481	Chlorodibromomethane
156606	1,2-Trans-dichloroethene
193395	Indeno(1,2,3-cd)pyrene
606202	2,6-Dinitrotoluene
1330207	Total xylenes
7221934	Endrin aldehyde/endrin
7440224	Silver
7440508	Copper
7664417	Ammonia
8001352	Toxaphene

Priority Group 4

51285	2,4-Diitrophenol
59507	p-Chloro-m-cresol
62533	Aniline
65850	Benzoic acid
67721	Hexachloroethane
74839	Bromomethane
75150	Carbon disulfide
75694	Fluorotrichloromethane
75718	Dichlorodifluoromethane
78933	2-Butanone
84662	Diethyl phthalate
85018	Phenanthrene
87683	Hexachlorobutadiene
95487	Phenol,2-methyl
95501	1,2-Dichlorobenzene
105679	2,4-Dimethylphenol
108101	2-Pentanone,4-methyl
120821	1,2,4-Trichlorobenzene
120832	2,4-Dichlorophenol
123911	1,4-Dioxane
131113	Dimethyl phthalate
206440	Fluoranthene
534521	4,6-Dinitro-2-methylphenol
541731	1,3-Dichlorobenzene
7440280	Thallium

REFERENCES

Andelman, J.B. 1990. Exposure to volatile chemicals from indoor uses of water. Pp. 300-311 in Proceedings of the EPA/A & WMA specialty conference, Total Exposure Assessment Methodology. Pittsburgh: Air & Waste Management Association.

Andelman, J.B., A. Couch, and W.W. Thurston. 1986. Inhalation exposures in indoor air to trichlorethylene from shower water. Pp. 201-211 in Environmental Epidemiology, F.C. Kopler and G.F. Craun, eds. Chelsea, Mich.: Lewis.

Anderson, H.A. 1985. Evolution of environmental epidemiologic risk assessment. Environ. Health Perpect. 62:389-392.

ATSDR (U.S. Public Health Service, Agency for Toxic Substances and Disease Registry). 1989. ATSDR Biennial Report to Congress: October 17, 1986–September 30, 1988. Atlanta: Agency for Toxic Substances and Disease Registry. 2 vols.

Bailar, J.C. 1989. Inhalation hazards: The interpretation of epidemiologic evidence. Pp. 39-48 in Assessment of Inhalation Hazards, D.V. Bates et al., eds. New York: Springer-Verlag.

Baker, D.B., S. Greenland, J. Mendlein, and P. Harmon. 1988. A health study of two communities near the Stringfellow Waste Disposal Site. Arch. Environ. Health 43:325-334.

Bramlett, J., C. Furman, A. Johnson, W.D. Ellis, and N. Nelson. 1987. Composition of Leachates from Actual Hazardous Waste Sites. Project report prepared for U.S. Environmental Protection Agency. EPA/600/2-87/043; available from NTIS as PB87-198743. Springfield: U.S. Department of Commerce, National Technical Information Service.

Breslow, L., Chairman of Commission on the health consequences of Casmalia resources facility operation, et al. 1989. Report of Santa Barbara Commission on Health Consequences of the Casmalia Resources Waste Disposal Facility. Report prepared for Santa Barbara Department of Health Services, California.

Budnick, L.D., D.C. Sokal, H. Falk, J.N. Logue, and J.M. Fox. 1984. Cancer and birth defects near the Drake Superfund site, Pennsylvania. Arch. Environ. Health 39:409-413.

Buffler, P.A., M. Crane, and M.M. Key. 1985. Possibilities of detecting health effects by studies of populations exposed to chemicals from waste disposal sites. Environ. Health Persp. 62:423-456.

Checkoway, H., N.E. Pearce, and D.J. Crawford-Brown. 1989. Research Methods in Occupational Epidemiology. New York: Oxford University Press.

Clark, C.S., C.R. Meyer, P.S. Gartside, V.A. Majeti, B. Specker, W.F. Balistreri, and V.J. Elia. 1982. An environmental health survey of drinking water contamination by leachate from a pesticide waste dump in Hardeman County, Tennessee. Arch. Environ. Health 37:9-18.

Cohen, D.B., and G.W. Bowes. 1984. Water Quality and Pesticides: A California Risk Assessment Program, Vol. 1. State Water Resources Control Board Report No. 84-6SP. Sacramento, Calif.: State Water Resources Control Board.

Dawson, B.V., P.D. Johnson, S.J. Goldberg, and J.B. Ulreich. 1990. Cardiac Teratogenesis of trichloroethylene and dichloroethylene in a mammalian model. J. Am. Coll. Cardiol. 16:1304-1309.

Day, R., E.O. Talbott, G.M. Marsh, and B.W. Case. 1990. A Comparative Ecological Study of Selected Cancers in Kanawha County, West Virginia. Paper presented at the Second Annual Meeting of the International Society for Environmental Epidemiology, August 12-15, 1990, Berkeley, California.

Deane, M., S.H. Swan, J.A. Harris, D.M. Epstein, and R. Neutra. 1989. Adverse pregnancy outcomes in relation to water contamination, Santa Clara County, California, 1980-1981. Am. J. Epidemiol. 129:894-904.

Droz, P.O., and M.M. Wu. 1991. Biological monitoring strategies. Pp. 251-270 in Exposure Assessment for Epidemiology and Hazard Control, S.M. Rappaport and T.J. Smith, eds. Boca Raton: CRC Press.

Duffee, R.A., and L.R. Errera. 1982. Final Report on the Air Quality and Odor Portions of the Environmental Investigation Program of the McColl Site. East Hartford, Conn.: TRC Environmental Consultants.

EHP (Environmental Health Perspectives). 1991. Lead in Bone: International Workshop on Lead in Bone: Implications for Dosimetry and Toxicology. Vol. 91, entire February issue.

EPA (U.S. Environmental Protection Agency). 1987a. National Water Quality Inventory: 1986 Report to Congress. EPA-440/4-87-008. Washington, D.C.: U.S. Government Printing Office.

EPA (U.S. Environmental Protection Agency). 1987b. Inert ingredients in pesticide products: Policy statement. Notices, April 22. Fed. Reg. 52(77):13305-13309.

EPA (U.S. Environmental Protection Agency, Office of Policy Planning and Evaluation). 1988. Environmental Progress and Challenges: EPA's update. EPA-230-07-88-033. Washington, D.C.: U.S. Government Printing Office.

Fagliano, J., M. Berry, F. Bove, and T. Burke. 1990. Drinking water contamination and the incidence of leukemia: An ecologic study. Am. J. Public Health 80:1209-1212.

Feldman, R.G., J. Chirico-Post, and S.P. Proctor. 1988. Blink reflex latency after exposure to trichloroethylene in well water. Arch. Environ. Health 43:143-148.

Froines, J.R. 1989. Worksite inspection and the control of occupational disease: The OSHA experience. Ann. N.Y. Acad. Sci. 572:177-183.

Froines, J.R., C.A. Dellenbaugh, and D.H. Wegman. 1986. Occupational health surveillance: A means to identify work-related risks. Am. J. Public Health 76:1089-1096.

Gann, P. 1986. Use and misuse of existing data bases in environmental epidemiology: The case of air pollution. Pp. 109-122 in Environmental Epidemiology, F. Kopfler and G.F. Craun, eds. Chelsea, Mich.: Lewis.

Gillette, J.R. 1987. Dose, species, and route extrapolation: General aspects. Pp. 96-158 in National Research Council, Pharmacokinetics in Risk Assessment, Drinking Water and Health, Vol. 8. Washington, D.C.: National Academy Press.

Goldberg, S.J., M.D. Lebowitz, E.J. Graver, and S. Hicks. 1990. An association of human congenital cardiac malformations and drinking water contaminants. J. Am. Coll. Cardiol. 16:155-164.

Goldman, L.R., B. Paigen, M.M. Magnant, and J.H. Highland. 1985. Low birth weight, prematurity and birth defects in children living near the hazardous waste site, Love Canal. Haz. Waste Haz. Materials. 2:209-223.

Grisham, J.W., ed. 1986. Health Aspects of the Disposal of Waste Chemicals. New York: Pergamon Press.

Hammond, S.K. 1991. The uses of markers to measure exposure to complex mixtures. Pp. 53-66 in Exposure Assessment for Epidemiology and Hazard Control, S.M. Rappaport and T.J. Smith, eds. Boca Raton: CRC Press.

Harris, R.H., J.H. Highland, J.V. Rodricks, and S.S. Papadopulos. 1984. Adverse health effects at a Tennessee hazardous waste disposal site. Hazardous Waste 1:183-204.

Hattis, D. 1987. A Pharmacokinetic/Mechanism-Based Analysis of the Carcinogenic Risk of Ethylene Oxide. CTIPD 87-1; available from NTIS as PB88-188784. Cambridge, Mass.: M.I.T. Center for Technology, Policy and Industrial Development.

Hattis, D. 1990. Pharmacokinetic principles for dose-rate extrapolation of carcinogenic risk from genetically active agents. Risk Anal. 10:306-316.

Hattis, D., and J.R. Froines. 1991. Uncertainties in Risk Assessment. Invited paper presented at the Conference on Chemical Risk Assessment in the DoD; Science, Policy and Practice. In press.

Hattis, D., and K. Shapiro. 1990. Analysis of dose/time/response relationships for chronic toxic effects: The case of acrylamide. Neurotoxicology 11:219-236.

Hattis, D., and J. Wasson. 1987. A Pharmacokinetic/Mechanism-Based Analysis of the Carcinogenic Risk of Butadiene. CTPID 87-3; available from NTIS as PB88-202817. Cambridge, Mass.: M.I.T. Center for Technology, Policy and Industrial Development.

Heath, C.W., Jr. 1983. Field epidemiologic studies of populations exposed to waste dumps. Environ. Health Perspect. 48:3-7.

Hertzman, C., M. Hayes, J. Singer, and J. Highland. 1987. Upper Ottawa Street Landfill Site health study. Environ. Health Perspect. 75:173-195.

Jo, W.K, C.P. Weisel, and P.J. Lioy. 1990a. Routes of chloroform exposure and body burden from showering with chlorinated tap water. Risk Anal. 10:575-580.

Jo, W.K, C.P. Weisel, and P.J. Lioy. 1990b. Chloroform exposure and the health risk associated with multiple uses of chlorinated tap water. Risk Anal. 10:581-585.

Lagakos, S.W., B.J. Wessen, and M. Zelen. 1986. An analysis of contaminated well water and health effects in Woburn, Massachusetts. J. Am. Stats. Assoc. 81:583-596.

Landrigan, P.J. 1983. Epidemiologic approaches to persons with exposures to waste chemicals. Environ. Health Perspect. 48:93-97.

Landrigan, P.J., J.R. Froines, and K.R. Mahaffey. 1985. Body lead burden: Epidemiology data and its relation to environmental sources and toxic effects. In Dietary and Environmental Lead: Human Health Effects. Amsterdam: Elsevier.

Leeden, F. van der, F.L. Troise, and D.K. Todd. 1990. The Water Encyclopedia. Chelsea, Mich.: Lewis.

Lioy, P.J. 1990. Assessing total human exposure to contaminants: A multidisciplinary approach. Environ. Sci. Technol. 24:938-945.

Lioy, P.L., J.M. Waldman, A. Greenberg, R. Harkov, and C. Pietarinen. 1988. The Total Human Environmental Exposure Study (THEES) to benzo(a)pyrene: Comparison of the inhalation and food pathways. Arch. Environ. Health 43:304-312.

Lipscomb, J.A., L.R. Goldman, K.P. Satin, D.F. Smith, W.A. Vance, and R.R. Neutra. In press. A follow-up study of the community near the McColl waste disposal site. Environ. Health Perspect.

Logue, J.N., and J. Fox. 1986. Residential health study of families living near the Drake Chemical Superfund Site in Lock Haven, Pennsylvania, U.S.A. Arch. Environ. Health 40:155-160.

MacKay, D.M., and L.A. Smith. 1990. Agricultural chemicals in groundwater: Monitoring and management in California. J. Soil Water Conserv. 45:253-255.

MacKay, D., M. Gold, and G. Leson. 1987. Current and prospective quality of California's groundwater. Pp. 97-110 in the Proceedings of the 16th Biennial Conference on Groundwater, J.J. Devries, ed. University of California Water Research Center Report No. 66.

MacKay, D.M., J.R. Froines, R.A. Mah, W. W.-G. Yeh, and W. Glaze. 1989. Nonconventional Pollutants in Raw and Treated Groundwater: Occurrence, Environmental Fate, Health Effects and Policy Implications. Final project report to the Toxic Substances Research and Teaching Program, University of California, Davis.

MacMahon, B. 1986. Comment. J. Am. Stats. Assoc. 81:597-599.

Marsh, G.M., and R.J. Caplan. 1987. Evaluating health effects of exposure at hazardous waste sites: A review of the state-of-the-art, with recommendations for future research. Pp. 1-80 in Health Effects from Hazardous Waste Sites, J.B. Andelman and D.W. Underhill, eds. Chelsea, Mich.: Lewis.

152   ENVIRONMENTAL EPIDEMIOLOGY

NRC (National Research Council). 1987. Pharmacokinetics in Risk Assessment. Drink-
ing Water and Health, Vol. 8. Washington, D.C.: National Academy Press.
NRC (National Research Council). 1988. Complex Mixtures: Methods for In Vivo Tox-
icity Testing. Washington, D.C.: National Academy Press.
NRC (National Research Council). 1991. Human Exposure to Airborne Pollutants.
Washington, D.C.: National Academy Press.
OTA (U.S. Congress, Office of Technology Assessment). 1989. Coming Clean: Superfund's
Problems Can Be Solved. OTA-ITE-433. Washington, D.C.: U.S. Government Print-
ing Office.
Ozonoff, D., M.E. Colten, A. Cupples, T. Heeren, A. Schatzkin, T. Mangione, M. Dresner,
and T. Colton. 1987. Health problems reported by residents of a neighborhood
contaminated by a hazardous waste facility. Am. J. Ind. Med. 11:581-597.
Paigen, B., L.R. Goldman, J.H. Highland, M.M. Magnant, and A.T. Steegman, Jr. 1985.
Prevalence of health problems in children living near Love Canal. Haz. Waste Haz.
Materials 2:23-43.
Paigen, B., L.R. Goldman, M.M. Magnant, J.H. Highland, and A.T. Steegman, Jr. 1987.
Growth of children living near the hazardous waste site, Love Canal. Hum. Biol.
59:489-508.
Pierce, T. 1985. The use of dermal absorption data in developing biological monitor-
ing standards. Ann. Am. Conf. Gov. Ind. Hyg. 12:331-337.
Rothman, K.J. 1990. A sobering start for the Cluster Busters' Conference. Keynote
Presentation. Am. J. Epidemiol. 132(Supp. 1):S6-S13.
Satin, K.P., M. Deane, A. Leonard, R. Neutra, M. Harnly, and R.R. Green. 1983. The
McColl Site Health Survey: An Epidemiologic and Toxicologic Assessment of the
McColl Site in Fullerton, California. Berkeley, Calif.: Special Epidemiological Studies
Program, California Department of Health Services.
Severn, D.J. 1987. Exposure assessment. Environ. Sci. Technol. 21(12):1159-1163.
Smith, T.J. 1988. Extrapolation of laboratory findings to risks from environmental ex-
posures: Male reproductive effects of ethylene oxide. Birth Defects 24(5):79-100.
Smith, L.A., K.P. Green, and M.M. MacKay. 1990. Quality of ground water in Califor-
nia: Overview and implications. Pp. 93-107 in Proc. Seventeenth Biennial Conf. on
Groundwater. Rpt. no. 72. Univ. Calif. Water Resources Center, Riverside.
Swan, S.H., G. Shaw, J.A. Harris, and R.R. Neutra. 1989. Congenital cardiac anomalies
in relation to water contamination, Santa Clara County, California, 1981-1983. Am.
J. Epidemiol. 129:885-893.
Travis, C.C., and H.A. Hattemer-Frey. 1987. Human exposure to 2,3,7,8-TCDD. Che-
mosphere 16(10-12):2331-2343.
Upton, A.C., T. Kneip, and P. Toniolo. 1989. Public health aspects of toxic chemical
disposal sites. Annu. Rev. Public Health 10:1-25.
U.S. Geological Survey. 1988. National Water Summary 1986: Hydrologic Events and
Groundwater Quality. U.S. Geological Survey Water Supply Paper 2325. Washing-
ton, D.C.: U.S. Government Printing Office
Vianna, N.J., and A.K. Polan. 1984. Incidence of low birth weight among Love Canal
residents. Science 226:1217-1219.
Viviano, F. 1991. U.S. toxics cleanup mired in lawsuits. San Francisco Chronicle (June
5):A1.
Waldorf, H., and R. Cleary. 1983. Water Distribution System, Woburn Massachusetts,
1964-1979. Engineering Draft Report, Massachusetts Department of Environmental
Quality.
Wallace, L.A., E.D. Pellizzari, T.D. Hartwell, R. Whitmore, C. Sparacino, and H. Zelon.
1986. Total exposure assessment methodology (TEAM) study: Personal exposures,

indoor-outdoor relationships, and breath levels of volatile organic compounds in New Jersey. Environ. Int. 12:369-387.

Wallace, L.A., E.D. Pellizzari, T.D. Hartwell, C. Sparacino, R. Whitmore, L. Sheldon, H. Zelon, and R. Perritt. 1987. The TEAM (Total Exposure Assessment Methodology) Study: Personal exposures to toxic substances in air, drinking water, and breath of 400 residents of New Jersey, North Carolina, and North Dakota. Environ. Res. 43:290-307.

Wallace, L.A., E.D. Pellizzari, T.D. Hartwell, R. Whitmore, H. Zelon, R. Perritt, and L. Sheldon. 1988. California TEAM study: Breath concentrations and personal air exposures to 26 volatile compounds in air and drinking water of 188 residents of Los Angeles, Antioch and Pittsburgh, California. Atmos. Environ. 22:2141-2163.

Whorton, M.D., R.W. Morgan, O. Wong, S. Larson, and N. Gordon. 1988. Problems associated with collecting drinking water quality data for community studies: A case example, Fresno County, California. Am. J. Public Health 78:43-46.

Wong, O., M.D. Whorton, N. Gordon, and R.W. Morgan. 1988. An epidemiologic investigation of the relationship between DBCP contamination in drinking water and birth rates in Fresno County, California. Am. J. Public Health 78:43-46.

Wong, O., R.W. Morgan, M.D. Whorton, N. Gordon, and L. Kheifets. 1989. Ecological analyses and case-control studies of gastric cancer and leukemia in relation to DBCP in drinking water in Fresno County, California. 1989. Br. J. Indust. Med. 46:521-528.

Wrensch, M., S. Swan, P.J. Murphy, J. Lipscomb, K. Claxton, D. Epstein, and R. Neutra. 1990a. Hydrogeologic assessment of exposure to solvent-contaminated drinking water: Pregnancy outcomes in relation to exposure. Arch. Environ. Health 45:21-216.

Wrensch, M., S. Swan, J. Lipscomb, D. Epstein, L. Fenster, K. Claxton, P.J. Murphy, D. Shusterman, and R. Neutra. 1990b. Pregnancy outcomes in women potentially exposed to solvent-contaminated drinking water in San Jose, California. Am. J. Epidemiol. 131:283-300.

Hazardous Wastes in Air, Water, Soil, and Food; Biologic Markers

4

Air Exposures

A N EXTENSIVE BODY OF literature exists on the epidemiology of air pollution. Rather limited information is available about airborne exposures from hazardous-waste sites. In order to improve the scientific basis for studying health effects of such exposures, this chapter reviews methodologic approaches to the study of air pollution, and discusses how these approaches may be applied to the study of airborne exposure to hazardous wastes. Also, relevant studies on airborne exposure to materials similar to those found at hazardous-waste sites are assessed, along with some evidence of exposures from hazardous-waste sites or other related exposures, such as may occur with the sick building syndrome.

This chapter is organized into four sections. The first part reviews longitudinal and cross-sectional studies of mortality. The second part details a variety of studies of morbidity. The third section discusses emerging evidence about the sick building syndrome, as similar constellations of symptoms have been reported at hazardous-waste sites. Conclusions are found in the fourth section. This chapter follows a methodologic sequence, but emphasizes questions, problems, and conclusions that apply to exposures from hazardous-waste sites and to exposures from single-point sources.

An increasing portion of recent epidemiologic studies involves studies of diseases with multifactorial causes, low relative risks, exposures to large populations, and therefore high attributable risks. This has also been true for the study of air pollution, because entire populations of cities or regions are exposed. In contrast, studies of hazardous-waste sites will often have to deal with risks from multi-factorial outcomes, and small populations are usually involved. Questions of analysis and sample size addressed in air pollution studies also must be addressed in any epidemiologic assessment of hazardous-waste exposure. Furthermore, exposure through air is recognized as a feature in the epidemiology of hazardous-waste sites, not only because lead dust can blow off such sites and volatile organic compounds can be encountered, but because the outgassing of volatile contaminants in domestic water is a recognized phenomenon (Andelman et al., 1986; McKone, 1987). As noted in Chapter 3, trichlorethylene, which has been shown to outgas in domestic water (Andelman et al., 1986), is the second most commonly found compound at hazardous-waste sites.

MORTALITY STUDIES

LONGITUDINAL ANALYSIS

Studies of trends over time in air pollution and disease patterns have produced a growing body of literature that has associated day-to-day fluctuations in air pollution with daily fluctuations in mortality across a wide range of exposures with no evidence of thresholds. The early studies of pollution and daily mortality in London examined discrete episodes (Great Britain Minstry of Health, 1954), and recent analyses show a strong and consistent association between daily particulate concentration and daily mortality across 14 years of data (Schwartz and Marcus, 1990). Figure 4-1 illustrates that relationship. In both cases, the relationship with particulates held independently of sulfur dioxide but not vice versa. One report that analyzes mortality in Steubenville, Ohio (Schwartz and Dockery, 1990), finds a significant association between mortality and airborne particulate matter at concentrations well below the ambient air quality standard of 150 micrograms per cubic meter. The consistency of findings in these studies is complemented by a consistency in the magnitude of the effect. Assuming a log linear model for mortality counts, the Steubenville analysis associates an increase of 100 micrograms per cubic meter in particle concentration with a 3.8 percent increase in the daily rate of mortality; in London it was associated with a 4 percent increase, and in New York with about a 3 percent increase. In separate analyses of the relationship between particu-

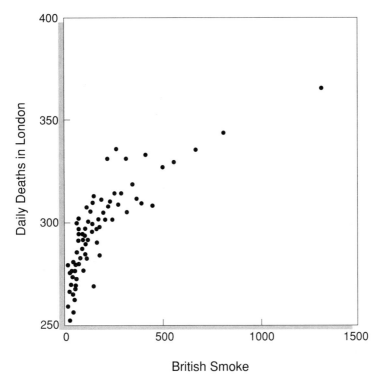

FIGURE 4-1 Mean daily deaths in London versus mean smoke ($\mu g/m^3$), 1958–1972. Source: Schwartz and Marcus, 1990, with permission.

lates and the daily rate of mortality for each year in London, the regression coefficients of particulates were consistent as well.

Acute mortality from exposure to hazardous industrial products occurred in Bhopal, India, in 1984. The analytical issues raised in studies of such acute events are relevant to the study of hazardous wastes. Longitudinal studies of such episodes within a single population are confounded by multiple factors that occur when different geographic regions are compared. These issues are discussed in more detail in the section on longitudinal studies of morbidity.

CROSS-SECTIONAL STUDIES OF MORTALITY

Cross-sectional studies provide epidemiologic snapshots or pulses of a given area at one point in time. Recent computer technology has permitted easier preparation of maps of comparative mortality data from different regions of the U.S. and Canada. Of more relevance to hazardous-waste studies are smaller scale comparisons of adjacent counties or Zip Codes. Although such indicators are relatively crude and insensitive, they have been used to compare mortality data in populations close to or more distant from point sources of emissions, such as smelters that emit arsenic. In one study in Sweden, Pershagen (1985) found significant small-scale regional differences in lung cancer rates that could be attributable to such air emissions, and Lloyd et al. (1984) suggest that changes in sex ratio of births might also be found in a similar polluted environment. In general, area studies of health patterns linked to hazardous-waste sites have been too small to permit significant mortality comparisons. Moreover, exposures in such studies certainly involve multiple routes and can induce multiple adverse effects.

At least one cross-sectional ecological study (Lave and Seskin, 1977) found associations between long-term airborne exposures to sulfate pollution and age-, race-, and sex-adjusted mortality rates in urban areas of the U.S. These studies were criticized because of their highly ecological nature and poor control for other factors that could explain geographic variations in mortality rates. Subsequent studies (Lipfert, 1980; Chappie and Lave, 1982) obtained better data on other relevant risk factors, such as smoking and industrial employment. A more recent study by Griffith et al. (1989) reports an association between the presence of hazardous-waste sites in counties in the U.S. and excess cancer mortality. No effort was made to control for cigarette sales by county, employment in high-risk industries, or presence of industrial facilities that might emit carcinogens. Without these controls, such studies may be of limited value.

Vinyl chloride (VC) is a substance found at many hazardous-waste sites (see Appendix 3-A of this volume). In the 1970s, several epidemiologic investigations indicated that occupational exposure to VC was associated with an increased risk of angiosarcoma of the liver as well as cancer of other sites (Infante, 1981). In addition, epidemiologic study and case reports associated angiosarcoma of the liver with community exposure to VC. Brady et al. (1977) reported the results of a New York State case control study of 26 confirmed cases of angiosarcoma of the liver. Controls were comprised of individuals who had an internal malignant tumor other than primary liver cancer; they were matched with cases on the basis of age at diagnosis, race, sex, place of residence and vital status. Of 10 women with angiosarcoma of the liver, five lived within one mile of VC polymerization or fabrication plants (1 case lived within 1700 feet for 62 years; 4 cases lived from 500 to 4500 feet for 8 to 27 years), whereas none of their matched controls lived as close. According to the authors, this observation added support to the hypothesis that exposure to VC outside the industrial setting may be an important factor in the etiology of angiosarcoma of the liver. In addition to the above study, Christine et al. (1974) noted six cases of angiosarcoma of the liver in Connecticut. Of these, one lived within two miles of a plant producing wire coated with polyvinyl chloride while a second lived within 0.5 mile of a plant producing vinyl sheets. None of the individuals was known to have had occupational exposure to VC or arsenic or diagnostic exposure to thorium dioxide. Rosenman et al. (1989) recently reported higher odds ratios for central nervous system birth defects in areas around two VC polymerization facilities in New Jersey.

One review of age-adjusted, sex-, race- and site-specific cancer mortality rates in U.S. counties for three time periods found significantly elevated rates of bladder cancer in males in counties surrounding the Drake Superfund site in Pennsylvania (Budnick et al., 1984). Elevations of birth defects also occurred, but were not statistically significant. This site, in Clinton County, Pennsylvania, included the volatile human carcinogens beta-naphthylamine, benzidine, and benzene dispersed over a 46-acre area. Airborne exposure was suspected to have occurred, given the nature of the chemicals involved. Subsequent investigation determined that males in these counties had between 20 and 30 times the rate of bladder cancer as nonexposed males; their primary employment was in the manufacture of beta-naphthylamine, a potent bladder carcinogen (Marsh et al., 1991). No general evidence of environmental effects was obtained, as Chapter 3 noted.

CHRONIC MORBIDITY STUDIES

LONGITUDINAL ANALYSIS

These studies have been of three types: long-term studies of actively exposed persons, prospective studies of a distinct group, and follow-up studies of exposed children.

Long-term studies of individuals acutely exposed to an initial single dose of a pollutant and then subjected to some chronic exposure have included a follow-up of the population exposed to dioxins at Seveso, Italy (Bertazzi et al., 1989). Follow-up studies of a small group of people acutely exposed to chlorine from an accidental release (Weill et al., 1969) have been published. These studies are required if long-term changes or risks are to be identified. In some instances, full recovery occurs; in others, involving sulfur dioxide, sulfuric acid, oxides of nitrogen, or ammonia, recovery may be very slow and incomplete (Bates, 1989). Where increased rates of cancer are involved, long-term follow-up will be needed.

One prospective study of a distinct group (such as Seventh Day Adventists—Euler et al., 1988—which have a stable population for which health outcomes can reliably be recorded) has been useful in identifying associations between total suspended particulates and respiratory symptoms and bronchitis, and between ozone levels and the incidence of asthma. Such studies are not applicable to hazardous-waste sites, however. Follow-up studies of residents of Love Canal, New York, chronically exposed for varying periods have been reported (Janerich et al., 1981). In general, these have not revealed striking long-term effects, although an increase in prevalence of low-birth-weight babies in Love Canal was linked to exposures from wastes deposited there (Vianna and Polan, 1984; Goldman et al., 1985).

There also are important data on children with chronic elevations of lead in their blood in whom subsequent effects have been detected with long-term follow-up studies. Follow-up studies of children known to have suffered from lead exposure showed that lead levels in umbilical cord blood predict a child's performance on the Bailey scales of mental development at 6 months and at 18 months of age (Bellinger et al., 1987). Exposure categories were in three groups, <5 µg/dL (micrograms per deciliter), 5-10 µg/dL, and >10 µg/dL. The fall-off in performance was significantly different between the lowest and highest exposure categories; in the middle it depended on economic circumstance, and poorer children performed worse than did others for the same lead level. Needleman et al. (1990) demonstrated that poorer school performance, reading problems, and deficits in intelligence tests persist into adolescence. Needleman's follow-up of children known to have been exposed to lead indicates an odds ratio of 5 for failure to graduate from high school and of 7 for reading disabilities (Needleman et al., 1990).

As noted in Chapter 3, lead is the commonest contaminant of hazardous-waste sites. It also is present in mining wastes, house paint, and urban soils contaminated by leaded gasoline and flaking house paint. Studies of the effects of lead are therefore clearly relevant to hazardous-waste site exposures, and they indicate the importance of ensuring that exposures of children to lead from hazardous-waste sites does not occur.

If adequate markers of exposure to developmental toxins can be secured (as was relatively easy in the case of lead), the outcome measurements can be sensitive enough to demonstrate significant long-term adverse effects. Unfortunately, markers of exposure often do not exist; where available they can provide reliable evidence of long-term effects.

CROSS-SECTIONAL STUDIES OF MORBIDITY

Community Studies

Cross-sectional community studies typically compare communities with different levels of air pollution or populations that live different distances from a hazardous-waste site. All such studies have several problems: Measurement error can occur when the same exposure is assumed for every subject within a group. There are undetected differences between communities for risk factors. There can be "recall bias" if one group knows it is in the high-exposure category. There is little standardization of the equipment used to measure exposure in different locations. Recent studies, such as that by Flessel et al. (1991), suggest that more detailed population exposure measurements over time, in this example to DNA adducts of polycyclic aromatic hydrocarbons, may permit more precise analyses of long-term consequences.

In spite of these difficulties, successful community studies have been done. In contrast to ecologic studies that lack information on potential confounders, community studies generally have collected individual data on nonpollution risk factors. One early study (Holland and Reid, 1965) compared lung function in groups of male postal workers in London and in a number of provincial towns where levels of particulate matter and sulfur dioxide were much lower. In all smoking categories, they found a significant decrement of pulmonary function, measured as Forced Expiratory Volume 1 (FEV1), in the London workers. A more recent study (Groupe Cooperatif PAARC, 1982) found significant regressions in men, women, and children of FEV1 against sulfur dioxide pollution levels in 10 French cities. In the U.S., the best example of such studies is the six-city study that found a strong association between respirable particles and prevalence of acute bronchitis in children, although no differences were found in FEV1 (Dockery et al., 1989).

Other studies of this kind, including one report from Israel (Goren and Hellman, 1988), document that different respiratory symptoms occur in communities with different pollutant exposures. A report from Finland (Jaakkola et al., 1990) indicates that malodorous emissions from kraft pulp mills are associated with eye, nasal, and respiratory symptoms, although reporting bias cannot be ruled out in this case. Schwartz (1989) presents an analysis of pulmonary performance, spirometric data from several thousand randomly selected children in the National Health and Nutrition Survey, which shows that those with greater chronic exposure to ozone experience reductions in lung capacity, as measured by forced vital capacity. An important aspect of most of these studies is that exposure was continuous, but to various levels, rather than dichotomous. This allows one to examine the dose-response relationship and to determine if the pattern suggests a direct linear, monotonic association, or some other dose-response relationship.

In addition to epidemiologic study results (Wagoner et al., 1980) and case reports (Sprince and Kazemi, 1980) among workers exposed to beryllium compounds, neighborhood cases of beryllium disease also have been observed in cross-sectional studies. Chronic beryllium disease is a pulmonary and systemic granulomatous disease caused by inhalation of beryllium. The interval between initial exposure and the clinical manifestation of disease varies from several months to years. Exertional dyspnea is the most common symptom. Other symptoms are cough, fatigue, weight loss, chest pain and arthralgia. Through the study of subjects admitted to the U.S. Beryllium Case Registry, specific criteria for the diagnosis of chronic beryllium disease have been established (Sprince and Kazemi, 1983). In 1948, Hardy reported chronic beryllium disease in persons who lived adjacent to a fluorescent lamp plant in Massachusetts. Additional cases of beryllium disease have been reported among persons living in the vicinity of a beryllium extraction plant (Eisenbud et al., 1949). Atmospheric pollution resulting from stack discharge was thought to be responsible for the latter diseases. By 1960, 47 cases of neighborhood beryllium disease were in the Beryllium Case Registry (Tepper et al., 1961); between 1966 and 1974, 76 new cases were added (Hasan and Kazemi, 1974).

Examples of cross-sectional morbidity studies that involve hazardous-waste sites include one on the Upper Ottawa Street Landfill in Hamilton, Ontario (Hertzman et al., 1987), in which significant differences in symptoms were found between an exposed and a control population, and a study (Baker et al., 1988) of 2039 persons in 606 households located near the Stringfellow Hazardous Waste Disposal Site in California. Both reports contain considerable discussion of how differences in symptom perception and recall can be reduced. A similar study involving a waste site in Lowell, Massachusetts, was reported by Ozonoff et al. (1987). The target population included all households within 400 meters of the site, and the control area was a ring of households between 800 meters and 1200 meters from the site. None of these studies found differences in reproductive outcome or cancer mortality, but all three documented significant differences in symptoms recording. The symptoms varied widely, with headache, irritability, and fatigue being common in all three studies. However, all of these symptoms may also increase due to other factors, such as perceived risk.

The authors of these reports drew somewhat different conclusions from their studies, based on the degree to which they believed recall bias accounted for differences in reported symptoms. Recall bias is difficult to avoid if a community is episodically exposed to a noxious agent (such as hydrogen sulfide) with a very powerful odor. Recent studies of such communities in Alberta report that symptoms were more common in exposed groups than in controls, but that there were no difference in objective data of morbidity or mortality (Dales et al., 1989). This paper includes considerable discussion of the problem of recall bias. Hopwood and Guidotti (1988) also show that recall bias operates in the recalling of incidents of acute exposure.

Although it might be concluded that recall bias explains the symptom differences in all of these studies, the real possibility nevertheless exists that the symptoms complained of are more sensitive as indicators of significant exposure than are more severe outcomes. In air pollution studies, recall bias cannot account for daily diary records of respiratory symptoms that relate to variations in air pollution. Longitudinal studies of recorded symptoms and exposure around hazardous-waste sites could similarly avoid much of the problem, although this has not so far, to our knowledge, been attempted.

A different example of the use of cross-sectional community studies is the use of data on birth defects from different localities separated by their proximity to known hazardous-waste sites or contaminated water supplies. The Lipari Landfill study (NJDOH, 1989) found low average birth weight in children born or conceived while the Gloucester County, New Jersey, landfill was operating. After the landfill closed, the differences disappeared, adding plausibility to the association between exposure to airborne pollutants and low birth weight. Follow-up studies of residents close to Love Canal yielded similar results with this end point, with some evidence of an effect that subsided in later years (Goldman et al., 1985).

Individual Studies

In community studies, the same exposure is assigned or assumed for all individuals. Individual cross-sectional studies use measures of individual rather than community levels of exposure and correlate them with differences in outcome variables across individuals rather than mean differences between communities. Many studies of the epidemiology of low-level lead toxicity fall into this category. Tooth lead levels in children have been related to intelligence and attention span deficits since the pioneering work of Needleman et al. (1972). Other studies have linked blood lead levels to children's stature (Schwartz et al., 1986), umbilical cord lead levels to congenital anomalies (Needleman et al., 1984), and identified bone demineralization as an internal source of lead exposure (Silbergeld et al., 1988).

It is clear that whenever one can use an individual marker of exposure, the power of such studies is greatly augmented. Monster and Smolders (1984) did an imaginative analysis of exhaled air for tetrachlorethane in teachers and their five-year-old pupils at a kindergarten near a factory with fugitive emissions. They then compared these levels to those found in a control group. Exhaled tetrachlorethane was then measured in a group of residents of an old people's home situated near a chemical-waste dump. Significant differences were found between the two groups of children, with those closer to the factory having higher levels. It was also shown that residents living on the first floor of the home (which is closer to the waste site) had significantly higher levels than did residents who lived on the second floor.

ACUTE MORBIDITY STUDIES

There are three categories of studies of acute morbidity: diary studies, population-based studies, and analysis of large data banks.

DIARY STUDIES

Diary studies of respiratory symptoms were first used in the 1950s as indicators of the pulmonary effects of air pollution (Lawther et al., 1970). These involved analyses of daily subjective records of respiratory symptoms, as they relate to pollution. There has recently been a resurgence of interest in this method, because it reduces the possibility of confounding by other factors that are difficult to control in cross-sectional studies, which compare rates of illness or symptoms across areas with different pollutant concentrations. In the longitudinal diary study, the population acts as its own control. Hence, variations between subjects in reporting rates due to subjective factors, differences in susceptibility, and passive smoke exposure are normalized and do not confound the pollution relationship.

Despite the inherent subjectivity of self-recorded data on symptoms, diaries of symptoms and medication use have been effective in identifying air pollution as a risk factor for respiratory illness in recent years. Most of these studies also demonstrate a lack of association between air pollution and nonrespiratory illness, giving credence to the primary findings. Monitoring of peak flow rates and symptoms was also useful in the analysis of occupational asthma in electronic workers employed in soldering (Burge et al., 1979).

Schwartz and Zeger (1990) re-examined an earlier diary study of student nurses in Los Angeles, California (Hammer et al., 1974), and found significant associations between exposure to ozone and the incidence of coughing, between exposure to nitrogen dioxide and daily incidence rates of sore throats, and between exposure to carbon monoxide and headaches. Analysis of the diary entries also proved a sensitive instrument for detecting the connection between chronic exposure to passive smoke and coughing with phlegm production.

A study in Utah of respiratory symptoms, medication use, and daily Peak Expiratory Flow (PEF) measurements of children and adults with asthma (Pope, 1991) finds a clear association between increased symptoms and decreased PEF values and levels of PM_{10} particulate pollution, which originated mostly from a nearby steel mill. This study was not complicated by the presence of other pollutants, such as ozone, sulfur dioxide, or sulfuric acid aerosol. Ozone has been associated with symptom reporting in persons with asthma (Whittemore and Korn, 1980). Ostro et al. (1991) report that symptoms worsened in a group of asthma patients studied in Denver, Colorado, in relation to daily aerosol hydrogen ion levels.

Studies reported by Lippman (1989), Raizenne et al. (1989), and Kinney et al. (1988) of children attending summer camps are a special case, because daily symptom reporting and daily measurements of lung function can be correlated to pollution levels measured continuously at the same site. The researchers found it difficult to attribute symptoms of function loss to specific pollutants, but they did show that combinations of pollutants, such as ozone, aerosol sulfates, and sulfuric acid, are associated with a variety of adverse respiratory effects. In these studies, daily measurements of lung function have generally been used as the outcome measurement.

Diary data might be useful in assessing the occurrence of symptoms when exposure to a single-point source (such as a factory) is intermittent because of changes in wind direction, and they would of course be much easier to interpret where the individuals have not been aware of fluctuations in the concentrations of the pollutants.

POPULATION-BASED STUDIES

Population-based studies assay all persons within a given region. They offer many of the advantages of diary studies because they deal with an entire community, and they allow the examination of rarer outcomes, such as physician visits or hospital admissions. Pope (1989) reports an association between hospitalization for respiratory illness and PM_{10} concentrations in Utah Valley, located in Utah County of central Utah. The relationship was found at levels well below the current ambient air quality standard (24-hour PM_{10} standard of 150 micrograms per cubic meter and an annual PM_{10} standard of an expected arithmetic mean of 50 $\mu g/m^3$). A particularly striking effect was seen for the opening, closing, and reopening of a local steel mill. Further analysis shows a significant association in Salt Lake County as well (Pope et al., in press). Bates and Sizto (1987) found a significant relationship between summer air pollutants and hospital admissions for acute respiratory disease in southern Ontario. Data from acute-care facilities in the region's 79 hospitals were taken over a nine-year observation period.

An example of a population-based case-control study relevant to airborne toxic substances, although not specific to hazardous-waste sites, is the one conducted by Linos et al. (1991). Mortality rates for leukemia and non-Hodgkin's lymphoma (NHL) have been rising in the central region of the U.S. Linos and colleagues were interested in the hypothesis that general environmental factors might account for this increase. Subjects consisted of white males in Iowa and Minnesota diagnosed between 1980 and 1983; there were 520 cases of leukemias and 572 of NHL, who were matched to 1130 controls. The relative risks (RR) were adjusted for factors associated with NHL and leukemia, e.g., pesticide exposure, occupational exposure, social class, use of hair dyes, smoking, and family history of hematopoietic malignancy. The authors found a statistically significant increase in the risk of developing NHL (RR=1.4) and a slight, nonsignificant excess for leukemia (RR=1.2) among men who lived 0.8-3.2 km (0.5-2 miles) from a factory. Petroleum or chemical factories were associated with the leukemia risk, while stone, clay, and glass factories correlated with NHL. The authors state: "These environmental associations may provide clues to the unexplained rising morality rates of leukemia and NHL in the central United States" (Linos et al., 1991, p. 73).

Other studies have reported a correlation between visits to hospital emergency departments and pollutant levels. Some of these have been positive (Levy et al., 1977; Bates et al., 1990); in another the association was present but weak (Samet et al., 1981), and in others no association was found (Richards et al., 1981; Goldstein and Weinstein, 1986). Because the mix of pollutants varies, and a number of other factors affect hospital emergencies, such results are not unexpected. Hospital studies that include all hospitals in the area can provide data comparable with those generated in population-based studies.

Hospital-based studies are very relevant to future research on hazardous wastes and point sources of pollution in several ways. First, they provide broad support for the use of systematic and longitudinal symptom reporting, or hospital visits, as valid outcome measurements and investigative tools. Such reports are easier to obtain than are physiologic measurements, and in the case of respiratory illness they appear to be as useful in some cases as are measurements of function test change. Second, the critical feature of such studies is their longitudinal nature. Many of the difficulties that arise from reporting bias in using data from questionnaires administered once for hazardous-waste exposures (detailed in the next section) could be avoided by using monitored data of temporal fluctuations in exposure in a population, together with diary information. This might be more effective than depending on cross-sectional comparisons between groups of subjects who probably are aware of their relative exposure ranking and who therefore are prone to recall bias.

LARGE DATA BANK ANALYSES

Recent analyses of the Health Interview Survey of the U.S. National Center for Health Statistics have permitted studies of associations between the number of days people report being restricted due to respiratory conditions and levels of air pollutants (Portney and Mullahy, 1986; Ostro and Rothschild, 1989). Strong associations were found with fine particles and weaker ones with ozone. The large numbers of subjects in these studies have permitted significant associations to be found. An important strength of their analyses is the random selection of the subjects.

SPECIAL CONSIDERATIONS

THE SICK BUILDING SYNDROME

Initial reports of the occurrence of mild symptoms in people working in sealed, usually recently constructed, office buildings were generally discounted. However, the syndrome has been firmly established for several reasons. First, a remarkable concordance has been found in the kinds of complaints made by workers in different locations and in different countries: Headaches, fatigue, inability to concentrate, and mild inflammation of the eyes and pharynx were the most common complaints (Mendell and Smith, 1990). The complaints were generally more common in air-conditioned buildings, and they could not be attributed to fungi (such as *Aspergillus*) known to be responsible for the infection "humidifier fever." Work from Denmark (Molhave, 1985; Kjaergaard et al., 1989) has not only identified a group of volatile organic compounds most commonly present when complaints are recorded, but has shown that controlled exposures to these compounds (and not to others) elicit the same symptoms in groups of subjects who might or might not have reported adverse symptoms previously. The recent controlled-exposure study of *n*-decane (common in building materials) from the Aarhus group (Kjaergaard et al., 1989) provides an excellent example of how subjective symptoms, such as eye irritation, can be objectively studied. Effects on humans were demonstrated at 1/500th of the exposure level that produced effects on rats. In the study, 63 healthy subjects randomly selected from the regular Danish population were exposed to *n*-decane in concentrations of 10, 35, or 100 microliters/liter in a controlled double-blind study. Subjects were exposed for 6 hours per exposure day for a total of 4 exposure days. Dose-dependent changes in irritation of mucous membranes (measured by decreased tear film stability and an increase in conjunctival polymorphs), as well as subjective observations of increased sensation of odor intensity and perception of reduced air quality, were documented.

Diary data also can be used to compare complaints of symptoms that arise from working in new office buildings (Mendell and Smith, 1990). Reports of similar symptoms (fatigue, headache, and inability to concentrate) by populations in North American and European cities lends credibility to the phenomenon being reported.

Although the unravelling of the genesis of this syndrome is not yet complete, it contains important lessons for studies of hazardous-waste-site epidemiology. In many cases involving hazardous-waste sites, the complaints are subjective and similar to those of the sick building syndrome. In addition, objective markers of exposure have not been identified. Furthermore, many of the volatile compounds found in sealed modern buildings, including formaldehyde, toluene, and trichlorethylene, also are common constituents of waste dumps.

It has recently been suggested that exposure to low levels of formaldehyde is followed by changes in cells that indicate that the immune system has been affected (Thrasher et al., 1987). Although the precise significance of such changes is unclear, the possibility must be considered that exposure to toxic substances from hazardous-waste dumps causes similar or related changes.

ASTHMA AND OTHER RESPIRATORY PROBLEMS

During the past decade, our knowledge of factors related to asthma and other examples of increased airway responsiveness has expanded greatly (NRC, 1989). Exposures to a wide range of substances (more than 200 are listed in a review (Taylor, 1980)) can induce airway responsiveness that can be specific for the substance. Asthma is a common and well-studied disturbance of the human immune system. More commonly, exposure leads to a nonspecific increase in airway responsiveness as measured by inhaled histamine or methacholine aerosols. This response is not always immunologic. Toluene diisocyanate, widely used in industry as a solvent, is a powerful inducer of asthma and adult-onset hypersensitivity (Paggiaro et al., 1986), as are platinum salts, anhydides, and some acids (NRC, 1989). Exposures to ozone can increase the sensitivity of the subject to a subsequent exposure to an allergen (Boushey, 1989) or to sulfur dioxide (Koenig et al., 1990); and asthma patients are much more sensitive to inhaled sulfur dioxide than are those who do not have asthma (Sheppard, 1989).

At the same time this knowledge was being secured, and when summer pollutant levels were being shown to be associated with respiratory morbidity as indicated by hospital admission data (Bates and Sizto, 1987), it became apparent that hospital admissions for asthma were increasing (Mao et al., 1987; Gergen and Weiss, 1990) and that increases in asthma mortality were occurring (Sly, 1988; Weiss and Wagener, 1990). Prevalence surveys also indicated an increase in asthma, both in the U.S. (Gergen et al., 1988) and in Britain (Burney et al., 1990).

A full discussion of these phenomena is beyond the scope of this volume; it is not yet established why these increases have occurred. A number of studies of hazardous-waste sites document complaints of "chest tightness" and "shortness of breath" or other respiratory symptoms (Ozonoff et al., 1987). Therefore, the possibility must be entertained that proximity to some of these sites has induced increased airway responsiveness. To our knowledge, this has not yet been specifically evaluated in hazardous-waste-site studies. One study found no evidence of an increased prevalence of asthma in people living close to a polyurethane factory in Finland (Nuorteva et al., 1987).

Although the role of ambient air pollution in asthma prevalence has not yet been determined, it seems likely that air pollution is an aggravating factor. It seems unlikely, however, that exposures from hazardous-waste sites could have played a part in the generally increased prevalence of asthma, given the relatively small size of the potentially exposed populations. The role of exposures from hazardous-waste sites in the development of respiratory symptoms cannot be readily evaluated.

MONITORING OF AIR POLLUTANTS

A crucial lesson from the recent history of environmental epidemiology has been the critical role played by the general availability of monitoring data for a number of air pollutants. Many of the analyses discussed above could not have been undertaken without this extensive data base on pollutants for which monitoring data are routinely acquired. The nature of the data base also has shaped epidemiologic studies. For example, fewer studies of daily exposure have been done for particulates, because these often are sampled only every sixth day. This has hindered the attempt to replicate the London mortality analyses, except in rare cases, such as Steubenville, Ohio, where sampling results were available on a daily basis (Schwartz and Marcus, 1990) or in the Utah studies (Pope, 1989; Pope et al., in press). Exposure to hydrocarbons in urban air has not been monitored routinely since the 1970s and there has been little work on their direct effects except in studies of the sick building syndrome (Molhave, 1985; Kjaergaard et al., 1989). Routine monitoring of ambient air around hazardous-waste sites is not feasible because of their number, the low likelihood of detection in most cases, and cost. In addition, the small size of the exposed populations in most cases makes the sites difficult to study with standard epidemiologic techniques. Nevertheless, more systematic assessments of where such monitoring and such studies might be appropriate needs to be done early in the process of identifying and describing sites for study. It might well be appropriate that one major site with a nearby exposed population should be intensively studied over a period of a year or so, to acquire data that might be applicable to similar sites.

CONCLUSIONS

A variety of methodological approaches have been taken to the study of air pollution epidemiology. These can be applied to the study of hazardous wastes, but are likely to vary as to their success.

Thus, studies of trends over time in air pollution and disease patterns have produced a growing body of literature that has associated day-to-day fluctuations in air pollution with daily fluctuations in mortality across a wide range of exposures with no evidence of thresholds. It is not likely to be worthwhile to conduct such studies at hazardous-waste sites, especially in light of the complex and changing nature of the pollutants, the absence of long-term records, such as exist for criteria air pollutants, and problems of determining the baseline, or expected rates, of a variety of subtle health end points of interest, such as neurological, behavioral, and reproductive problems.

Lessons that have been learned in air pollution studies are relevant to epidemiologic studies of hazardous-waste sites. Of particular importance are the need to measure exposure as precisely as possible, and the value of obtaining longitudinal data on exposures and disease outcomes in order to strengthen time-series analyses. The recent symposium organized by the National Academy of Sciences (NRC, 1991) stressed the paramount importance (and difficulties) of exposure measurement.

Symptom reports appear to be sensitive indicators of adverse health effects. Simultaneous use of air monitoring and diary records could reduce the problem of recall bias, and are particularly valuable when small changes in pollutant levels cannot be detected by the subjects in a study. It is likely that air emissions from hazardous-waste sites have caused a variety of symptoms indicating low-level interference with normal function. These are often comparable to the symptoms reported in the sick building syndrome. There are insufficient data to determine whether or not airborne exposure to toxics from hazardous-waste sites has resulted in nationwide increases in cancer mortality, or adverse pregnancy outcomes. However, the limited number and low power of studies, and the long latency of some cancers and other chronic diseases, mean that these effects cannot be completely ruled out in most areas.

It is not easy to decide whether to launch an epidemiologic study. With more detailed assessment of exposure, the extent of possible adverse effects will be better understood. We think it is important to draw attention to resource needs for adequate study designs. While a decision to conduct an epidemiologic study of hazardous-waste sites must take account of expressed public concern, this concern should, especially in an era of scarce resources, be balanced by the best available scientific evidence, including the quality of exposure and outcome data and the probability that an answer could be obtained that would be interpretable per se or after combination with the data from multiple studies.

REFERENCES

Andelman, J.B., A. Couch, and W.W. Thurston. 1986. Inhalation exposures in indoor air to trichlorethylene from shower water. Pp. 201-213 in Environmental Epidemiology, F.C. Kopfler and G.F. Craun, eds. Chelsea, Mich.: Lewis.

Baker, D.B., S. Greenland, J. Mendlein, and P. Harmon. 1988. A health study of two communities near the Stringfellow Waste Disposal site. Arch. Environ. Health 43:325-334.

Bates, D.V., M. Baker-Anderson, and R. Sizto. 1990. Asthma attack periodicity: A study of hospital emergency visits in Vancouver. Environ Res. 51:51-70.

Bates, D.V. 1989. Respiratory Function in Disease. Third Edition. Philadelphia: W.B. Saunders. 558 pp.

Bates, D.V., and R. Sizto. 1987. Hospital admissions and air pollutants in Southern Ontario: The acid summer haze effect. Environ Res. 43:317-331.

Bellinger, D., A. Leviton, C. Waternaux, H. Needleman, and M. Rabinowitz. 1987. Longitudinal analyses of prenatal and postnatal lead exposure and early cognitive development. N. Engl. J. Med. 316(17):1037-1043.

Bertazzi, P.A., C. Zocchetti, A.C. Pesatori, S. Guercilena, M. Sanarico, and L. Radice. 1989. Ten-year mortality study of the population involved in the Seveso incident in 1976. Am. J. Epidemiol. 129:1187-1200.

Boushey, H.A. 1989. Ozone and asthma. Pp. 214-217 in Susceptibility to Inhaled Pollutants, M.J. Utell and R. Frank, eds. ASTM STP 1024. Philadelphia: American Society for Testing and Materials.

Brady, J., F. Liberatore, P. Harper, P. Greenwald, W. Burnett, J.N.P. Davies, M. Bishop, A. Polan, and N. Vianna. 1977. Angiosarcoma of the liver: An epidemiologic survey. J. Natl. Cancer Inst. 59:1383-1385.

Budnick, L.D., D.C. Sokal, H. Falk, J.N. Logue, and J.M. Fox. 1984. Cancer and birth defects near the Drake Superfund site, Pennsylvania. Arch. Environ. Health 39:409-413.

Burge, P.S., W.H. Perks, I.M. O'Brien, A. Burge, R. Hawkins, D. Brown, and M. Green. 1979. Occupational asthma in an electronics factory: A case control study to evaluate aetiological factors. Thorax 34:300-307

Burney, P.G.J., S. Chinn, and R.J. Rona. 1990. Has the prevalence of asthma increased in children? Evidence from the national study of health and growth 1973-1986. Br. Med. J. 300:1306-1310.

Chappie, M., and L. Lave. 1982. The health effects of air pollution: A reanalysis. J. Urban Econ. 12:346-376.

Christine, B.W., H.S. Barrett, and D.S. Lloyd. 1974. Epidemiologic notes and reports. Angiosarcoma of the liver—Connecticut. Morbid. Mort. Weekly Rep. 23:210-211.

Dales, R.E., W.O. Spitzer, S. Suissa, M.T. Schechter, P. Tousignant, and N. Steinmetz. 1989. Respiratory health of a population living downwind from natural gas refineries. Am. Rev. Respir. Dis. 139:595-600.

Dockery, D.W., F.E. Speizer, D.O. Stram, J.H. Ware, J.D. Spengler, and B.G. Ferris, Jr. 1989. Effects of inhalable particles on respiratory health of children. Am. Rev. Respir. Dis. 139:587-594.

Eisenbud, M., R.C. Wanta, C. Dustan, L.T. Steadman, W.B. Harris, and B.S. Wolf. 1949. Non-occupational berylliosis. J. Ind. Hyg. Toxicol. 31:282-294.

Euler, G.L., D.E. Abbey, J.E. Hodgkin, and A.R. Magie. 1988. Chronic obstructive pulmonary disease symptom effects of long-term cumulative exposure to ambient levels of total oxidants and nitrogen dioxide in California Seventh-Day Adventist residents. Arch. Environ. Health 43:279-285.

Flessel, P., Y.Y. Wang, K.I. Chang, J.J. Wesolowski, G.N. Guirguis, I.-S. Kim, D. Levaggi, and W. Siu. 1991. Seasonal variations and trends in concentrations of filter-collected polycyclic aromatic hydrocarbons (PAH) and mutagenic activity in the San Francisco Bay area. J. Air Waste Manage. Assoc. 41:276-281.

Gergen, P.J., and K.B. Weiss. 1990. Changing patterns of asthma hospitalization among children: 1979 to 1987. J. Am. Med. Assoc. 264:1688-1692.

Gergen, P.J., D.I. Mullally, and R. Evans III. 1988. National survey of prevalence of asthma among children in the United States, 1976 to 1980. Pediatrics 81:1-7.

Goldman, L.R., B. Paigen, M.M. Magnant, and J.H. Highland. 1985. Low birth weight, prematurity and birth defects in children living near the hazardous waste site, Love Canal. Haz. Waste Haz. Materials 2:209-223.

Goldstein, I.F., and A.L. Weinstein. 1986. Air pollution and asthma: Effects of exposures to short-term sulfur dioxide peaks. Environ. Res. 40:332-345.

Goren, A.I., and S. Hellman. 1988. Prevalence of respiratory symptoms and diseases in schoolchildren living in a polluted and in a low polluted area in Israel. Environ. Res. 45:28-37.

Great Britain Ministry of Health. 1954. Mortality and Morbidity During the London Fog of December 1952. Report on Public Health and Medical Subjects, Vol. 95. London: Her Majesty's Stationery Office. 60 pp.

Griffith, J., R.C. Duncan, W.B. Riggan, and A.C. Pellom. 1989. Cancer mortality in U.S. counties with hazardous waste sites and ground water pollution. Arch. Environ. Health 44:69-74.

Groupe Cooperatif PAARC. 1982. Air pollution and chronic or repeated respiratory diseases. II. Results and Discussion. Bull. Eur. Physiopath. Respir. 18:101-116.

Hammer, D.I., V. Hasselblad, B. Portnoy, and P.F. Wehrle. 1974. Los Angeles students nurse study. Daily symptom reporting and photochemical oxidants. Arch. Environ. Health 28:255-260.

Hardy, H.L. 1948. Delayed chemical pneumonitis in workers exposed to beryllium compounds. Am. Rev. Tuberc. 57:547-556.

Hasan, F.M., and H. Kazemi. 1974. Chronic beryllium disease: A continuing epidemiologic hazard. Chest 65:289-293.

Hertzman, C., M. Hayes, J. Singer, and J. Highland. 1987. Upper Ottawa Street Landfill Site health study. Environ. Health Perspect. 75:173-195.

Holland, W.W., and D.D. Reid. 1965. The urban factor in chronic bronchitis. Lancet 1:445-448.

Hopwood, D.G., and T.L. Guidotti. 1988. Recall bias in exposed subjects following a toxic exposure incident. Arch. Environ. Health 43:234-237.

Infante, P.F. 1981. Observations of the site-specific carcinogenicity of vinyl chloride to humans. Environ. Health Perspect. 41:88-94.

Jaakkola, J.J.K., V. Vilkka, O. Marttila, P. Jappinen, and T. Haahtela. 1990. The South Karelia Air Pollution Study: The effects of malodorous sulfur compounds from pulp mills on respiratory and other symptoms. Am. Rev. Respir. Dis. 142:1344-1350.

Janerich, D.T., W.S. Burnett, G. Feck, M. Hoff, P. Nasca, A.P. Polednak, P. Greenwald, and N. Vianna. 1981. Cancer incidence in the Love Canal area. Science 212:1404-1407.

Kinney, P.L., J.H. Ware, and J.D. Spengler. 1988. A critical evaluation of acute ozone epidemiology results. Arch. Environ. Health 43:168-173.

Kjaergaard, S., L. Molhave, and O.F. Pedersen. 1989. Human reactions to indoor air pollutants: n-decane. Environ. Int. 15:473-482.

Koenig, J.Q., D.S. Covert, Q.S. Hanley, G. van Belle, and W.E. Pierson. 1990. Prior exposure to ozone potentiates subsequent response to sulfur dioxide in adolescent asthmatic subjects. Am. Rev. Respir. Dis. 141:377-380.

Lave, L.B., and E.P. Seskin. 1977. Air Pollution and Human Health. Baltimore: Published by Johns Hopkins University Press for Resources for the Future. 368 pp.

Lawther, P.J., R.E. Waller, and M. Henderson. 1970. Air pollution and exacerbations of bronchitis. Thorax (England) 25:525-539.

Levy, D., M. Gent, and M.T. Newhouse. 1977. Relationship between acute respiratory illness and air pollution levels in an industrial city. Am. Rev. Respir. Dis. 116:167-173.

Linos, A., A. Blair, R.W. Gibson, G. Everett, S. Van Lier, K.P. Cantor, L. Schuman, and L. Burmeister. 1991. Leukemia and non-Hodgkin's lymphoma and residential proximity to industrial plants. Arch. Environ. Health 46:70-74.

Lipfert, F.W. 1980. Sulfur oxides, particulates, and human mortality: Synopsis of statistical correlations. J. Air Pollut. Control Assoc. 30:366-371.

Lippmann, M. 1989. Health effects of ozone: A critical review. J. Air Pollut. Control Assoc. 39:672-695.

Lloyd, O.L., M.M. Lloyd, and Y. Holland. 1984. An unusual sex ratio of births in an industrial town with mortality problems. Br. J. Obstet. Gynaecol. 91:901-907.

Mao, Y., R. Semenciw, H. Morrison, L. MacWilliam, J. Davies, and D. Wigle. 1987. Increased rates of illness and death from asthma in Canada. Can. Med. Assoc. J. 137:620-624.

Marsh, G.M., L.C. Leviton, E.O. Talbott, C. Callahan, D. Pavlock, G. Hemstreet, J.N. Logue, J. Fox, and P. Schulte. 1991. Drake Chemical Workers' Health Registry Study: 1. Notification and medical surveillance of a group of workers at high risk of developing bladder cancer. Am. J. Ind. Med. 19:291-301.

McKone, T.E. 1987. Human exposure to volatile organic compounds in household tap water: The indoor inhalation pathway. Environ. Sci. Technol. 21:1194-1201.

Mendell, M.J., and A.H. Smith. 1990. Consistent pattern of elevated symptoms in air-conditioned office buildings: A reanalysis of epidemiologic studies. Am. J. Pub. Health 80:1193-1199.

Molhave, L. 1985. Volatile organic compounds as indoor air pollutants. Pp. 403-414 in Indoor Air & Human Health, R.B. Gammage and S.V. Kaye, eds. Chelsea, Mich.: Lewis.

Monster, A.C., and J.F.F. Smolders. 1984. Tetrachloroethane in exhaled air of persons living near pollution sources. Int. Arch. Occup. Environ. Health 53:331-336.

Needleman, H.L., O.C. Tuncay, and I.M. Shapiro. 1972. Lead levels in deciduous teeth of urban and suburban American children. Nature. 235(5333):111-112.

Needleman, H.L., M. Rabinowitz, A. Leviton, S. Linn, and S. Schoenbaum. 1984. The relationship between prenatal exposure to lead and congenital anomalies. J. Am. Med. Assoc. 251:2956-2959.

Needleman, H.L., A. Schell, D. Bellinger, A. Leviton, and E.N. Allred. 1990. The long-term effects of exposure to low doses of lead in childhood. An 11-year follow-up report. N. Engl. J. Med. 322:83-88.

NJDOH (New Jersey Department of Health). 1989. A Report on the Health Study of Residents Living Near the Lipari Landfill. Environmental Health Service. 120 pp.

NRC (National Research Council). 1989. Biologic Markers in Pulmonary Toxicology. Washington, D.C.: National Academy Press.

NRC (National Research Council). 1991. Frontiers in Assessing Human Exposures to Environmental Toxicants. Washington, D.C.: National Academy Press.

Nuorteva, P., T. Assmuth, T. Haahtela, J. Ahti, E. Kurvonen, T. Nieminen, T. Saarainen, K. Seppala, P. Veide, and S. Viholainen. 1987. The prevalence of asthma among inhabitants in the vicinity of a polyurethane factory in Finland. Environ. Res. 43:308-316.

Ostro, B.D., and S. Rothschild. 1989. Air pollution and acute respiratory morbidity: An observational study of multiple pollutants. Environ. Res. 50:238-247.

Ostro, B.D., M.J. Lipsett, M.B. Weiner, and J.C. Selner. 1991. Asthmatic responses ot airborne acid aerosols. Am. J. Public Health 81:694-702.

Ozonoff, D., M.E. Colten, A. Cupples, T. Heeren, A. Schatzkin, T. Mangione, M. Dresner, and T. Colton. 1987. Health problems reported by residents of a neighborhood contaminated by a hazardous waste facility. Am. J. Ind. Med. 11:581-597.

Paggiaro, P.L., A. Innocenti, E. Bacci, O. Rossi, and D. Talini. 1986. Specific bronchial reactivity to toluene diisocyanate: Relationship with baseline clinical findings. Thorax 41:279-282.

Pershagen, G. 1985. Lung cancer mortality among men living near an arsenic-emitting smelter. Am. J. Epidemiol. 122:684-694.

Pope, C.A. 1989. Respiratory disease associated with community air pollution and a steel mill, Utah Valley. Am. J. Public Health 79:623-628.

Pope, C.A. 1991. Respiratory hospital admissions associated with PM_{10} pollution in Utah, Salt Lake, and Cache valleys. Arch. Environ. Health 46:90-97.

Pope, C.A., D.W. Dockery, J.D. Spengler, and M.E. Raizenne. In press. Respiratory health and PM_{10} pollution: A daily time series analysis. Am. Rev. Respir. Dis.

Portney, P.R., and J. Mullahy. 1986. Urban air quality and acute respiratory illness. J. Urban Economics 20:21-38.

Raizenne, M.E., R.T. Burnett, B. Stern, C.A. Franklin, and J.D. Spengler. 1989. Acute lung function responses to ambient acid aerosol exposures in children. Environ. Health Perspect. 79:179-185.

Richards, W., S.P. Azen, J. Weiss, S. Stocking, and J. Church. 1981. Los Angeles air pollution and asthma in children. Ann. Allergy 47:348-354.

Rosenman, K.D., J.E. Rizzo, M.G. Conomos, and G.J. Halpin. 1989. Central nervous system malformations in relation to two polyvinyl chloride production facilities. Arch. Environ. Health 44:279-282.

Samet, J.M., Y. Bishop, F.E. Speizer, J.D. Spengler, and B.G. Ferris, Jr. 1981. The relationship between air pollution and emergency room visits in an industrial community. J. Air Pollut. Control Assoc. 31:236-240.

Schwartz, J. 1989. Lung function and chronic exposure to air pollution: A cross-sectional analysis of NHANES II. Environ. Res. 80:309-321.

Schwartz, J., and D.W. Dockery. 1990. Particulate air pollution and daily mortality in Steubenville, Ohio. Am. Rev. Respir. Dis. 141:A74.

Schwartz, J., and A. Marcus. 1990. Mortality and air pollution in London: A time series analysis. Am. J. Epidemiol. 131:185-194.

Schwartz, J., and S. Zeger. 1990. Passive smoking, air pollution, and acute respiratory symptoms in a diary study of student nurses. Am. Rev. Respir. Dis. 141:62-67.

Schwartz, J., C. Angle, and H. Pitcher. 1986. The relationship between childhood blood lead levels and stature. Pediatrics 77:281-288.

Sheppard, D. 1989. Mechanisms of airway hyperresponsiveness. Pp. 47-52 in Susceptibility to Inhaled Pollutants, M.J. Utell and R. Frank, eds. ASTM STP 1024. Philadelphia: American Society for Testing and Materials.

Silbergeld, E.K., J. Schwartz, and K. Mahaffey. 1988. Lead and osteoporosis: Mobilization of lead from bone in postmenopausal women. Environ. Res. 47:79-94.

Sly, R.M. 1988. Mortality from asthma, 1979-1984. J. Allergy Clin. Immunol. 82:705-717.

Sprince, N.L., and H. Kazemi. 1980. U.S. beryllium case registry through 1977. Environ. Res. 21:44-47.

Sprince, N.L., and H. Kazemi. 1983. Beryllium disease. Pp. 481-490 in Environmental and Occupational Medicine, W. Rom, ed. 1st edition. Boston: Brown, Little.

Taylor, A.J. Newman. 1980. Editorial: Occupational asthma. Thorax 35:241-245.

Tepper, L.B., H.L. Hardy, and R.I. Chamberlin. 1961. Pp. 25-29 in Toxicity of Beryllium Compounds. New York: Elsevier Pub.

Thrasher, J.D., A. Wojdani, G. Cheung, and G. Heuser. 1987. Evidence of formaldehyde antibodies and altered cellular immunity in subjects exposed to formaldehyde in mobile homes. Arch. Environ. Health 42:347-350.

Vianna, N.J., and A.K. Polan. 1984. Incidence of low birth weight among Love Canal residents. Science 226(4679):1217-1219.

Wagoner, J.K., P.F. Infante, and D.L. Bayliss. 1980. Beryllium: An etiologic agent in the induction of lung cancer, nonneoplastic respiratory disease, and heart disease among industrially exposed workers. Environ. Res. 21:15-34.

Weill, H., R. George, M. Schwarz, and M. Ziskind. 1969. Late evaluation of pulmonary function after acute exposure to chlorine gas. Am. Rev. Respir. Dis. 99:374-379.

Weiss, K.B., and D.K. Wagener. 1990. Changing patterns of asthma mortality. J. Am. Med. Assoc. 264:1683-1687.

Whittemore, A.S., and E.L. Korn. 1980. Asthma and air pollution in the Los Angeles area. Am. J. Public Health 70:687-696.

5

Domestic Water Consumption

I N THE LATE NINETEENTH AND early twentieth centuries, industrial wastes contaminated many rivers and streams (Tarr, 1985). These waterways often supplied drinking water for urban populations, so gross contamination of many sources of drinking water became widespread. This eventually led to laws initially passed by state legislatures and later Congress (such as the Federal Water Pollution Control Act of 1948), that required intervention by the U.S. Public Health Service and subsequently by the U.S. Environmental Protection Agency (EPA) to ensure the safety of the nation's water supply. In general, water supplies are now safe bacteriologically, and usually free of gross contamination or obvious chemical pollution. However, drinking water can still be a source of harm to human health, particularly in areas where there are chemical dumps and where aquifers have been contaminated (Ram and Schwartz, 1987). Runoff from fields after nitrate and pesticide use for agricultural purposes also can contaminate drinking water, as can aromatic and aliphatic compounds that leak from underground gasoline storage tanks. Moreover, exposure is not limited to ingestion, but occurs through outgassing or volatilization in other uses of domestic water, as discussed in Chapter 3.

Marsh and Caplan (1987) point out that the existence of abandoned hazardous-waste sites largely stems from the strong sanctions that were enacted between 1952 and 1977 to control air and water pollution. Because of the Federal Water Pollution Control Act (1952), the Clean Air Act (1963), and the Clean Water Act (1977) surface water and ambient air were no longer considered acceptable outlets for the disposal of wastes. Consequently, industries and municipalities turned increasingly to the land for waste disposal. Contamination of groundwater and aquifers occurred where the waste dumps were poorly constructed or managed, or where wastes were disposed of improperly.

This chapter reviews evidence about some compounds commonly found at hazardous-waste sites that have been shown to cause adverse effects in humans exposed to these materials from consumption of domestic water. First it discusses studies of cancer risk posed by trihalomethanes (THMs) as an indicator of the sort of effects that can be anticipated from contamination of drinking water by such compounds. Then it assesses the relatively scanty literature on adverse effects that can be linked to the contamination of drinking water from toxic dump sites, including congenital anomalies, cancer, and other chronic diseases. As the importance of lead in drinking water is currently the subject of extensive analysis and regulatory attention, this chapter does not review this topic.

Epidemiologic evidence on the risk to health from contaminated water from hazardous-waste sites or other sources of contamination, such as pesticide runoff, has largely been derived from ecologic or descriptive studies, and therefore is seldom conclusive as to cause. The ecologic studies involving broad-scale comparisons of available data are unable to control for important confounding variables, such as smoking or other relevant exposures. Recent literature on the contamination of drinking water include a number of ecologic and case-control studies that evaluate the cancer risk of by-products of chlorination on human health (Jolley et al., 1990). Some chlorination by-products, particularly halogenated hydrocarbons or THMs, occur in greater quantities in drinking water if large amounts of organic matter are present (Burke et al., 1983). Two of these, chloroform and carbon tetrachloride, have been commonly found in the chemical mixtures at some toxic dump sites. Chloroform tends to be readily identified because it is more easily measured. Whether or not they, or other chemicals also present, increase the risk of cancer for exposed residents is unclear (Crump and Guess, 1982).

Several case-control studies based on examinations of death certificates have found an increased risk for cancers of the colon, rectum, bladder, breast, brain, and lung in persons who have consumed chlorinated drinking water (Velema, 1987). However the results have not always been consistent and causality cannot reliably be inferred.

THMs AND OTHER WATER QUALITY VARIABLES

Several hypothesis-generating ecologic studies have been based on cancer incidence data provided by the Iowa cancer registry for 1969 to 1978. The data were taken from municipalities that had populations of at least 1000 and public water supplied by a single source that had remained stable for a minimum of 14 years. Rates for cancers of the lung and rectum among males and females were higher for municipalities using chlorinated surface water compared to those with groundwater sources (Bean et al., 1982a). Subsequently Isacson et al. (1985) studied cancer incidence data for the years 1969-1981 from the Iowa cancer registry for towns with a public water supply from a single stable ground source and the levels of volatile organic compounds and metals found in the finished drinking water of these towns in 1979. This study lessened one of the problems common to ecologic investigations, namely, misclassification of exposure. Early studies of cancer and drinking water associated consumption of water and rates of cancer by comparing the proportion of county or parish residents supplied by surface water sources with overall cancer mortality rates for the total area. In these early studies, the lack of data on individual consumption patterns hampered interpretation of the results. Isacson et al. (1985) used cancer incidence by municipality, along with a survey on drinking water habits, in order to reduce misclassification of exposure. Associations between 1,2-dichloroethane and the incidence of cancers of the colon and rectum and between nickel and cancers of the bladder and lung were most clearly seen in males. Although nickel, 1,2-dichloroethane and trichloroethane are known to be carcinogens, the levels of these materials found in this study were well below the nondetectable-response level estimated from the experimental literature on these compounds. The researchers concluded that one plausible explanation of their result is that the mere presence of these industrial effluents in groundwater indicates that exposures have occurred from anthropogenic sources. Thus, the measured substances do not necessarily account for the increased rate of cancer, but rather indicate the presence of other materials.

In an earlier report from the Iowa cancer registry, Bean et al. (1982b) considered the contribution of waterborne radioactivity to differences in cancer incidence. They found that incidence rates of cancers of the lung and bladder among males and of cancers of the breast and lung among females were higher in towns where the water supply contained more than 5.0 picocuries per liter of radium-226. A gradient of increasing incidence associated with rising radioactivity levels for three periods also was seen for lung cancer among males. These findings were not explained by smoking patterns or water treatment methods.

A nationwide ecologic study examined cancer mortality from 1950 to 1969 and organic contamination of drinking water, using the data on carbon chloroform extract (CCE) and carbon alcohol extract (CAE), available through monitoring for varying periods between 1957 and 1972 at 129 stations throughout the U.S. (Clark et al., 1986). The researchers found strong associations of CCE and CAE with total cancer mortality and mortality from grouped gastrointestinal and urinary tract cancers (Clark et al., 1986). However, scattergrams reveal that much of the associations result from a small number of outliers where mortality rates or pollution levels were unusually high. Although the regression coefficients are statistically significant, they might not represent causal associations, given these outliers.

A similar study in Canada evaluated mortality rates in 66 cities between 1973 and 1979 and selected drinking-water characteristics with adjustment for socioeconomic factors (Wigle et al., 1986). Water source, chlorine dose, and the concentrations of asbestos, chloroform, total THMs except chloroform, and total THMs were not significantly correlated with any of the disease categories examined, which comprised all causes of death, all cancers, various cancer sites, and coronary heart disease mortality. When dose of total organic carbon was substituted for chlorine dose in a multivariate analysis, there was a significant association with large intestine cancer among males. One possible reason for the findings could be that in the total data age-standardized mortality rates for overall mortality (males), all cancers combined (males), and stomach cancer (both sexes) had a strong correlation with lower average level of education. The analysis was adjusted for low education in the examination for possible associations with the water variables, as lower education and socioeconomic status are strongly associated with increased cancer risk.

In Houston, Texas, an opportunity arose to assess the effect of changing from a lightly chlorinated drinking water source to one that was heavily chlorinated after the construction in 1954 of Lake Houston, which became the source of drinking water for a sizable portion of the city's population (Cech et al., 1987). The concentrations of THMs ranged from below detectable limits to more than 200 micrograms per liter (twice the level allowed by U.S. drinking water standards) in treated lake water. These exposures were described by census tract, and the trends in mortality from urinary tract cancer from 1940 through 1974 were compared with the trends for three other causes of death— respiratory cancer, bronchitis and emphysema, and homicide. Although an increase in urinary tract mortality in white females was noted for those exposed to treated lake water by 1970-1974, no increase was noted in white males or in the nonwhite population. It was concluded that a detrimental effect of the switch to chlorinated surface water had not been demonstrated.

The largest individual- and population-based case-control study of cancer with evaluations of exposure to by-products of chlorination in drinking water was performed in 1978 in 10 areas of the U.S. (Cantor et al., 1987). These by-products include THMs generated by chlorination, as well as chloroform. A group of 2982 persons with bladder cancer and 5782 control subjects were interviewed in the original study and individual year-by-year profiles of water source and treatment were developed by linking lifetime residential information with historical water utility data from an ancillary survey of 2805 cases and 5258 controls. Risk of bladder cancer increased with intake of beverages made with tap water. The odds ratio for the highest versus the lowest quintile of tap water consumption was 1.43 (95 percent CI 1.23-1.67). The increased risk was largely restricted to persons with at least a 40-year exposure to chlorinated surface water and was not found among long-term users of nonchlorinated groundwater. There was no evidence of confounding by other causes of bladder cancer, including smoking. In particular, women and nonsmokers of both sexes, who consumed chlorinated surface water at rates above the median for 60 or more years, had rates of bladder cancer that were more than three times the rates of those who had not consumed treated surface water.

In an analysis of the Iowa portion of a national bladder case-control study on bladder cancer, the effect of misclassification on estimates of years of exposure to chlorinated drinking water was investigated (Lynch et al., 1989). It was shown that only with detailed information of the type used by Cantor et al. (1987) would it be possible to derive a significant association of duration of consumption of chlorinated surface water with bladder cancer, while taking account of potential confounders.

A case-control study of colon cancer (366 cases, 785 cancer controls, and 654 population controls) in Wisconsin did not find an increased risk associated with an index of THM exposure (Young et al., 1987). Only a small risk of marginal significance was found for exposure to chlorinated water for 0-10 years before diagnosis. The authors noted that the majority of water supplies in Wisconsin contain low levels of THMs and that it is unlikely that a small risk, if present, could have been detected.

A case-control study that used interviews with informants of 614 individuals who had died of bladder cancer and 1074 individuals who had died of other causes found that the rate of death from bladder cancer among individuals who resided only in communities supplied with chlorine-disinfected drinking water relative to those who resided only in communities supplied with chloramine-disinfected drinking water was 1.6 (95 percent CI 1.2-2.1) (Zierler et al., 1988a). Chloramination of drinking water is a process that results in lower amounts of THMs than result from chlorine disinfection.

The effect of contamination of drinking water with arsenic has been investigated in an area of Taiwan with endemic blackfoot disease, a peripheral vascular disease related to continuous exposure to arsenic in artesian well water. Elevated mortality from cancers of the bladder, kidney, skin, lung, liver, and colon was found in association with such exposure (Chen et al., 1985). A subsequent study related arsenic levels in well water in 1964-1966 to age-adjusted mortality rates for 1973-1986 (Wu et al., 1989). A significant dose-response relationship was found for cancers of the bladder, kidney, skin, and lung in both sexes and for cancers of the prostate and liver in males. Another study examined ecologic correlations between arsenic content in well water and mortality from various neoplasms in 314 precincts and townships of Taiwan as a whole (Chen and Wang, 1990). A significant association with the arsenic level in well water was observed for cancers of the liver, nasal cavity, lung, skin, bladder, and kidney in males and females and for prostate cancer in males. Although arsenic is regarded as a cause of blackfoot disease, there has been speculation that other factors in artesian well water, such as humic acid, are involved in what is probably a multistage, multifactorial disease that results from chronic progressive arteriosclerosis (Chen and Wang, 1990).

The relationship between chlorinated water and serum cholesterol (SC) levels has also been investigated (Zeighami et al., 1990). Significantly higher SC levels were found in females from chlorinated communities.

TOXIC DUMP SITE EXPOSURES

CANCER AS THE END POINT

Love Canal, New York, is perhaps the best known of toxic dump sites. Human exposure there to chemicals was through contaminated water, although not strictly through drinking water. Rather, contaminated water seeped into the basements of homes and subsequently exposure was largely through inhalation; contaminated soil also played a role. The possibility that Love Canal residents could develop cancer was raised because benzene and γ-hexachlorobenzene, both carcinogens, were found in the wastes at the site. Janerich et al. (1981) published a report that compared cancer incidence for census tracts in the Love Canal area with cancer incidence throughout the state except for New York City. No significant elevation of rates was found among Love Canal residents for any cancer, including those selected a priori for special attention—liver cancer, lymphoma, and leukemia— though the numbers of cancers in the Love Canal census tracts were very small. Thus the standardized incidence ratio for liver cancer was 2.0 in males and 2.9 in females, but this was based on only two observed cases for each sex and was not significant. A further difficulty relates to the fact that numerous other hazardous-waste sites exist in the state. Comparing Love Canal to this area may have produced some dilution of effect, as both populations have incurred exposures from hazardous waste sites.

New Jersey also has a large number of toxic dump sites. Najem et al. (1983, 1985) conducted ecologic studies that related cancer mortality at the county and municipal level to environmental variables, including the location of chemical toxic-waste-disposal sites. At the county level they found associations with most gastrointestinal cancers (Najem et al., 1983). In addition, an analysis of age-adjusted female reproductive organ and breast cancer mortality showed significant positive associations between breast cancer mortality and proximity to toxic disposal sites among whites in 21 New Jersey counties (Najem and Greer, 1985). At the municipal level, statistically significant positive associations were found for 8 of 12 cancers considered, with stomach, colon, and rectal cancer clusters being particularly noted (Najem et al., 1985). The clusters of excess cancer mortality were confined for the most part to the highly urban and industrial northeastern part of the state, and air pollution and lack of information on other possible confounders complicated interpretation of the results.

In a reinvestigation of health effects potentially arising from two contiguous wells supplying part of the drinking water for Woburn, Massachusetts, Lagakos et al. (1986) found positive associations between access to domestic water from two contaminated wells and the incidence of childhood leukemia. The wells were contaminated with trichloroethylene, tetrachloroethylene, and chloroform. Large pits of buried animal hides, solvents, and other chemical wastes were discovered as was an abandoned lagoon that was heavily contaminated with lead, arsenic, and other metals. However, Woburn has been an industrial site for more than 130 years, and at the time of this study, EPA had not yet determined the precise sources of the contamination. The wells were closed in 1979, and the leukemia cases studied were diagnosed between 1964—the year the wells began pumping—and 1983. It had previously been determined that 12 cases diagnosed between 1969 and 1979 were in excess—only 5.3 were expected—and these 12 were included in the 20 evaluated by Lagakos et al. (1986). The authors confirm that the 20 cases were significantly higher than the 9.1 expected from national rates. They used two different methods for estimating exposure. A cumulative estimate of exposure from the two wells from birth until age t; and a binary indicator of whether there had been any exposure by age t. Each of these exposure metrics was associated with the incidence of childhood leukemia. The cumulative metric statistically explained about four cases, while the "ever-never" metric explained about six cases. This leaves an excess of five or six cases for which no explanation may be inferred from the reconstructions of well water exposure. Four of the recent leukemia cases occurred in West Woburn, where exposures to contaminated water did not occur, confounding the determination of causality. Analyses of time trends since the wells were closed suggests that the rate of leukemia has fallen significantly, strengthening the inference of a causal association with past exposures. However, this finding does not rule out the possibility that other unrecognized factors may also have been involved in explaining the leukemia cluster, or the possibility that the cluster was a random event. In a commentary, MacMahon (1986) noted that a more complex exposure metric (which might have been expected to more precisely measure exposure than an "ever-never" comparison) in fact led to a lesser degree of association with leukemia. Perhaps the major difficulty with this study is that it was unable to overcome problems in exposure assessment already discussed in Chapter 3. Nevertheless, because the exploration of the incidence of leukemia followed the identification of the contamination of the wells, this study avoids the pitfalls that can arise when many of the cases of leukemia are first identified as part of an original "index" set. Therefore, the same cases did not contribute to the derivation but only to the testing of the hypothesis.

The New Jersey Department of Health (Fagliano et al., 1987, 1990) conducted an ecologic study to determine whether there was a relationship between incidence of leukemia and contamination of public drinking-water supplies with volatile organic compounds (trichloroethylene, tetrachloroethylene, 1,1,1-trichloroethane, and related chlorinated solvents) known to have been derived from improper disposal. These compounds are used in metal degreasing, dry cleaning, and in some household products. An excess of leukemia among females, but not among males, was found in towns in the highest of three exposure categories in the study years 1979-1984. The standardized incidence ratio for females was 1.53 (95 percent CI 1.02-2.21); for males it was 1.00. The authors were unable to explain this gender difference, but it would seem to weaken the argument that the leukemia was caused by exposure to the toxins. However, for males other exposures, such as those in the workplace, could be more important determinants of leukemia than environmental exposures.

A nationwide ecologic study was conducted by Griffith et al. (1989) using the National Priorities Listing (NPL) of hazardous-waste sites developed by EPA and cancer mortality data for 13 major cancer sites by county for 1970-1979. The NPL identified 593 waste sites in 339 U.S. counties in 49 states with analytical evidence of contamination in groundwater that provided a sole source of potable water supply. Significant associations between excess deaths and all counties with hazardous-waste sites were shown for cancers of the lung, bladder, esophagus, stomach, large intestine, and rectum for white males and for cancers of the lung, breast, bladder, stomach, large intestine, and rectum for white females, when compared with the counties that did not have hazardous-waste sites. No adjustment was possible for the effect of industrialization or other confounders at the individual level, such as factors related to lifestyle, including cigarette smoking. Many of the associations were strong and of a similar order in both sexes; there were odds ratios of 5.9 in males and 4.3 in females for cancer of the large intestine. The odds ratio for lung cancer was higher in females (5.2) than it was in males (2.0). These associations could have resulted from factors not considered in the analysis or from other problems with the method of the studies. For example, Greenland (1990) has shown that ecologic estimates can be more sensitive to misspecification and misclassification than are individual-level estimates, primarily because ecologic estimates are based on assumptions and inferences rather than on direct measurements.

Wong et al. (1989) conducted ecologic and case-control analyses to evaluate the possibility that contamination of drinking water in Fresno County, California, with dibromochloropropane (DBCP) increased mortality from gastric cancer and leukemia. The study was conducted because a previous ecologic analysis by the California Department of Health Services for 1970 to 1979 found such an association. Mortality data for 1960-1983 were included in the ecologic analyses, and deaths for the period 1975 to mid-1984 were used in the case-control studies; nongastric cancer or leukemia deaths served as controls. The only positive association was an increased risk of leukemia for farm workers. No relationship was found for gastric cancer or leukemia with DBCP contamination of drinking water.

Evaluation of the cancer maps by county produced by the National Cancer Institute for 1950 through 1979 reveals areas of high mortality from bladder cancer in several northwestern Illinois counties. This led to an incidence study of bladder cancer cases diagnosed between 1978 and 1985 in those counties (Mallin, 1990). A cluster in males and females was identified by zip code within Winnebago County, a county that had been known in advance of the study to be at risk of groundwater contamination because of the dumping of solid and liquid waste in water supply zones over the last 100 years. It was found that one of four public water wells had been closed due to contamination; two wells were within a half-mile of a landfill site that had ceased to operate in 1970. Tests of these two wells revealed traces of trichloroethylene, tetrachloroethylene, and other solvents.

Concern by residents led to the evaluation of another cancer cluster in North Carolina (Osborne et al., 1990). Comparison of cancer deaths for the rural community of Bynum with those expected for the state as a whole showed no increase in the proportion of deaths due to cancer between 1947 and 1964 (range, 9-14 percent), but thereafter there was a steady increase to 58 percent in 1980-1985. Standardized proportionate mortality ratios for cancer for 1957 to 1985 were 2.4 to 2.6 times greater than expected. The number of cancer deaths was small, and the cancers were diverse. The hypothesized cause was the consumption of raw river water by a majority of residents from 1947 to 1976. The river was contaminated with pollutants, including known carcinogens, from industrial and agricultural contamination upstream of the town.

Cancer clusters like those investigated by Mallin (1990) and Osborne et al. (1990) often are reported under circumstances that are difficult to evaluate, and it seems likely that few with negative outcomes are reported in the literature. One exception is a study by Day et al. (1989). The investigation was prompted by public concern in Randolph, Massachusetts, that led to a survey of households, with data on cancer supplemented by records from the town, the state, and the Massachusetts cancer registry. Although a cancer cluster was confirmed, overall cancer incidence and mortality in the neighborhood were not elevated. No unusual feature of the cancer data was identified and no environmental hazard was suspected.

From 1980 through 1982, 183 patients with esophageal cancer, or 17 percent of all such cases referred to the King Faisal Specialist Research Center, came from the Gassim region of Saudi Arabia, compared with 5 percent of the total cancer patient referrals from this region (Amer et al., 1990). This observation prompted a case-control study of cases diagnosed between 1983 and 1987. The regional disparity in referrals persisted, and the only differences noted with referrals from other regions were for sources of drinking water. Traces of petroleum oil were found in five of six water samples from the Gassim region during 1983, compared with 3 of 49 from other areas. Mutagenicity tests on 12 water samples from Gassim showed significant activity in two-thirds of the samples, with up to a 26-fold increase in mutagenic activity in the TA98 bacterial system. The authors also note that aromatic hydrocarbons can occur at higher levels in groundwater than in surface water, due to the lack of evaporation. They point to corroborating evidence on the importance of petroleum and petrochemical exposures. Gottlieb and Carr (1981) report that workers in these industries have more than three times the average rate of esophageal cancer. The authors suggest that contamination of drinking water combined with malnutrition could promote esophageal cancer in the Gassim region. Although this is a reasonable inference from the data presented, it is unclear whether other differences between the regions can explain the differences seen. There are marked variations in esophageal cancer incidence in many areas, some of which could be attributable to differences in nutrition or use of opium. Few data were collected in the study on nutrition, and no data were reported on opium use.

ADVERSE PREGNANCY OUTCOMES

Following the identification of a cluster of central nervous system defects in the Mount Gambier area of South Australia, a case-control study was performed of 218 pairs from the period 1951-1979 (Dorsch et al., 1984). Compared with women who drank only rainwater, women who consumed principally groundwater had an increase in the risk of bearing a malformed child (RR=2.8, 95 percent CI 1.6-4.4). The malformations in excess of expected rates were of the musculoskeletal central nervous systems. An even stronger association was found after reanalysis for estimated water nitrate concentration (a fourfold increase in risk for those consuming >15 parts per million nitrate). It was recognized that other, as-yet-undetected chemicals could have been responsible for the excess. These might include brominated phenols, which occasionally have been detected in one of the groundwater sources, believed to have resulted from aerial contamination from nearby timber preservation plants.

In the investigation of health effects associated with the two wells that supplied part of the drinking water for Woburn, Massachusetts, Lagakos et al. (1986) found positive associations between access to water from the contaminated wells and perinatal deaths, two of five categories of congenital anomalies (central nervous system, eye, ear, chromosomal, and oral cleft), and two of nine categories of childhood disorders (infections of the kidney and urinary tract and disorders of the respiratory tract). There was no positive association with spontaneous abortions or low birth weight. The wells, which were closed in 1979, were contaminated with trichloroethylene, tetrachloroethylene, and chloroform. The health outcomes evaluated were identified by a telephone sample survey conducted in 1982 of 4936 pregnancies and 5018 residents of Woburn aged 18 or younger. Several of these outcomes were grouped according to "assertions in the literature of potential links with chemicals, pesticides or trace elements," a grouping that was subsequently criticized (MacMahon, 1986). MacMahon (1986) also commented on the lack of correction for the multiple comparisons made as a result of the health survey and the fact that six of the interviewers were from families of the leukemia patients.

Several studies have reported low birth weight as a consequence of exposure to toxins at Love Canal (Vianna and Polan, 1984; Goldman et al., 1985; Paigen and Goldman, 1987). The timing and extent of the effect differed in these studies. Vianna and Polan (1984) evaluated the cohort of infants born in the Love Canal area from 1940 through 1978. As a surrogate for exposure, they considered whether or not a family resided in an area known to have more water that percolated up to the ground through swales. Such homes arguably could be expected to incur greater exposure to contaminants in these swales and to outgassing emissions from them that could enter basements, especially during times of sewer overflows. Using a five-year moving average, they found a significant excess of low-birth-weight babies occurred during the time when dumping was estimated to be most active in the area, namely 1940 through 1953. No such excess was evident for later years.

Goldman et al. (1985) studied a larger population and a somewhat different cohort of births. Using single family homes in the entire Love Canal neighborhood—an area three times as large as that included in Vianna and Polan—they found an excess of low birth weight between the years 1963 and 1980. The adjusted odds ratio was 3.0 (range, 1.3 to 7.0) for 131 exposed and 357 controls, with a prevalence of low-birth-weight babies of 16 percent for the swale area, 10 percent for the nonswale area, and 4.8 percent for the controls. Paigen and Goldman (1987) defined exposure in two ways: distance of the home from the canal and proximity of the homes to possible paths of chemical migration, inferred from hydrogeological information about the migration of groundwater pollutants from the abandoned site into homes and basements, via swales, or large subterranean, wet paths via which pollutants can move. However, there remains a possibility of misclassification of exposure that could have biased the findings toward the null (Paigen and Goldman, 1987). No significant difference in prematurity was found. Birth defects also were more common among the exposed than the unexposed children born to homeowners or renters living in Love Canal, with odds ratios of 1.95 (95 percent CI 1.03-3.72) and 2.87 (95 percent CI 1.15-7.18), respectively. A study conducted by Vianna and Polan (1984) of all children born in single-family houses on a series of parallel streets in the area between 1940 and 1978 found that the significant rates of low birth weight in infants born in the same areas between 1954 and 1978, after dumping of chemical wastes had ceased, were similar to those of upstate New York as a whole. However, from 1940 through 1953, the period when various chemicals were dumped in the site, there was a significant excess of low birth weight among infants born in the Love Canal swale area, an area of natural, low-lying drainage depressions that traverse the dump site.

An ecologic study was performed to evaluate the relationship between dibromochloropropane (DBCP) contamination of drinking water and birth ratios between 1978 and 1982 in Fresno County, California (Wong et al., 1988). No relationship between birth ratios and DBCP contamination in drinking water was found.

A case-control study of residents of Massachusetts born alive between April 1, 1980, and March 31, 1983, with severe congenital heart disease has been reported (Zierler et al., 1988b). Controls were randomly selected from birth certificates filed with the Massachusetts Division of Health Statistics during the study period. Of 440 identified cases, 170 were excluded for various reasons, as were 264 of 929 controls. The toxins of interest were chemicals routinely monitored in public water supplies (arsenic, barium, cadmium, chromium, lead, mercury, selenium, fluoride, nitrate, and sodium); these were assigned according to the maternal residential history obtained by telephone interview. There was no indication of any association of exposure to the chemicals of concern above the minimal detectable limit for congenital heart disease as a whole. Only for coarctation of the aorta was there any association, a prevalence odds ratio of 3.4 (95 percent CI 1.3-8.9) for exposure to arsenic. Given the large number of comparisons made, at least one would have been expected to be significant by chance. The authors comment that non-differential errors in the measurement and classification of exposures, as well as the paucity of contaminant levels above the minimal detectable limits, could explain the lack of positive findings.

A series of studies conducted in Santa Clara County, California, followed discovery of a leak of toxic chemicals in November 1981. The point source was an underground waste solvent storage tank at a semiconductor plant, 0.7 kilometers from a well that supplied drinking water to nearby industrial and residential areas (Swan et al., 1989). The well was removed from service in December 1981 after contamination with solvents (predominantly 1,1,1-trichloroethane or methyl chloroform) was discovered. Because of the concern of residents, the California Department of Health Services conducted two studies. In one, there was an increased prevalence of major cardiac anomalies in children born to persons who lived in the service area of the water company that operated the contaminated well (Swan et al., 1989). A relative risk of 2.2 (95 percent CI 1.2-4.0) was determined for the contaminated area in comparison with the remainder of the county. No excess was observed for the period between September 1982 and December 1983. However, on the assumption that the greatest degree of chemical contamination of drinking water occurred in the three-month period before the leak was discovered, it was expected that the excess cases would be found in children born between May and August 1982. Cases were not found in excess of the expected rate. Therefore, it seemed that the chemical contamination of the drinking water could not explain the excess of cardiac anomalies in children. This conclusion was reinforced by a follow-up telephone interview of 145 mothers of children born with severe cardiac anomalies and 176 mothers of children without such anomalies (Shaw et al., 1990). However, longer-term analyses were not conducted. Although there was a positive association between a mother's consumption of tap water during the first trimester of pregnancy and cardiac anomalies in her infant for the year 1981 that was not present for 1982 or 1983, this appeared unrelated to the source of water and to the incident of contamination. Chlorination by-products should be considered further, given recent studies of TCE and cardiac anomalies discussed below. Consumption of bottled water appeared protective, however. The data could not be used to distinguish between a potential causal agent in the water and differential reporting of exposure by study subjects.

In the second study, a cluster of adverse pregnancy outcomes, including spontaneous abortions, low birth weight, and congenital malformations, was identified (Deane et al., 1989). An odds ratio of 2.3 for spontaneous abortion was found in comparison to a census tract free of contaminated water, while the odds ratio for congenital malformations was 3.1. In a subsequent study, Wrensch et al. (1990a) also investigated adverse pregnancy outcomes during 1980-1985 in two communities where solvents had leaked from the underground storage tank to contaminate local drinking water. Two demographically similar unexposed communities also were studied. The period 1980-1981 was considered as that of exposure; 1982-1985 was the post-contamination period. The study did not produce internally consistent results. Thus, the odds ratio (OR) for the original study area of those exposed versus those unexposed for 1980-1981 was 3.5. This may have been due to a low rate of spontaneous abortions in the unexposed community for 1982-1985. This rate for 1982-1985 was substantially below the rate in the same community and that in the exposed community for the same period (the OR for 1982-1985 was 1.0). The rate for spontaneous abortions in 1980-1981 in the exposed community was only marginally higher than that in the same community for 1982-1985. Similarly, the OR for 1980-1981 in the new study area for exposed versus unexposed persons was 0.3, due to a low rate of spontaneous abortions in the new exposed study area. Further, exposure estimates based on hydrogeologic modeling and contaminant distribution within the exposed areas (Wrensch et al., 1990b) also indicate that the leak was not likely to have caused the observed excesses of adverse pregnancy outcomes in the originally studied area. The adverse pregnancy outcomes occurred in areas with lower exposure levels, as opposed to those with higher exposure levels; causes remain unknown.

An association has been reported between congenital heart disease and contamination of groundwater in the Tucson valley of Arizona (Goldberg et al., 1990). It had been noted that approximately one-third of patients with congenital heart disease lived in a small area of the Tucson valley in 1973. In 1981, groundwater for a nearly identical area was found to be contaminated with trichloroethylene and to a lesser extent with dichloroethylene and chromium. It was believed that contamination began in the 1950s, and the affected wells were closed after the contamination was discovered. Interviews with parents of 707 children with congenital heart disease, who between 1969 and 1987 had conceived the children in and resided in the Tucson valley for the first trimester of pregnancy, revealed that 35 percent had work or residential contact with the contaminated water. Two random telephone surveys showed that 10.5 percent of the Tucson valley population had such contact. The OR for children with congenital heart disease born to parents where there was active water contamination was 3 compared to those without contact with contaminated water; the ratio decreased to near unity for those who arrived in the contaminated water area after the wells closed. A recent report from the Centers for Disease Control Birth Defects Monitoring Program indicates that cardiac defects made up almost half the malformations that showed increasing trends from 1979 to 1987 (Edmonds and James, 1990). Recorded time trends for such anomalies are likely to include artifacts, such as improved case finding and other improvements in diagnosis, but merit further study.

Although causality cannot be assumed from a single study, a study that used a rat model identified a variety of cardiac defects caused by the administration of trichloroethylene and dichloroethylene in solutions delivered through a catheter into the gravid uterus from an intraperitoneal osmotic pump (Dawson et al., 1990). There was a dose-response relationship: 9 percent and 12.5 percent of congenital cardiac anomalies were found in the lower-dose trichloroethylene and dichloroethylene groups; 14 percent and 21 percent, respectively, were found in the higher-dose groups compared with 3 percent in the control group. Experimental studies have also found that TCE applied through a catheter directly into the gravid uterus during the period of heart development induces cardiac anomalies in both chicks (Loeber et al., 1988) and rats (Dawson et al., 1990). Dichloroacetic acid (DCA) and trichloroacetic acid (TCA) are both by-products of chlorine disinfection of water containing natural organic material; TCA is a metabolite of TCE. DCA or TCA exposure of pregnant Long-Evans rats by oral intubation produced dose-related cardiac malformations in fetuses (Smith et al., 1989a,b).

Taken together the preceding evidence strengthens the empirical basis for concluding that TCE induces cardiac anomalies in humans. The grounds for this inference include evidence that the relationship is biologically plausible, in that exposure to TCE or its metabolites experimentally induces cardiac teratogenesis in exposed animals (Loeber et al., 1988; Dawson et al., 1990). Moreover, these same effects have been significantly detected in exposed humans, with some evidence of a dose-response relationship in the animal studies. In addition, markers of exposure to TCE have been detected in humans and animals, and the findings are statistically significant. Thus, a chain of evidence links TCE to cardiac anomalies, although additional studies need to be conducted to confirm the association. In addition, extensive studies in animals demonstrate a range of other effects of TCE from reproductive impairment to effects on DNA (ATSDR, 1989), for which corroborating human data do not exist.

One cross-sectional study of health problems compared rates of morbidity and mortality from 1980-1985 for a number of chronic diseases, including heart disease, anemia, skin cancer, hypertension, stroke, and chronic kidney disease, in residents of three towns surrounding an abandoned Superfund site in Galena, Kansas, with those of residents in two control towns (Neuberger et al., 1990). Environmental exposures to lead and cadmium and other mine wastes occurred chiefly through domestic water use. Some surface soils may also have provided airborne exposure. Significant elevations in rates of a number of causes of death and disease were evident in persons over age 44. Among residents of the three towns who had lived there at least five years, there was either a statistically significant or borderline excess in women for chronic kidney disease (aged 65), heart disease (aged 45 and older), and anemia (aged 45 and above). This sex difference may reflect the fact that factors such as smoking, work, and drinking are more important determinants of some of these diseases in men than women. A significant excess of mortality also occurred from ischemic heart disease in males and females (aged 65 and older). The authors conclude that environmental agents in Galena City may have contributed to the causation of several chronic diseases in residents.

OTHER HEALTH END POINTS

An environmental health survey of residents who had consumed drinking water contaminated with leachate from a waste dump where a pesticide plant had deposited large amounts of liquid and solid waste between 1964 and 1972 was conducted in Hardeman County, Tennessee (Clark et al., 1982). Twelve chlorinated organic compounds were found in wells that served individuals living near the dump site. Carbon tetrachloride was the most abundant, and residents had complained of a number of symptoms, including eye and skin irritation; upper respiratory infection; and gastrointestinal symptoms including nausea, diarrhea, and abdominal cramping. The survey used a health questionnaire, a clinical examination, and biochemical screening for liver and kidney dysfunction. Results of the physical examination of 118 individuals found six of 48 individuals in the exposed group had slight hepatomegaly (enlargement of the liver), compared to one of 24 in an intermediate exposed group and none in the 46-member group of unexposed control subjects. The difference between the groups was significant ($p=.034$) with the Pearson chi-square test. Elevated concentrations of alkaline phosphatase and serum glutamic oxaloacetic transaminase, measures of liver function, were found more often in the exposed group than in the controls. The concentrations fell significantly in follow-up testing two months after use of the contaminated water had ceased. The authors conclude that the clinical and biochemical observations were consistent with transitory liver injury. In a subsequent independent study, Rhamy (1982, cited by Harris et al., 1984) collected health histories and conducted physical examinations on 112 persons who then lived or had formerly lived within three miles of the site. Analyses were restricted to 102 persons who claimed to be exposed. A large number of symptoms was reported, as were liver, eye, and neurological abnormalities on examination. The Rhamy study is almost impossible to interpret because there was no control group, questions on symptoms were asked repeatedly during examinations, and the study was conducted after the contamination had been widely publicized. Thus, recall bias may well explain much of the reported symptomatology. However, after a comprehensive evaluation of this same exposed population, Meyer (1983) reported evidence of hepatomegaly and elevated liver function tests (alkaline phosphatase and serum glutamic oxaloacetic transaminase (SGOT) were elevated at levels of 0.016 and 0.010, respectively, when compared to the control population; albumin and total bilirubin levels were significantly lower) that he attributed to ingestion of organic chemicals, including hepatotoxins. The second larger and more comprehensive study, performed three months after the wells had been closed, showed no difference between the control, intermediate, and exposed groups.

Rothenberg (1981) reported on a cross-sectional health survey of residents near a Hyde Park, New York, landfill. The landfill was inactive, but exposure through groundwater to diverse chemicals, including chlorinated hydrocarbons, was suspected. Nine positive associations were found among the 180 variables assessed. With multiple comparisons, such results may chiefly be due to chance variations.

It was noted above that the exposures that caused concern in the Love Canal area were not derived from drinking water per se, which came from an uncontaminated municipal source, but from contaminated groundwater from the site that seeped into the basements of homes and led to exposure through sump pumps, soil, and air inside the homes. To evaluate general health effects from such exposures Paigen et al. (1985) conducted a general health survey with interviewers inquiring about physician-diagnosed complaints of the parents of 523 Love Canal and 440 control children. An excess of seizures, learning problems, hyperactivity, eye irritation, skin rashes, abdominal pain, and incontinence was found in Love Canal children. It was not possible to eliminate the effects of respondent bias, recall bias, or stress in this study, although the authors believe that the true differences had been under- rather than overestimated. The same group reported on factors related to growth in 493 Love Canal and 428 control children (Paigen et al., 1987), using technicians (who were unaware of the children's place of residence) to conduct the measurements. Of the Love Canal children, the 172 born there who had spent at least 75 percent of their lives in the Love Canal area were significantly shorter for age percentile than were the control children. Mean weight for age percentile also was less in the Love Canal group. These differences could not be accounted for by various potential confounders.

Some of the chemicals that contaminate drinking water, such as trichloroethylene (TCE), are known to have neurotoxic effects, although specific neuropsychological testing of potentially exposed subjects has rarely been performed. Feldman et al. (1988) administered a questionnaire and performed clinical testing, nerve-conduction studies, and neuropsychological testing on 28 members of 8 families who had alleged chronic exposure to industrial chemicals as a result of contamination of two public drinking-water wells in Woburn, Massachusetts. Electrophysiological measurement of the blink reflex was used to quantify damage to two cranial nerves known to be affected by TCE exposure. Of the 28 potentially exposed subjects, 4 were not tested because they were too young. The results for three of the subjects were not used because of potential confounders (diabetes, working with TCE, and treatment for leukemia). The results from the remaining 21 were compared with those from 27 laboratory controls. There was a highly significant difference in the conduction latency means of the blink reflex, or the speed with which nerves responded, between the test subjects and the controls, suggesting a subclinical alteration of cranial nerve function due to exposure to TCE.

Substantial environmental contamination with chemicals in drinking water has occurred in a number of places in Eastern Europe and in developing countries. One study of pesticide contamination was done in a village in Nicaragua, where children from a community in the path of rainwater runoff from a large crop-dusting airport were tested for cholinesterase levels in comparison with children from an unexposed community (McConnell et al., 1990). Six of 17 children from the exposed community had low cholinesterase levels, the mean level for the 17 being 0.5 international units/milliliter/minute lower (95 percent CI 0.24-0.76) than that for 43 children from the unexposed community. A sample of water from a well in the exposed community showed contamination with toxaphene and chlordimeform at levels above the U.S. Food and Drug Administration's Recommended Acceptable Daily Intake. However, the children also were exposed because they played barefoot in grossly contaminated rainwater runoff from the airport, and the authors believe this was the more important source of exposure.

CONCLUSIONS

We have commented elsewhere in this report that complete accounts of investigations of cancer and other risks in relation to human exposure to hazardous-waste sites are not generally available because of legal restrictions. Hence, the available literature on the epidemiology of drinking-water contamination and adverse health outcomes is scanty and not conclusive. Nevertheless, several factors lead us to conclude that drinking-water contamination with a number of chemicals is injurious to human health, although the magnitude of the risk cannot be determined. Perhaps the most persuasive evidence now derives from studies of drinking-water contamination with trihalomethanes linked to increased risk of bladder cancer (Cantor et al., 1987). Bladder cancer also has been associated in a large ecologic study with exposure to contaminated drinking water from hazardous-waste sites (Griffith et al., 1989). Bladder cancer is well recognized as chemically induced, and the fact that individual studies have not found an increased incidence of bladder cancer in persons exposed to toxic-waste sites could result from the long latency period generally anticipated for this cancer, and the fact that multiple causes are likely to be involved. Continued surveillance of exposed populations for this sentinel cancer are well justified. Osborne et al. (1990) found a cancer cluster for all cancers with an exceptionally high rate; moreover, the period of the excess corresponded to the estimated time of peak exposure to contaminated domestic water, taking into account the normal latency for cancer.

Where increased risk might be anticipated after solvent contamination of drinking water, leukemia and lymphoma are of obvious concern. Unfortunately, the rarity of these diseases and the greater likelihood that a rare cancer will come to notice if clusters occur have resulted in a dearth of studies with sufficient power to detect an increase in risk. Neutra (1990) advocates restricting studies of clusters to those where very high risks are anticipated. However, the number of heavily exposed individuals that might be expected to show an increase in risk of fivefold or more is generally so small that with a cancer as rare as leukemia or lymphoma such risks would be difficult to detect. Meta-analysis might overcome the limitations resulting from the small numbers. This will be discussed in the next report of the committee.

A limited number of reports in the peer-reviewed scientific literature have linked spontaneous abortion, low birth weight, and birth defects to drinking-water contamination. The studies in Santa Clara County have been inconclusive as to the cause of the cluster observed. Indeed, it seems likely that the study population was too small to prevent chance variation in frequency of events (as appears to have occurred) from obfuscating the issue. In Love Canal, low birth weight was clearly linked to exposures from the hazardous wastes, although the extent of the time during which it continued is unclear. Such outcomes should continue to be monitored because there is far less difficulty with the latency period for reproductive effects than for cancer.

Concerning other health effects, there is evidence that neurologic, hepatic, and immunologic function can be damaged by exposure to drinking water contaminated with toxic chemicals. The long-term consequences of the abnormalities detected, however, are largely unknown and must be the subject of further research, on which the committee will comment in more detail in its next report.

REFERENCES

Amer, M.H., A. El-Yazigi, M.A. Hannan, and M.E. Mohamed. 1990. Water contamination and esophageal cancer at Gassim region, Saudi Arabia. Gastroenterology 98:1141-1147.

ATSDR (U.S. Public Health Service, Agency for Toxic Substances and Disease Registry). 1989. Toxicological Profile for Trichloroethylene. ATSDR/TP-88/24. Atlanta: Agency for Toxic Substances and Disease Registry.

Bean, J.A., P. Isacson, W.J. Hausler, and J. Kohler. 1982a. Drinking water and cancer incidence in Iowa. I. Trends and incidence by source of drinking water and size of municipality. Am. J. Epidemiol. 116:912-923.

Bean, J.A., P. Isacson, R.M.A. Hahne, and J. Kohler. 1982b. Drinking water and cancer incidence in Iowa. II. Radioactivity in drinking water. Am. J. Epidemiol. 116:924-932.

Burke, T.A., J. Amsel, and K.P. Cantor. 1983. Trihalomethane variation in public drinking water supplies. Pp. 1343-1351 in Water Chlorination: Environmental Impact and Health Effects, Vol. 4. Book 2: Environment, Health, and Risk, R.L. Jolley et al., eds. Ann Arbor, Mich.: Ann Arbor Science.

Cantor, K.P., R. Hoover, P. Hartge, T.J. Mason, D.T. Silverman, R. Altman, D.F. Austin, M.A. Child, C.R. Key, L.D. Marrett, M.H. Myers, A.S. Narayana, L.I. Levin, J.W. Sullivan, G.M. Swanson, D.B. Thomas, and D.W. West. 1987. Bladder cancer, drinking water source, and tap water consumption: A case-control study. J. Natl. Cancer Instit. 79:1269-1279.

Cech, I., A.H. Holguin, A.S. Littel, J.P. Henry, and J. O'Connell. 1987. Health significance of chlorination byproducts in drinking water: The Houston experience. Int. J. Epidemiol. 16:198-207.

Chen, C.-J. 1990. Blackfoot disease [letter]. Lancet 336(8712):442.

Chen, C.-J., and C.-.J Wang. 1990. Ecological correlation between arsenic level in well water and age-adjusted mortality from malignant neoplasms. Cancer Res. 50:5470-5474.

Chen, C.-J., Y.-C. Chuang, T.-M. Lin, and H.-Y. Wu. 1985. Malignant neoplasms among residents of a blackfoot disease-endemic area in Taiwan: High-arsenic artesian well water and cancers. Cancer Res. 45:5895-5899.

Clark, C.S., C.R. Meyer, P.S. Gartside, V.A. Majeti, B. Specker, W.F. Balisteri, and V.J. Elia. 1982. An environmental health survey of drinking water contamination by leachate from a pesticide waste dump in Hardeman County, Tennessee. Arch. Environ. Health 37:9-18.

Clark, R.M., J.A. Goodrich, and R.A. Deininger. 1986. Drinking water and cancer mortality. Sci. Total Environ. 53:153-172.

Crump, K.S., and H.A. Guess. 1982. Drinking water and cancer: Review of recent epidemiological findings and assessments of risk. Ann. Rev. Public Health 3:339-357.

Dawson, B.V., P.D. Johnson, S.J. Goldberg, and J.B. Ulreich. 1990. Cardiac teratogenesis of trichloroethylene and dichloroethylene in a mammalian model. J. Am. Coll. Cardiol. 16:1304-1309.

Day, R., J.H. Ware, D. Wartenberg, and M. Zelen. 1989. An investigation of a reported cancer cluster in Randolph, Massachusetts. J. Clin. Epidemiol. 42:137-150.

Deane, M., S.H. Swan, J.A. Harris, D.M. Epstein, and R.R. Neutra. 1989. Adverse pregnancy outcomes in relation to water contamination, Santa Clara County, California, 1980-1981. Am. J. Epidemiol. 129:894-904.

Dorsch, M.M., R.K.R. Scragg, A.J. McMichael, P.A. Baghurst, and K.F. Dyer. 1984. Congenital malformations and maternal drinking water supply in rural South Australia: A case-control study. Am. J. Epidemiol. 119:473-486.

Edmonds, L.D., and L.M. James. 1990. Temporal trends in the prevalence of congenital malformations at birth based on the Birth Defects Monitoring Program, United States, 1979-1987. Morbid. Mortal. Week. Rep. 39(SS-4):19-23.

Fagliano, J., M. Berry, F. Bove, and T. Burke. 1987. Drinking Water Contamination and the Incidence of Leukemia: An Ecologic Study. New Jersey Department of Health, Division of Occupational and Environmental Health.

Fagliano, J., M. Berry, F. Bove, and T. Burke. 1990. Drinking water contamination and the incidence of leukemia: An ecologic study. Am. J. Public Health 80:1209-1212.

Feldman, R.G., J. Chirico-Post, and S.P. Proctor. 1988. Blink reflex latency after exposure to trichloroethylene in well water. Arch. Environ. Health 43:143-148.

Goldberg, S.J., M.D. Lebowitz, E.J. Graver, and S. Hicks. 1990. An association of human congenital cardiac malformations and drinking water contaminants. J. Am. Coll. Cardiol. 16:155-164.

Goldman, L.R., B. Paigen, M.M. Magnant, and J.H. Highland. 1985. Low birth weight, prematurity, and birth defects in children living near the hazardous waste site, Love Canal. Haz. Waste Haz. Materials 2:209-223.

Gottlieb, M.S., and J.K. Carr. 1981. Mortality studies on lung, pancreas, esophageal and other cancers in Louisiana. Pp. 195-204 in R. Peto and M. Schneiderman, eds. Banbury Report 9, Quantification of Occupational Cancer, Cold Spring Harbor Laboratory.

Greenland, S. 1990. Divergent Biases in Ecologic and Individual-Level Studies. Invited paper for the Second Annual Meeting of the International Society for Environmental Epidemiology, August 12-15, 1990. University of California, Berkeley.

Griffith, J., R.C. Duncan, W.B. Riggan, and A.C. Pellom. 1989. Cancer mortality in U.S. counties with hazardous waste sites and ground water pollution. Arch. Environ. Health 44:69-74.

Harris, R.H., J.H. Highland, J.V. Rodricks, and S.S. Papadopulos. 1984. Adverse effects at a Tennessee hazardous waste disposal site. Hazardous Waste 1:183-204.

Isacson, P., J.A. Bean, R. Splinter, D.B. Olson, and J. Kohler. 1985. Drinking water and cancer incidence in Iowa. III. Association of cancer with indices of contamination. Am. J. Epidemiol. 121:856-869.

Janerich, D.T., W.S. Burnett, G. Feck, M. Hoff, P. Nasca, A.P. Polednak, P. Greenwald, and N. Vianna. 1981. Cancer incidence in the Love Canal area. Science 212:1404-1407.

Jolley, R.L., L.W. Condie, J.D. Johnson, S. Katz, R.A. Minear, J.S. Mattice, and V.A. Jacobs, eds. 1990. Water Chlorination: Chemistry, Environmental Impact and Health Effects, Vol. 6. Chelsea, Mich.: Lewis.

Lagakos, S.W., B.J. Wessen, and M. Zelen. 1986. An analysis of contaminated well water and health effects in Woburn, Massachusetts. J. Am. Stat. Assoc. 81:583-596.

Loeber, C.P., M.J.C. Hendrix, S. Diez de Pinos, and S.J. Goldberg. 1988. Trichloroethylene: A cardiac teratogen in developing chick embryos. Pediatr. Res. 24:740-744.

Lynch, C.F., R.F. Woolson, T. O'Gorman, and K.P. Cantor. 1989. Chlorinated drinking water and bladder cancer: Effect of misclassification on risk estimates. Arch. Environ. Health 44:252-259.

MacMahon, B. 1986. Comment. J. Am. Stat. Assoc. 81:597-599.

Mallin, K. 1990. Investigation of a bladder cancer cluster in northwestern Illinois. Am. J. Epidemiol. 132:S96-S106.

Marsh, G.M., and R.J. Caplan. 1987. Evaluating health effects of exposure at hazardous waste sites: A review of the state-of-the-art, with recommendations for future research. Pp. 3-80 in Health Effects from Hazardous Waste Sites, J.B. Andelman and D.W. Underhill, eds. Chelsea, Mich.: Lewis.

McConnell, R., F. Pacheco, K. Wahlberg, W. Klein, O. Malespin, R. Magnotti, M. Akeblom, and D. Murray. 1990. Health effects of environmental pesticide contamination in a third world setting: Cholinesterase depression in children. In preparation.

Meyer, C.R. 1983. Liver dysfunction in residents exposed to leachate from a toxic waste dump. Environ. Health Perspect. 48:9-13.

Najem, G.R., and T.W. Greer. 1985. Female reproductive organs and breast cancer mortality in New Jersey counties and the relationship with certain environmental variables. Prev. Med. 14:620-635.

Najem, G.R., D.B. Louria, M.A. Lavenhar, and M. Feuerman. 1985. Clusters of cancer mortality in New Jersey municipalities: With special reference to chemical toxic waste disposal sites and per capita income. Int. J. Epidemiol. 14:528-537.

Najem, G.R., I.S. Thind, M.A. Lavenhar, and D.B. Louria. 1983. Gastrointestinal cancer mortality in New Jersey counties, and the relationship with environmental variables. Int. J. Epidemiol. 12:276-289.

Neuberger, J.S., M. Mulhall, M.C. Pomatto, J. Sheverbush, and R.S. Hassanein. 1990. Health problems in Galena, Kansas (USA): A heavy metal mining Superfund site. Sci. Total Environ. 94:261-272.

Neutra, R.R. 1990. Counterpoint from a cluster buster. Am. J. Epidemiol. 132:1-8.

NRC (National Research Council). 1986. Data on humans: Clinical and epidemiological studies. Pp. 226-249 in Drinking Water and Health, Vol. 6. Washington, D.C.: National Academy Press.

Osborne, J.S., III, C.M. Shy, and B.H. Kaplan. 1990. Epidemiologic analysis of a reported cancer cluster in a small rural population. Am. J. Epidemiol. 132(Suppl. 1): S87-S95.

Paigen, B., and L.R. Goldman. 1987. Lessons from Love Canal, New York, U.S.A.: The role of the public and the use of birth weights, growth, and indigenous wildlife to evaluate health risk. Pp. 177-192 in Health Effects from Hazardous Waste Sites, J. B. Andelman and D.W. Underhill, eds. Chelsea, Mich.: Lewis.

Paigen, B., L.R. Goldman, J.H. Highland, M.M. Magnant, and A.T. Steegman. 1985. Prevalence of health problems in children living near Love Canal. Haz. Wastes Haz. Materials 2:23-43.

Paigen, B., L.R. Goldman, M.M. Magnant, J.H. Highland, and A.T. Steegman. 1987. Growth of children living near the hazardous waste site Love Canal, New York, USA. Hum. Biol. 59:489-508.

Ram, B.J., and H.E. Schwartz. 1987. Bedford, Massachusetts case study. Pp. 341-367 in Planning for Groundwater Protection, G.W. Page, ed. Orlando, Fla.: Academic Press.

Rhamy, R. 1982. Testimony in the United States District Court for the Western District of Tennessee, Eastern Division, Woodrow Sterling et al. vs. Velsicol Chemical Corporation, Transcript of Evidence, September 29, pp. 2976-3092.

Rothenberg, R. 1981. Morbidity study at a chemical dump - New York. Morbid. Mortal. Weekly Rep. 30:293-294.

Shaw, G.M., S.H. Swan, J.A. Harris, and L.H. Malcoe. 1990. Maternal water consumption during pregnancy and congenital cardiac anomalies. Epidemiology 1:206-211.

Smith, M.K., J.L. Randall, E.J. Read, J.A. Stober, and R.G. York. 1989a. Developmental effects of dichloroacetic acid in Long-Evans rats. Teratrology 39:482.

Smith, M.K., J.L. Randall, E.J. Read, and J.A. Stober. 1989b. Teratogenic activity of trichloroacetic acid in the rat. Teratology 40:445-451.

Swan, S.H., G. Shaw, J.A. Harris, and R.R. Neutra. 1989. Congenital cardiac anomalies in relation to water contamination, Santa Clara County, California, 1981-1983. Am. J. Epidemiol. 129:885-893.

Tarr, J.A. 1985. Industrial wastes and public health: Some historical notes, Part I, 1876-1932. Am. J. Public Health 75:1059-1067.

Velema, J.P. 1987. Contaminated drinking water as a potential cause of cancer in humans. Envir. Carcino. Revs. (J. Environ. Sci. Health) C5:1-28.

Vianna, N.J., and A.K. Polan. 1984. Incidence of low birth weight among Love Canal residents. Science 226:1217-1219.

Wigle, D.T., Y. Mao, R. Semenciw, M.H. Smith, and P. Toft. 1986. Contaminants in drinking water and cancer risks in Canadian cities. Can. J. Public Health 77:335-342.

Wong, O., M.D. Whorton, N. Gordon, and R.W. Morgan. 1988. An epidemiologic investigation of the relationship between DBCP contamination in drinking water and birth rates in Fresno County, California. Am. J. Public Health 78:43-46.

Wong, O., R.W. Morgan, M.D. Whorton, N. Gordon, and L. Kheifets. 1989. Ecological analyses and case-control studies of gastric cancer and leukemia in relation to DBCP in drinking water in Fresno County, California. Br. J. Ind. Med. 46:521-528.

Wrensch, M., S. Swan, J. Lipscomb, D. Epstein, L. Fenster, K. Claxton, P.J. Murphy, D. Shusterman, and R. Neutra. 1990a. Pregnancy outcomes in women potentially exposed to solvent-contaminated drinking water in San Jose, California. Am. J. Epidemiol. 131:283-300.

Wrensch, M., S. Swan, P.J. Murphy, J. Lipscomb, K. Claxton, D. Epstein, and R. Neutra. 1990b. Hydrogeologic assessment of exposure to solvent-contaminated drinking water: Pregnancy outcomes in relation to exposure. Arch. Environ. Health 45:210-216.

Wu, M.-M., T.-L. Kuo, Y.-H. Hwang, and C.-J. Chen. 1989. Dose-response relation between arsenic concentration in well water and mortality from cancers and vascular diseases. Am. J. Epidemiol. 130:1123-32.

Young, T.B., D.A. Wolf, and M.S. Kanarek. 1987. Case-control study of colon cancer and drinking water trihalomethanes in Wisconsin. Int. J. Epidemiol. 16:190-197.

Zeighami, E.A., A.P. Watson, and G.F. Craun. 1990. Chlorination, water hardness, and serum chlolesterol in forty-six Wisconsin communities. Int. J. Epidemiol. 19:49-58.

Zierler, S., L. Feingold, R.A. Danley, and G. Craun. 1988a. Bladder cancer in Massachusetts related to chlorinated and chloraminated drinking water: A case-control study. Arch. Environ. Health 43:195-200.

Zierler, S., M. Theodore, A. Cohen, and K.J. Rothman. 1988b. Chemical quality of maternal drinking water and congenital heart disease. Int. J. Epidemiol. 17:589-594.

6

Soil and Food as Potential Sources of Exposure at Hazardous-Waste Sites

A T TIMES IT IS DIFFICULT TO identify completely the routes of exposure when ill health effects are suspected from hazardous-waste sites. The same problem of determining precisely who is exposed to what compounds and in what concentrations exists for exposure through ingestion of soil as it does for exposure through domestic water consumption, in that direct ingestion is not likely to constitute the sole route. Soil ingestion suffers from an additional complexity. Except among small children, it is unusual for soil to be ingested directly, although adults do ingest modest amounts of soil nonetheless (Calabrese et al., 1990). Unless a chemical is extremely potent, the exposure is unusually direct as with certain occupations, or there is extensive dust contamination of food and residences (the contaminated dust being available to be resuspended in the air and inhaled), contamination due chiefly to exposure to soil is unusual. However, contaminated soil and domestic water can act as vehicles for contamination of plant or animal foods that are subsequently ingested—as is the case for mercury and pesticide contamination of fish and heavy metal or pesticide contamination of fruits and vegetables. The questions of the effects of pesticide residues on foods and the subsequent health risks for children are the subject of study by another National Research Council committee, and they will not be considered here.

This chapter reviews the health effects linked to exposure to contaminants in soil or food, other than those resulting from direct pesticide applications to crops. These include home gardening in contaminated soil, some exposures involving work with soil, and consumption of fish from contaminated waters. Although heavily exposed persons could have a high risk of disease, in general, small numbers of persons have been exposed directly or indirectly through ingestion of foods that have absorbed contaminants from soil or water, or through avocational or vocational exposures to contaminated materials. Studies of soil and food contamination usually encompass many individuals with relatively low or negligible exposure in the "exposed" group. Accordingly, low estimates of risk, as well as low attributable risks in the general population, can be discerned, although some highly exposed individuals can incur serious risks, especially when contaminated soil has been used as topsoil in building construction.

CHEMICAL EXPOSURE THROUGH FISH AND OTHER FOODS

In accordance with Figure 1-1 of this report, animal studies on the consumption of contaminated fish are relevant to this discussion. Animals experimentally exposed to fish contaminated with polychlorinated biphenyl (PCB) congeners and other pollutants display a range of neurologic, immunologic, and enzymatic impairments. Hertzler (1990) reports that rats fed different concentrations of Lake Ontario salmon consistently evidence lower activity, rearing, and other behaviors, when compared to rats fed ocean salmon or rat chow. Studies of the levels of two common pesticides, Mirex and PCBs in rat brain and fish, found dose-related neurobehavioral effects. Cleland et al. (1989) similarly report that mice fed diets of Lake Ontario salmon had reduced immune function, including lowered immunoglobulin, which correlated with elevated PCB levels in the ingested salmon. An earlier study by Cleland et al. (1987) produced both hepatomegaly and suppression of important detoxifying enzymes in mice fed Lake Ontario coho salmon, compared to unexposed control mice.

Regarding environmental contamination of finfish and shellfish and other freshwater species, inadequate harvest management and control is in effect for environmental chemicals such as mercury, lead, cadmium, PCBs, dioxin, and pesticides, according to a recent report of the Institute of Medicine (1991). Regional agricultural or industrial pollution varies considerably and can be substantial in some small areas. One fifth of the fish and shellfish eaten in the United States comes from recreational or subsistence fishing, and is not subject to health-based control or monitoring. One study reported that regular fish eaters have dichlorodiphenyl trichloroethane (DDT) and PCB levels significantly higher than those who are not regular fish eaters (Fiore et al., 1989). In addition, well over half of the U.S. supply of seafood is imported (Institute of Medicine, 1991). Seafood may also be contaminated by bacterial, viral, and other biologic agents (Teitelbaum, 1990). Whether these may be affected by environmental agents is unclear.

MERCURY CONTAMINATION

In 1953, a severe neurological disorder was first recognized among persons living in several villages near Minamata Bay, Japan. Mercury-containing effluent from a vinyl chloride production process emptied into the bay from a nearby chemical factory was responsible for the contamination of fish and shellfish consumed by inhabitants of small villages along the shore. The onset of Minamata disease usually began with a progressive numbness in the fingers and toes and often in the lips and tongue (Kurland et al., 1960). This was followed by lack of muscle coordination, clumsiness, difficulty in swallowing, deafness, and blurring of vision. Spasticity and muscle rigidity often were present. Most cases ended in death or severe, permanent disability. The incidence of the disease for the period 1953-1960 in the total of about 10,000 inhabitants varied from 4 percent for those in a village near the industrial facility to 0.2 percent for those in a distant village. Cats and fish-eating birds were affected, and laboratory animals fed fish and shellfish from Minamata Bay also developed the disease (Tsubaki and Irukayama, 1977).

In the U.S., mercury contamination of fish is especially prevalent in the Great Lakes region; for example, the State of Michigan has issued advisories based on its monitoring of mercury and other contaminants in sport fish (Institute of Medicine, 1991). Since 1983, levels of methylmercury exceeded levels of concern in about 3 out of 4 of the 60 Michigan inland lakes tested. Because of methylmercury contamination the state advised pregnant women, nursing mothers, women who intended to have children, and children over age 15 to eat no large-mouth bass, walleye, northern pike, or muskie from these lakes and to eat no more than one meal per month of rock bass, crappie, and yellow perch over 5 inches in length (Institute of Medicine, 1991). No advisory was issued for men who may wish to reproduce, despite evidence that sperm may be vulnerable to subtle effects as well (NRC, 1989).

CADMIUM CONTAMINATION

The mining and refining of metals such as zinc, copper, lead, and cadmium from ore have given rise to substantial cadmium pollution in several areas of the world. Cadmium emissions in water from mines upstream of farming areas and deposition of atmospheric emissions from zinc smelters have resulted in pollution of soil. Basic food-stuffs, such as rice and wheat, constitute major hazards when they are grown in such polluted areas. The best-known example is the case of contaminated rice grown in cadmium-polluted areas of Japan (Friberg et al., 1985a). River water used for irrigation had been pol-luted by cadmium-containing wastes from a nearby mine. In 1946, *Itai-Itai byo*, the "ouch-ouch disease," was first identified. Its symp-toms were later recognized to be the result of osteomalacia—a soften-ing of the bones caused by a deficiency of vitamin D or of calcium and phosphorous—from chronic cadmium poisoning that developed through the consumption of the contaminated rice (Friberg et al., 1985b). Nakagawa et al. (1990) recently found that both definitely diagnosed and suspected Itai-Itai subjects showed a significantly lower cumulative survival rate than the controls. In the past three decades, a number of epidemiologic studies demonstrated that cadmium soil pollution is associated with a number of diseases. A dose-response relationship between cadmium in rice and the prevalence of tubular proteinuria (an excess of serum proteins in the urine) has been dem-onstrated (Nogawa and Ishizaki, 1979). Further, pH of the water supply can directly or indirectly affect the levels of a number of heavy metals, including mercury, lead, and cadmium that may leach into domestic water (Graham et al., 1990).

DDT

The widespread distribution and recycling of DDT, a heavily used pesticide in the 1950s and 1960s, illustrates how hazards to humans can remain in the food chain. High levels of metabolites of DDT in fish caught for subsistence eating near Triana, Alabama, in 1978 were mirrored in similarly high levels in the persons eating those fish. An initial study of 12 residents showed blood levels of metabolites of DDT among the highest ever recorded (Anonymous, 1979). A subse-quent cross-sectional study of residents of Triana and the surround-ing rural area used a questionnaire and blood and urine analysis for DDT residues. It found a positive association of elevated serum trig-lyceride with DDT (Kreiss et al., 1981). There were no associations with other health effects. Other studies of residents also detected elevated levels of PCB, presumably ingested from fish as well (Kreiss, 1985). Levels were linked with elevations in blood pressure and a host of other indications of altered systemic effects, as discussed in the following chapter. The route of exposure was believed to be to DDT, PCB, and related chemicals derived from industrial waste dumped into a stream. The case was the subject of intense litigation, and after its settlement, no efforts were made to obtain additional health data. This highlights a general problem, which will be discussed further in the next report of the committee.

DIOXIN

Recent research shows that humans who regularly consume fish from certain regions of the U.S. have higher levels of dioxin than those who do not regularly eat fish (Kuehl et al., 1989; Schwartz et al., 1983). A European study (Svennsson et al., 1991) has shown a statistically significant association between reported amount of fish eaten (from polluted waters) and plasma levels of dioxin. Fries and Paustenbach (1990) reviewed potential food sources of dioxins. They conclude that beef is a more important pathway than milk for dioxins.

On the matter of the toxicity to humans from dioxin, the published literature is uneven. In animals, dioxin remains one of the most potent carcinogens ever studied. In humans, the evidence remains mixed, although the burden of proof has recently shifted. A study of the largest cohort of exposed workers ever studied finds that workers exposed to dioxin have increased death rates from overall cancer, as well as from soft-tissue sarcoma and non-Hodgkin's lymphoma (Fingerhut et al., 1991). Many of the previous studies of this problem have been plagued with errors in classification of exposed and unexposed groups, according to some reports, and hence have been biased toward a finding of no effect. Thus, Zack and Gaffey (1983) reported no increase in cancer in a series of studies on a subgroup of the same workers in which the positive finding has just been noted by Fingerhut et al. (1991). However, their study excluded workers in maintenance and repair from the exposed study group; these workers are, in fact, likely to have had high intermittent exposures when repairing product machinery.

Studies of agricultural and forest workers directly exposed to pesticides have also found elevations in non-Hodgkin's lymphoma and other cancers (Alavanja et al., 1989; Wigle et al., 1990). The net result of these studies has been to strengthen the case for considering that dioxin, a common contaminant of some pesticides, does increase the risk of cancer in humans. Although a number of issues remain to be resolved, the risk involved for humans is likely to be substantially less than that predicted by animal studies. Bailar (1991) notes that while the results on the Fingerhut et al. (1991) study are equivocal, they do effectively shift the burden on proof. "The hypothesis that low exposures [to dioxin] are entirely safe for humans is distinctly less tenable now than before" (Bailar, 1991, p. 262).

PCBS

Reports of increasing incidence of tumors in fish in the Great Lakes and other bodies of water (Baumann, 1984) were regarded as indicators of a potential human hazard, especially to groups such as sport fishermen and their families. Subpopulations that consume fish taken from contaminated waters, such as Lake Michigan and near Triana, Alabama, have mean serum polychlorinated biphenyl (PCB) levels several times those found in other general population groups in ranges that extend into concentrations found in industrial populations involved in capacitor manufacture (Kreiss, 1985). Because of concerns over prenatal exposure to PCBs and related contaminants, 236 children born to women who had consumed Lake Michigan fish were assessed at four years of age (Jacobson et al., 1990a,b). Prenatal exposure (indicated by umbilical cord serum PCB level) was associated with lower weight (Jacobson et al., 1990a). The children with the greatest exposure weighed 1.8 kilograms less on the average than did the least exposed children. In addition, tests showed a dose-response relationship for prenatal exposure that led to poorer short-term memory function on verbal and quantitative tests. The effects were not attributable to a range of confounding factors, including lead exposure.

In 1985, Rogan et al. (1988) examined 117 children born to women affected by the 1979 mass poisoning of cooking oil with thermally degraded PCBs in Taiwan, and 108 exposed controls. The exposed children were shorter and lighter than the controls, and had more frequent abnormalities of gingiva, skin, nails, teeth, and lungs. The exposed also showed higher frequency of delay of developmental milestones, deficits on developmental testing, and abnormalities of behavioral assessment.

EXPOSURE TO PCBS THROUGH OTHER ROUTES

PCBs were widely used in the U.S. for two decades, and are now restricted. Manufacture is prohibited, but exposure continues from PCBs used in the past, primarily in electric capacitors. Capacitor fires can produce emissions of PCBs, along with dioxin (2,3,7,8-tetrachlorodibenzodioxin, a common contaminant of incomplete combustion of PCBs). Further, PCBs are a major contaminant at Superfund sites, as noted in Chapter 3.

As an indicator of the types of effects that might be sought in those potentially exposed to PCBs from hazardous waste sites, data from those exposed to PCBs under other circumstances are potentially relevant. Kilburn et al. (1989) studied 14 firemen 6 months after exposure to PCBs and their by-products generated in a transformer fire. Comparison with other firemen not involved in the fire showed that those exposed had significant neurobehavioral (cognitive function) impairment. No relationship, however, was found between the firemen's serum or fat levels of PCBs such as Arochlor 1258 and their type or degree of neurobehavioral impairment. These levels varied widely and were within the ranges described for environmentally exposed populations. There were improvements in some signs after a detoxification program. It is possible that much of this symptomatology was related to toxic by-products of PCBs generated in the fire.

After an office building electrical transformer fire in Binghamton, New York, in 1981, a medical surveillance program was established for 482 fire fighters, police, clean-up workers and others involved (Fitzgerald et al., 1989). Of those followed, 33 percent had never worked in the building but were in the vicinity and were included as a low-exposure control. Over a three-year period there was no reduction in fertility, fetal loss, or excess cancer incidence in comparison to that expected from New York state rates. However, there was an excess of reported unexplained weight loss, muscle pain, frequent coughing, skin color changes, and nervousness or sleep problems in the heavily exposed compared to the low-exposure group. Many of the subjects knew their exposure status and possible health effects, so recall bias could not be excluded as an explanation for these differences. Nevertheless, there were higher mean serum PCB levels measured immediately after the fire in those who subsequently reported excessive weakness, skin color changes, or loss of appetite compared to those without such symptoms.

In a case report, Shalat et al. (1989) described three kidney adenocarcinomas in men who worked for a public utility company and were exposed to PCBs. The authors commented on the relatively young age of the subjects (34, 43, and 56) but gave no details of the population from which the cases were drawn, or the time period of observation.

In a series of studies, Rogan and his colleagues at the National Institute of Environmental Health Sciences (NIEHS) have studied the effects of transplacental exposure to PCBs and DDE (dichlorodiphenyl dichloroethene). The routes of exposure are unknown, but believed to include contaminated soil. In a study of 912 infants born in North Carolina, samples of placenta, maternal and cord serum, and milk/colostrum were obtained and analyzed for PCB and DDE levels (Rogan et al., 1986). No relationship was found between birth weight, head circumference, or neonatal jaundice and PCB or DDE levels. However, higher PCB levels were associated with hypotonicity and hyporeflexia and higher DDE levels with hyporeflexia. In a subsequent follow-up of 858 of these children, examinations were conducted at 6 months and 1 year (Gladen et al., 1988). Psychomotor testing using a scale of infant development was related to the estimated PCB and DDE body burden of the mother at birth. Low psychomotor development index (PDI) scores were related to higher transplacental exposure to PCBs at 6 and 12 months of age, but no relationship was found for the mental index (MDI) score. For high DDE levels there was no relationship to the PDI at either 6 or 12 months, while for the MDI higher transplacental exposure to DDE was associated with higher scores at 6 months, but there was no association at 12 months. No association was found for breast milk PCB or DDE levels and either score. There is evidence that prenatal exposure to PCBs shortens gestational age (Taylor et al., 1984).

In a review, Tilson et al. (1990) point to the similarity of effects from perinatal exposure to PCBs in a variety of species (rodents, rhesus monkeys, and humans). However, humans appear to be the most sensitive species to show adverse effects on development and behavior in the young in terms of measured levels of PCBs. It is also worth noting that such effects were detected after exposure of mothers to PCBs at levels below both the relevant standards for occupational exposure and those for food contamination.

DIRECT EXPOSURE FROM DUMPS

ARSENIC

ATSDR (1989) conducted a human exposure study to determine whether adults or children living near an abandoned arsenic production site who frequented the area had elevated levels of urinary arsenic, and if so whether time spent at the site was correlated with elevated urinary arsenic levels. The only indication of unusual exposure was the finding that three children had elevated levels of urine arsenic. These levels fell after residents were cautioned to stay away from contaminated and potentially contaminated areas.

The Anaconda Company Smelter in Montana operated from 1884 to 1980, extracting copper from ore. Wastes from the smelter contaminated the area surrounding it, including the upwind town of Anaconda (population 10,000) and the closer, downwind community of Mill Creek (population 100). The site was listed on the National Priorities List final list in 1983 (EPA, 1990). Binder et al. (1987) conducted a population-based survey of the Anaconda area, studying the relation of arsenic soil contamination levels with urinary arsenic levels in children. It was known that the children had elevated arsenic levels when the smelter was operating, and they were interested in seeing whether new exposure data would verify several exposure models that predicted that the children would have continuing significant and measurable exposure to arsenic. Soil levels (measured in 1985) of arsenic ranged from 140-1950 ppm (mean = 715 ppm) for Mill Creek, 27-345 ppm (mean = 144 ppm) for Anaconda, to 19-146 ppm (mean = 44 ppm) for Livingston, the control community that was demographically similar to Anaconda but had no history of mining or smelting industries; housedust levels were also measured. Urinary arsenic levels of the Mill Creek children were significantly higher than the Livingston children for both March (66.1 µg/l to 10.6 µg/l) and July (54 µg/l to 16.6 µg/l). Surprisingly, the urinary arsenic levels for Anaconda and Opportunity (6 kilometers from the smelter stack) were not significantly higher than Livingston, thereby contradicting the prediction of the exposure models. EPA (1990) decided to temporarily relocate all Mill Creek residents between 1986 and 1987; by 1988 all residents were permanently relocated.

LEAD EXPOSURE

Mined and processed since antiquity, lead remains a ubiquitous, persistent environmental pollutant that is also one of those most common at Superfund sites. Lead enters the environment through a broad range of pathways, reflecting the diverse uses to which industrial societies have put this heavy metal. These range from automobile and industrial emissions to paint pigments and solder. In addition, lead enters drinking water through old lead pipes, common in many older northeastern cities, through leaching of lead solder applied to water pipes in homes prior to 1988, or through brass faucets that contain some lead. Once lead is emitted into the air, it ultimately settles by means of wet and dry deposition as soil dust and into waterways, where it can be recycled through the environment and into humans.

Natural sources of lead provide a minimal contribution to the total human burden. Levels of lead in the atmosphere now are estimated to be 10 to 20 thousand times higher in some urban areas compared to more remote regions of the globe. Lead deposited on soils can bind to a number of other naturally occurring materials, including other dusts, clays, hydrous oxides, and humic and fulvic acids. Soil is logically the most common repository, or sink, for airborne lead, but it cannot be considered a permanent sink. As with other soil contaminants, once lead pollutes soil, opportunities are enhanced for lead to be absorbed and recycled into the human food chain through grazing animals, home gardening, and general agricultural activity. Also, lead exposure can occur directly from soil exposure to young children who play outdoors, mouth objects on the ground, or engage in extensive pica. In addition, millions of children are at risk of exposure to lead dust from old lead paint in their homes and schools. The amount of lead that can be toxic to a young child is quite small. The average toddler should consume no more than 100 micrograms per day of lead, according to the World Health Organization. In the 1970s, a person running her hand along a table top could acquire more than that amount on her fingertip because of deposits from ambient air. Because such small amounts of lead can be toxic, efforts are continuing to reduce exposures.

ATSDR is conducting a number of studies involving mining wastes. A study of residential surface soils in Leadville, Colorado, located near the California Gulch Superfund site, found that more than 60 percent of the residential soil levels were higher than 1000 ppm and more than 80 percent had levels higher than 500 ppm (CDOH et al., 1990). Soil lead levels of more than 500-100 ppm are associated with increased in blood lead concentrations, especially in young children (CDC, 1985). The Leadville study found that 41 percent of the children had blood lead levels greater than 10 µg/dl and 15 percent had greater than 15 µg/dl. The authors note that the Bunker Hill Superfund site in Idaho had similar findings of 41 percent of the children having levels of 10 µg/dl and above, and 14 percent had greater than 15 µg/dl; the Silver Creek (Utah) mine tailings exposure study found a mean blood lead level of 7.8 µg/dl compared to the 4.0 µg/dl of their control population (CDOH, 1990). EPA uses a level of 1.4 µg/dl as its estimate of background blood level. This indicated that at all these sites, children have elevated levels of lead.

Studies of community residents living near metal smelters have found that their blood lead levels correlate directly with the distance that they live from these facilities (Landrigan et al., 1975; Baker et al., 1977), as have studies of children living near major highways (Mahaffey, 1983). For those Superfund sites that involve previously operating waste incinerators, similar patterns of exposure may also have occurred. ATSDR issued a health advisory for the Caldwell incinerator, located in Lenore, North Carolina, based on a health assessment that found significant elevations of blood lead both in workers at the small incinerator and in residents of the community (ATSDR, 1990). In addition, more than half of the 80 workers had advanced neuropathies. Although this advisory has not been published in the literature that this report generally reviews, we cite it here as an illustration of the fact that such community effects have been documented. Soil lead levels in these circumstances can be an important reservoir for continuous re-exposure of the population.

MIXED CHEMICAL EXPOSURE

Under many circumstances, the route of exposure is unclear. This applies to potential chemical exposures from many toxic-waste sites. One example is a study of residents near a landfill site in Hamilton Ontario, used from the early 1950s until 1980 for disposal of solid and liquid industrial wastes (Hertzman et al., 1987). The study of residents was preceded by a study of workers to help focus on relevant symptomatology. Both groups exhibited mood, narcotic, skin, and respiratory disorders. Although perception of exposure could explain the results of the study, it was the authors' conclusion that the adverse effects seen were more likely than not the result of chemical exposure.

DETECTION OF CONTAMINANTS

Where residents near hazardous-waste sites have engaged in home gardening, residues in their foods need to be carefully evaluated. In order to evaluate these residues, background levels need to be determined. The Food and Drug Administration (FDA) Market Basket Survey consists of four samples of grocery products purchased annually in each of four regions of the U.S., and prepared for eating. In the Total Diet Study, 234 different food items are collected and analyzed four times each year in three cities in each of four regions. Analyses are conducted on chemical residues in this market basket, in some cases evaluating contaminants in samples as small as three raisins, and extrapolated to the general food supply. Comparisons are made between the residues measured and the Acceptable Daily Intakes (ADI) established for individual contaminants. The ADI is established by panels of scientific experts at the FDA and other international organizations and are estimated to be the daily amount of a chemical that can be safely ingested, without substantially increasing an individual's lifetime risk. The FDA Total Diet Study includes very few seafood samples. Those included, such as haddock, pollock and fish sticks, are among the products least likely to include significant lipophilic pesticide or other chemical contamination (Institute of Medicine, 1991). A number of analysts have questioned the validity of applying such a limited sampling strategy to generalizations about the nation's overall food supply (Institute of Medicine, 1991). ADIs are set for individual compounds; the cumulative effect cannot be calculated by such means. In addition, the market basket survey cannot estimate contributions from either imported or home grown produce.

PESTICIDE CONTAMINATION OF FOOD

Accidental or illegal pesticide contamination of food can result in acute epidemics of illness. This is demonstrated by a study of one such episode in California in 1985 (Goldman et al., 1990). Aldicarb, a carbamate pesticide, can be incorporated into the flesh of fruits, and was found to be the source of an extensive outbreak of illness associated with contaminated watermelons. As in restaurant food-poisoning episodes, detection of the contamination was aided by the fact that watermelon was consumed by a group of persons, which made it easier to trace the cause of the multiple illnesses.

Several hazardous-waste sites contain pesticide residues and therefore could be potential sources of foodborne exposure if they were to contaminate nearby areas. To the committee's knowledge, such episodes have not been reported. For example, the Hardeman County, Tennessee site (discussed in Chapter 5) contained pesticide wastes, but the studies focussed on groundwater as the route of exposure (Clark et al., 1982; Harris et al., 1984). While it is probable that chronic exposure of the general population to pesticides is mainly through the food chain (Kutz et al., 1991), accurate exposure assessment of this route is difficult (McKone and Ryan, 1989).

ANIMALS AS SENTINELS

Studies on animals provide a useful additional source of information with which to evaluate chemical contamination in soil. Rowley et al. (1983) studied the natural vole population at Love Canal. Voles were trapped in three areas: I-the immediate Love Canal area, II-very close to Love Canal, and III-an area about one kilometer away, whose vole population served as the control. They found significant differences in mortality. The mean life expectancy after weaning for voles in areas I and II being 23.6 and 29.2 days, respectively, compared to 48.8 days for the control animals from area III. Liver and adrenal weights in females and seminal vesicle weights in males were also significantly reduced in area I compared to area III voles. Also, levels of contaminants such as hexachlorocyclohexane and other chlorinated hydrocarbons were detected in voles from areas I and II, but not in those from the control area.

Another relevant study in this regard was recently completed by Hayes et al. (1990). They conducted a case-control study of Military Working Dogs (MWD) that served in Vietnam during the war, compared with control dogs that served in the continental U.S. during the same time period. They found a statistically significant elevation in the risk of testicular tumors for MWD from Vietnam. Other laboratory studies have also detected a link between exposure to some of the chemicals used in Vietnam, which include dioxin as a contaminant, and a variety of cancers.

These studies of wildlife may be useful indicators of potential exposure at hazardous waste sites, especially for those sites that have previously been used as playgrounds or sites for other recreational activities involving extensive contact with soil. For further exploration of this topic, see the recent National Research Council report on the use of animals as sentinals of environmental health hazards (NRC, 1991).

CONCLUSIONS

Soil provides a usually unrecognized source of exposure to contaminants. Models indicate that adults may be exposed directly or indirectly, through the food chain, and that children incur greater exposures per unit of body weight. Home gardening and ingestion of subsistence or recreational fish can be important sources of these contaminants, according to a number of sources. In addition, commercial shellfish and finfish may also be contaminated. Epidemiologic studies of hazardous-waste sites need to incorporate consideration of soil as a route of exposure.

REFERENCES

Alavanja, M.C.R., A. Blair, S. Merkle, J. Teske, B. Eaton, and B. Reed. 1989. Mortality among forest and soil conservationists. Arch. Environ. Health 44:94-101.
Anonymous. 1979. High serum concentrations of DDT residues: Triana, Alabama. Morbid. Mortal. Week. Rep. 28:123-124.
ATSDR (Agency for Toxic Substances and Disease Registry). 1989. The Crystal Chemical

Company Arsenic Exposure Study, Houston Texas. Atlanta, Ga.: Epidemiology & Medicine Branch, Agency for Toxic Substances and Disease Registry.

ATSDR (Agency for Toxic Substances and Disease Registry). 1990. Public Health Advisory for Caldwell Systems, Inc., Caldwell County, Lenore, North Carolina. July 25, 1990.

Bailar, J.C. 1991. How dangerous is dioxin? N. Engl. J. Med. 324:260-262.

Baker, E.L., Jr., C.G.Hayes, P.J. Landrigan, J.L. Handke, R.T. Leger, W.J. Houseworth, and J.M. Harrington. 1977. A nationwide survey of heavy metal absorption in children living near primary copper, lead, and zinc smelters. Am. J. Epidemiol. 106:261-273.

Baumann, P.C. 1984. Cancer in wild freshwater fish populations with emphasis on the Great Lakes. J. Great Lakes Res. 10:251-253.

Binder, S., D. Forney, W. Kaye, and D. Paschal. 1987. Arsenic exposure in children living near a former copper smelter. Bull. Environ. Contam. Toxicol. 39:114-121.

Calabrese, E.J., E.J. Stanek, C.E. Gilbert, and R. M. Barnes. 1990. Preliminary adult soil ingestion estimates: Results of a pilot study. Regul. Toxicol. Pharmacol. 12:88-95.

CDC (Centers for Disease Control). 1985. Preventing Lead Poisoning in Young Children: A Statement by the Centers for Disease Control, January 1985. DHHS Publication No. 99-2230. Atlanta: U.S. Department of Health and Human Services, Public Health Service.

CDOH (Colorado Department of Health), University of Colorado at Denver, and Agency for Toxic Substances and Disease Registry. 1990. Leadville Metals Exposure Study. [n.p.]: State of Colorado.

Clark, C.S., C.R. Meyer, P.S. Gartside, V.A. Majeti, B. Specker, W.F. Balisteri, and V.J. Elia. 1982. An environmental health survey of drinking water contamination by leachate from a pesticide waste dump in Hardeman County, Tennessee. Arch. Environ. Health 37:9-18.

Cleland, G.B., J.F. Leatherland, and R. A. Sonstegard. 1987. Toxic effects in C57B1/6 and DBA/2 mice following consumption of halogenated aromatic hydrocarbon-contaminated Great Lakes coho salmon (*Oncorhynchus kisutch* Walbaum). Environ. Health Perspect. 75:153-157.

Cleland, G.B., P.J. McElroy, and R.A. Sonstegard. 1989. Immunomodulation in C57Bl/6 mice following consumption of halogenated aromatic hydrocarbon-contaminated coho salmon (*Oncorhynchus kisutch*) from Lake Ontario. J. Toxicol. Environ. 24:477-486.

EPA (U.S. Environmental Protection Agency). 1990. National Priorities List Sites: Montana. EPA/540/4-90/027. Washington, D.C.: United States Environmental Protection Agency.

Fingerhut, M.A., W.E. Halperin, D.A. Marlow, L.A. Picitelli, P.A. Honchar,, M.H. Sweeney, A. L. Greifa, P.A. Dill, K. Streenland, and A.J. Suruda. 1991. Cancer mortality in workers exposed to 2,3,7,8-tetrachlorodibenzo-p-dioxin. N. Engl. J. Med. 324:212-218.

Fiore, B.J., H.A. Anderson, L.P. Hanrahan, L.J. Olson, and W.C. Sonzogni. 1989. Sport fish consumption and body burden levels of chlorinated hydrocarbons: A study of Wisconsin anglers. Arch. Environ. Health 44:82-88.

Fitzgerald, E.F., A.L. Weinstein, L.G. Youngblood, S.J. Standfast, and J.M. Melius. 1989. Health effects three years after potential exposure to the toxic contaminants of an electrical transformer fire. Arch. Environ. Health 44:214-221.

Friberg, L., C.-G. Elinder, T. Kjellstorm, and G.F. Nordberg, eds. 1985a. Cadmium and Health: A Toxicological and Epidemiological Appraisal, I. Exposure, Dose and Metabolism. Boca Raton: CRC Press.

Friberg, L., C.-G. Elinder, T. Kjellstrom, and G.F. Nordberg, eds. 1985b. Cadmium and Health: A Toxicological and Epidemiological Appraisal, II. Effects and Response. Boca Raton: CRC Press.

Fries, G.F., and D. J. Paustenbach. 1990. Evaluation of potential transmission of 2,3,7,8-tetrachlorodibenzo-p-dioxin-contaminated incinerator emissions to humans via foods. J. Toxicol. Environ. Health 29:1-43.

Gladen, B.C., W.J. Rogan, P. Hardy, J. Thullen, J. Tingelstad, and M. Tully. 1988. Development after exposure to polychlorinated biphenyls and dichlorodiphenyl dichloroethene transplacentally and through human milk. J. Pediatr. 113(6):991-995.

Goldman, L.R., D.F. Smith, R.R. Neutra, L.D. Saunders, E.M. Pond, J. Stratton, K. Waller, R.J. Jackson, and K.W. Kizer. 1990. Pesticide food poisoning from contaminated watermelons in California, 1985. Arch. Environ. Health 45:229-236.

Graham, J.A., L.D. Grant, L.J. Folinsbee, D.E. Gardner, R.B. Schlesinger, J.H. Overton, S.W. Lounsbury, T.R. McCurdy, V. Hasselblad, D.J. McKee, H.M. Richmond, B.V. Polkowsky, and A.H. Marcus. 1990. Direct Health Effects of Air Pollutants Associated With Acidic Precursor Emissions. NAPAP SOS/T Report 22, in Acidic Deposition, State of Science and Technology, Vol. III. Washington, D.C.: National Acid Precipitation Assessment Program.

Harris, R.H., J.H. Highland, J.V. Rodricks, and S.S. Papadopulos. 1984. Adverse effects at a Tennessee hazardous waste disposal site. Hazardous Waste 1:183-204.

Hayes, H.M., R.E. Tarone, H.W. Casey, and D.L. Huxsoll. 1990. Excess of seminomas observed in Vietnam services U.S. military working dogs. J. Natl. Cancer Instit. 82:1042-1046.

Hertzler, D.R. 1990. Neurotoxic behavioral effects of Lake Ontario salmon diets in rats. Neurotoxicol. Teratol. 12:139-143.

Hertzman, C., M. Hayes, J. Singer, and J. Highland. 1987. Upper Ottawa Landfill Site health study. Environ. Health Perspect. 75:173-195.

Institute of Medicine. 1991. Seafood Safety. Washington, D.C.: National Academy Press.

Jacobson, J.L., S.W. Jacobson, and H.E.B. Humphrey. 1990a. Effects of exposure to PCBs and related compounds on growth and activity in children. Neurotoxicol. Teratol. 12:319-326.

Jacobson, J.L., S.W. Jacobson, and H. Humphrey. 1990b. Effects of in utero exposure to polychlorinated biphenyls and related contaminants on cognitive functioning in young children. J. Pediatr. 116:38-45.

Kilburn, K.H., R.H. Warsaw, and M.G. Shields. 1989. Neurobehavioral dysfunction in firemen exposed to polychlorinated biphenyls (PCBs): Possible improvement after detoxification. Arch. Environ. Health 44:345-350.

Kreiss, K, 1985. Studies on populations exposed to polychlorinated biphenyls. Environ. Health Perspect. 60:193-199.

Kreiss, K., M.M. Zack, R.D. Kimbrough, L.L. Needham, A.L. Smrek, and B. T. Jones. 1981. Cross-sectional study of a community with exceptional exposure to DDT. J. Am. Med. Assoc. 245:1926-1930.

Kuehl, D.W., B.C. Butterworth, A. McBride, S. Kroner, and D. Bahnick. 1989. Contamination of fish by 2,3,7,8-tetrachlorodibenzo-p-dioxin: A survey of fish from major watersheds in the United States. Chemosphere 18:1997-2014.

Kurland, L.T., S.N. Faro, and H. Siedler. 1960. Minamata disease. World Neurol. 1:370-395.

Kutz, F.W., P.H. Wood, and D.P. Bottimore. 1991. Organochlorine pesticides and polychlorinated biphenyls in human adipose tissue. Rev. Environ. Contam. Toxicol. 120:1-82.

Landrigan, P.J., R.H. Whitworth, R.W. Baloh, N.W. Staehling, W.F. Barthel, and B.F. Rosenblum. 1975. Neuropsychological dysfunction in children with chronic low-level lead absorption. Lancet 1(7909):708-712.

Mahaffey, K.R. 1983. Sources of lead in the urban environment. Am. J. Public Health 73:1357-1358.

McKone, T.E., and P.B. Ryan. 1989. Human exposures to chemicals through food chains: An uncertainty analysis. Environ. Sci. Technol. 23:1154-1163.

Nakagawa, H., M. Tabata, Y. Morikawa, M. Senma, Y. Kitagawa, S. Kawano, and T. Kido. 1990. High mortality and shortened life-span in patients with itai-itai disease and subjects with suspected disease. Arch. Environ. Health 45:283-287.

Nogawa, K., and A. Ishizaki. 1979. A comparison between cadmium in rice and renal effects among inhabitants of the Jinzu River Basin. Environ. Res. 18:410-420.

NRC (National Research Council). 1989. Biologic Markers in Reproductive Toxicology. Washington, D.C.: National Academy Press.

NRC (National Research Council). 1991. Animals as Sentinels of Environmental Health Hazards. Washington, D.C.: National Academy Press.

Rogan, W. J., B.C. Gladen, J.D. McKinney, N. Carreras, P. Hardy, J. Thullen, J. Tingelstad, and M. Tully. 1986. Polychlorinated biphenyls (PCBs) and dichlorodiphenyl dichloroethene (DDE) in human milk: Effects of maternal factors and previous lactation. Am. J. Public Health 76:172-177.

Rogan, W.J., B.C. Gladen, K.-L. Hung, S.-L. Koong, L.-Y. Shin, J.S. Taylor, Y.-C. Wu, D. Yang, N.B. Ragan, and C.-C. Hsu. 1988. Congenital poisoning by polychlorinated biphenyls and their contaminants in Taiwan. Science 241:334-336.

Rowley, M.H., J.J. Christian, D.K. Basu, M.A. Pawlikowski, and B. Paigen. 1983. Use of small mammals (voles) to assess a hazardous waste site at Love Canal, Niagara Falls, New York. Arch. Environ. Contam. Toxicol. 12:383-397.

Schwartz, P.M., S.W. Jacobson, G. Fein, J.L. Jacobson, and H.A. Price. 1983. Lake Michigan fish consumption as a source of polychlorinated biphenyls in human cord serum, maternal serum, and milk. Am. J. Public Health 73:293-296.

Shalat, S.L., L.D. True, L.E. Fleming, and P.E. Pace. 1989. Kidney cancer in utility workers exposed to polychlorinated biphenyls (PCBs). Br. J. Ind. Med. 46:823-824.

Svennsson, B.G, A. Nilsson, M. Hansson, C. Rappe, B. Akesson, and S. Skerfving. 1991. Exposure to dioxins and dibenzofurans through the consumption of fish. N. Engl. J. Med. 324:8-12.

Taylor, P.R., C.E. Lawrence, H.L. Hwang, and A.S. Paulson. 1984. Polychlorinated biphenyls: Influence on birthweight and gestation. Am. J. Public Health 74:1153-1154.

Tilson, H.A., J.L. Jacobson, and W.J. Rogan. 1990. Polychlorinated biphenyls and the developing nervous system: Cross-species comparisons. Neurotoxicol. Teratol. 12:239-248.

Tsubaki, T., and K. Irukayama, eds. 1977. Minamata Disease: Methylmercury Poisoning in Minamata and Niigata, Japan. Tokyo: Kodansha. 317 pp.

Wigle, D.T., R.M. Semenciw, K. Wilkins, D. Riedel, L. Ritter, H.I. Morrison, and Y. Mao. 1990. Mortality study of Canadian male farm operators: Non-Hodgkin's lymphoma mortality and agricultural practices in Saskatchewan. J. Natl. Cancer Inst. 82:575-582.

Zack, J.A., and W.R. Gaffey. 1983. A mortality study of workers employed at the Monsanto Company plant in Nitro, West Virginia. Environ. Sci. Res. 26:575-591.

7

Biologic Markers in Studies of Hazardous-Waste Sites

THE EPIDEMIOLOGIC STUDY of hazardous-waste sites can benefit by incorporating into study designs analyses of biologic specimens collected from people potentially at risk. In accord with the framework in Figure 1-1, this chapter reviews studies of biologic markers in persons exposed to materials like those commonly encountered at hazardous-waste sites and the few studies of persons directly exposed at such sites. Examples of markers of exposure, effect, and susceptibility are provided, and methodologic or other important considerations in their use are presented. The final section discusses some of the ethical and legal issues in the use of biologic markers in studies at hazardous-waste sites.

TYPES OF MARKERS

As defined by the NRC Board on Environmental Studies and Toxicology, a "biologic marker" is any cellular or molecular indicator of toxic exposure, adverse health effects, or susceptibility (NRC, 1987).

It is useful to classify biologic markers into three types—exposure, effect, and susceptibility. A biologic marker of exposure is an exogenous substance or its metabolites or the product of an interaction between a xenobiotic agent and some target molecule or cell that is measured in a compartment within an organism. A biologic marker

219

of effect is a measurable biochemical, physiologic, or other alteration within an organism that, depending on magnitude, can be recognized as an established or potential health impairment or disease. A biologic marker of susceptibility is an indicator of an inherent or acquired limitation of an organism's ability to respond to the challenge of exposure to a specific xenobiotic substance (NRC,1987).

Biologic markers have been discussed extensively in the scientific literature in the past ten years but rarely with regard to hazardous-waste research (Perera and Weinstein 1982; Fowle, 1984; CEQ, 1985; Underhill and Radford, 1986; Harris et al., 1987; Perera, 1987a,b; Hatch and Stein, 1987; NRC, 1987; Schulte, 1987, 1989; Hulka and Wilcosky, 1988; Hulka et al., 1990).

Biologic markers are not new. Markers such as blood lead, urinary phenol levels in benzene exposure, and liver function assays after solvent exposure have long been used in occupational and public health research and practice to indicate recent exposures to these compounds. What distinguishes the current generation of research on markers from previous markers is the greater degree of analytical sensitivity available to detect markers and the ability these markers offer researchers to describe events that occur all along the continuum between exposure and clinical disease. There are domains of biologic response and levels of resolution that were unknown 20 years ago (Schulte, 1990). For instance, within the past few years more than 400 proteins have been identified on sperm. In theory, chemical adducts to these can form and they have already been detected in protamine, hemoglobin, and other vital human proteins (NRC, 1987).

Accompanying these advances in sensitivity is the requirement to consider that numerous factors can influence the appearance of biological markers. All people with similar exposures do not develop disease or markers indicative of exposure or disease. Various acquired and hereditary host factors are responsible for this variation in responses.

Biologic markers may represent signals in a continuum or progression of events between a causal environmental exposure and resultant disease (NRC, 1987). Current technological advances and developments in basic sciences allow for detection of smaller signals at diverse points in the continuum. These markers are generally biochemical, molecular, genetic, immunologic, or physiologic signals of an event. The current method for estimating risks by relating exposure to clinical disease (morbidity and mortality) can now be supplemented by a fuller method, one that identifies intervening relationships more precisely or with greater detail than in the past. As a result, health events are less likely to be viewed as binary phenomena (presence or absence of disease) than they are to be seen as a series of changes on a continuum—through homeostatic adaptation, dysfunction, to disease and death.

The progression from exposure to disease has been characterized by a number of authors and scientific committees (NRC, 1987, 1991; Perera, 1987a,b; Hatch and Stein, 1987; Schulte, 1989) and is shown in Figure 7-1. Along the progression from exposure (E) in the environment to the development of clinical disease (CD), four generic component classes of biologic markers can be delineated: those that show the internal dose (ID), and those that show the biologically effective dose (BED), early biologic effects (EBE), and altered structure and function (ASF). Clinical disease also can be represented by biologic markers for the current disease as well as by markers for prognostic significance (PS). Internal dose (ID) is the amount of a xenobiotic substance found in a biologic medium; the biologically effective dose (BED) is the amount of that xenobiotic material that interacts with critical subcellular, cellular, and tissue targets or with an established surrogate tissue. A marker of early biologic effect represents an event that is correlated with, and possibly predictive of, health impairment. Altered structure and function (ASF) are precursor biologic changes more closely related to the development of disease. Markers of clinical disease (CD) and of prognostic significance (PS) show the presence and predict the future of developed disease, respectively. Markers of susceptibility are indicators of increased (or decreased) risk for any component in the continuum.

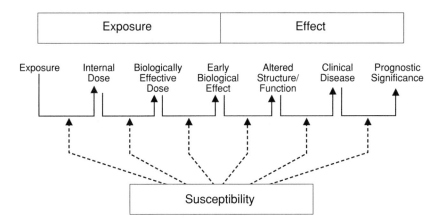

FIGURE 7-1 Relationship between biomarkers of susceptibility, exposure, and effect.

The relationship among the markers that represent events in the continuum is influenced by various factors that reflect susceptibility for occurrence (such as genetic or other host characteristics). These can also be represented by markers. The definition of all the marked events has been elaborated elsewhere (NRC, 1987; Hulka and Wilcosky, 1988).

Some biologic markers of exposure, such as DNA or protein adducts, can be specific. DNA adducts, hemoglobin adducts, and other directly altered proteins indicate both the presence of the xenobiotic substance and its interaction with a critical macromolecule or the macromolecule's surrogate. Validated markers of effect also can be used to resolve questions of whether a constellation of signs and symptoms does or does not indicate a disease or early pathologic process. Moreover, recognition of markers of effect can allow for timely or prudent interventions.

It now appears possible that where valid markers can be found in exposed persons it will not be necessary to wait for disease to occur before an association can be made between exposure and disease. If, for example, a preclinical change predictive of disease is identified, then the same clinical and epidemiologic methods used in traditional epidemiology can be used to determine an association between an exposure and a marker representing the disease. For instance, Hemstreet et al. (1988) found that DNA hyperploidy correlated with disease risk in workers exposed to 2-naphthylamine, a compound known to cause bladder cancer.

Eventually, as an optimistic goal, it should be possible to identify markers of effect that appear very early in the exposure-disease continuum, that is, closer to the time of exposure. Similarly, exposure characterization no longer needs to be chiefly an ecologic assessment, that is, the lumping of subgroups of individuals into a single category or into a few categories of presumed exposure (Hulka and Wilcosky, 1988). For instance, with biologic markers of lead exposure, it is usually possible to distinguish workers and community residents by evaluating the dose to target tissues: This is the true "exposure" that occurs in people with different lifestyles, work practices, physiologic and metabolic characteristics, and levels of exposure. Hence, from the exposure end of the continuum, using biologic markers of dose makes it possible to move forward in time toward the disease end. The classic epidemiologic paradigm of a dichotomous classification of exposure and disease (exposed or not, diseased or not) worked well in the past when exposures were large and effects were detectable by alert clinicians and epidemiologists. However, because it is difficult to characterize exposure accurately by using such categorical descriptors, epidemiologic analyses can misclassify people in terms of exposure. Biologic markers encompass all the exposure that occurs by various routes and from various sources and are thus of great utility for environmental epidemiology.

Exposures to complex mixtures and multiple substances are characteristic of hazardous-waste sites. Perera et al. (1990) have presented a stepwise approach for separating the effects of specific constituents of a mixture. First, external exposure is characterized as completely as possible through ambient or personal monitoring and questionnaires. This provides an estimate of the level and pattern of exposure both to the mixture and to its individual components. The next step is to analyze the relationship between integrated and specific exposure variables on the one hand and total genotoxic and procarcinogenic effect, the broad spectrum of DNA adducts (by the postlabeling assay), class-specific adducts (e.g., polycyclic aromatic hydro carbons by immunoassay), and individual chemical-specific adducts (e.g., 4-ABP-Hb or BP-DNA) on the other. For substances that do not form adducts, other indicators of biologically effective dose can be used. Correlations between biologic markers are also examined. Of interest is the proportion of the total genotoxic and procarcinogenic effect of exposure to complex mixtures that is attributable to specific constituents in the mixture. Also, there is need to know whether there is an interaction between individual constituents or whether the effects are to be additive. The answers could allow identification of the major pathogenic agents present in a chemical mixture.

USE OF BIOLOGIC MARKERS IN STUDIES OF HAZARDOUS SUBSTANCES

Biologic markers have been used occasionally in epidemiologic studies of hazardous-waste sites (Levine and Chitwood, 1985; Phillips and Silbergeld, 1985; Buffler et al., 1985; Upton et al., 1989), predominantly as indicators of effect. In a comprehensive review of the literature, Buffler et al. (1985) identified an array of dermatologic, behavioral, and neurological symptoms that might provide markers of exposure to toxic chemicals, or early indicators of effect. Not counting symptoms or frank signs of morbidity, changes in liver enzymes, which indicate liver function, are among the most commonly used, presumably because of their nonspecificity and ease of analysis. Sometimes these effects are transitory, as with a study of elevated liver function tests (alkaline phosphatase) in persons exposed to chlorinated chemicals in domestic water. After exposure ceased, liver function returned to normal in persons exposed to a variety of pollutants in

Hardeman County, Tennessee (Clark et al., 1982). The possible long-term effects of temporary alterations in liver enzymes are unknown.

Other multiphasic tests to find markers of exposure or effect in blood and urine also have been used, but to a lesser extent. For example, serum cholesterol, gamma-glutamyl transpeptidase level (an indicator of enzyme induction in the liver), and blood pressure have been studied as markers of effect in residents of Triana, Alabama who were exposed to polychlorinated biphenyls (PCBs) from eating fish (Kreiss et al., 1981). Eighty to ninety percent of the levels of PCB found in the Triana study population fell within the range found in other community groups. Results indicated that serum PCB levels were positively associated with all the preceding measures, independent of age, sex, body mass, and social class. Similar findings of an effect of PCB exposure on blood pressure have been reported in studies of workers exposed to PCBs from capacitor manufacturing (Fischbein et al., 1979).

Other studies of environmental exposure to PCB have identified additional markers of effect in children exposed transplacentally (Rogan et al., 1988) or through nursing or eating contaminated foods (Jacobson et al., 1990a,b). Children born to mothers in Taiwan who previously consumed contaminated oil have characteristic skin lesions and pigmentation, lower birth weights, impeded neurobehavioral development, and reduced head circumference (Rogan et al., 1988). Children with PCB levels that fall in the range of background for the U.S. in their cord blood at birth were more likely to be developmentally retarded than children with lower PCB levels (Rogan and Miller, 1989). Jacobson et al. (1990a) found that the highest exposed children on average weighed 1.8 kg less than the least exposed. Follow up studies of these children at age 4 showed that serum PCB levels were associated with reduced activity and some decrements in neurobehavioral performance (Jacobson et al., 1990b).

The development of markers of exposure and markers of effect is proceeding rapidly in the field of neurotoxicology (NRC, in press). Studies that use nerve conduction velocity as a marker of potential neurotoxic effects have been conducted on persons exposed to mixtures from some dump sites (Schaumburg et al., 1983); they found significant impedance of normal conduction linked to such exposures.

More recently, researchers at Boston University have studied markers of neurological function in persons from Woburn, Massachusetts, six years after exposure ceased to trichloroethylene (TCE) (Feldman et al., 1990). TCE levels in domestic water had been from 30 to 80 times higher than the recommended EPA Maximum Contamination Levels (MCL) of 5 ppb. As Chapter 3 noted, TCE is one of the most common pollutants at Superfund sites and also is emitted by drycleaners, household cleaning agents, and degreasers. Exposed and control subjects were studied with a neurobehavioral evaluation protocol that included clinical tests, nerve conduction studies, blink reflex measurements, and extensive neuropsychological testing. The blink reflex indicates the physiological integrity of the afferent and efferent circuitry of the Vth (trigeminal) and VIIth (facial) cranial nerves. A physician using electromyographic equipment, quantitatively evaluated reflex latency responses with an automated oscilloscope for several modalities of stimulation. Highly significant differences were detected between the two groups, with a level of significance of 0.0001. Feldman et al. (1990) conclude that the blink reflex measurement appears useful in evaluating a population group with a history of chronic low-dose exposure to TCE, providing a sensitive method for evaluating subclinical neurotoxic effects on the Vth-VIIth cranial nerve circuitry.

While not commonly thought of as constituting markers, neurobehavioral tests can provide a diverse range of measures of toxic exposures and effects. A battery of neurobehavioral tests has been applied to the study of persons exposed to materials that occur at hazardous-waste sites (Table 7-1). This battery includes numerous expressions of neurotoxic central and peripheral neuropathy and covers a wide array of functions. A comprehensive review of developing techniques in neurobehavioral assessment found consistent and significant neurobehavioral effects and a range of other subtle neurological alterations in persons exposed to metals, solvents, and insecticides, with some indication of greater effects in those with greater estimated exposures (White et al., 1990). Animal studies reveal that TCE inhalation also induces a range of neurotoxic effects in rodents (Dorfmueller et al., 1979).

As discussed in Chapter 6, biologic monitoring for neurotoxic chemicals such as TCE has also identified specific markers of exposure. Levels of metabolites of TCE in urine have been determined in persons exposed environmentally and in human volunteers. About 60 percent of TCE is metabolized and excreted in the urine as one of three compounds, di- and trichloroacetic acid, trichloroethanol, and trichloroethanol glucuronide; a small amount (about 10 percent) is exhaled by the lungs as TCE. The typical kinetics and compartments for excretion or uptake of the remaining 30 percent of TCE are unknown, according to studies that have used human volunteers (Monster et al., 1979). There is no evidence of saturation in humans, that is, an exposure above and beyond which there is no uptake; but studies in mice and rats exposed to TCE in water or air indicate metabolic saturation in those species (ATSDR, 1989). Dichloroacetic acid (DCA) is both a by-product of chlorine disinfection of water containing natural organic material and a key metabo-

TABLE 7-1 Neuropsychological Test Battery

Test	Description	Function
1. Wechsler Adult Intelligence Scale, Wechsler Adult Intelligence Scale—Revised		
Subtests:		
Information	Questions of an academic nature	Basic academic verbal skills
Digit span	Digits forward and backward	Attention
Vocabulary	Word definitions	Verbal concept formation
Arithmetic	Oral calculations	Attention, calculation
Comprehension	Questions involving problem solving, judgment, social knowledge, proverb interpretation	Verbal concept formation
Similarities	Deduction of similarities between nouns	Verbal concept formation
Picture completion	Identification of missing parts of pictures	Visuospatial (analysis)
Picture arrangement	Sequencing pictures to tell a story	Sequencing, visuospatial (reasoning)
Block design	Replicating designs of red & white blocks	Visuospatial (organization)
Object assembly	Puzzle assembly	Visuospatial (organization)
Digit symbol (with incidental learning tast)	Coding	Motor speed (visual short-term memory)

TABLE 7-1 *Continued*

Test	Description	Function
2. Weschler Memory Scale, Weschler Memory Scale—Revised		
Information	Personal information and political names	
Orientation	Time and place	
Mental control	Count backwards 20-1; recite alphabet; count by 3's beginning with 1	Cognitive tracking, attention
Digit span	Digits forward and backward	Attention
Visual spans	Pointing Span on visual array	Attention (visual)
Logical memories with delayed recall	Recall of narrative material presented in 2 paragraphs	Verbal memory acquisition, retention
Visual reproductions with delayed recall	Drawing visual designs from immediate recall	Visual memory acquisition, retention
Verbal paired associates	Learning of 10 paired associates	Verbal memory acquisition, retention
Visual paired associates	Recognition memory for colors paired with designs	Visual memory
Figural memory	Multiple-choice memory for visual designs	Visual memory
3. Continuous Performance Testing	Subject sees rapidly presented letters, must press button when X appears	Attention reaction time

TABLE 7-1 *Continued*

Test	Description	Function
4. Trails	Connecting numbered dots, then alternating between numbered and lettered dots	Attention, tracking sequencing
5. Wisconsin Card Sorting Test	Categorical sorting of cards	Concept formation
6. FAS-Verbal Fluency	Production of words with F, A, and S in 1' each	Language (fluency)
7. Boston Naming Test	Naming objects depicted in line drawings	Language
8. Reading Comprehension Subtest, Boston Diagnostic Aphasia Examination	Screening test of reading comprehension	Language (reading)
9. Wide Range Achievement Test	Reading, spelling, arithmetic	Basic academic skills
10. Boston Visuospatial Quantitative Battery	Drawing objects spontaneously and to copy, clocks, U.S. map locations	Visuospatial
11. Santa Ana Form Board Test	Turn pegs 90 degrees with each hand separately and both hands	Motor speed
12. Milner Facial Recognition Test	Matching and remembering similar unknown faces	Visual memory, visuospatial (analysis)
13. Benton Visual Retention Test	Multiple choice recall of visual designs	Visual memory
14. Difficult Paired Learning	10 paired associates low in associative value	Verbal memory
15. Albert's Famous Faces Test	Recall of famous faces from past decades	Retrograde memory

TABLE 7-1 *Continued*

Test	Description	Function
16. Profile of Mood States	Mood testing on 6 dimensions: anger, vigor, tension, depression, fatigue, confusion	Affect
17. Minnesota Multiphasic Personality Inventory, MMPI-R	Personality test	Personality, affect
18. Interview	Extensive clinical interview re: medical and cognitive symptoms, psychiatric symptoms, personal background, and work and educational history	

Source: Adapted from draft of White et al., 1990, with permission of the authors.

lite of TCE. DCA exposure of pregnant Long-Evans rats by oral intubation produced dose-related cardiac malformations in fetuses (Smith et al., 1990). Other studies of environmental exposures to TCE have found significant associations between exposures to TCE in workers in chemical or paint manufacturing facilities plants and levels of TCE in exhaled breath (Wallace et al., 1986).

There is a growing literature on cytogenetic changes and somatic mutations as markers that indicate either exposures to carcinogens or as potential early effects predictive of cancer (Albertini, 1982; Marx, 1989). Cytogenetic markers, sister chromatid exchanges, and chromosome aberrations were assessed in residents of Love Canal, New York (Heath et al., 1984), but otherwise use of these markers in epidemiologic studies of hazardous-waste sites has been limited.

One potentially useful marker is the T-cell assay for the hypoxanthine-guanine phosphoribosyltransferase (HPRT) gene as a mutation indicator. This assay has been shown to detect HPRT mutations in human T-cells of atomic bomb survivors 40 years after the explosion (Hakoda et al., 1988). To assess the mutational impact of various types of environmental exposures, an HPRT Mutational Spectra Repository has been established (Marx, 1989). This could assist in assessing hazardous-waste exposures. In addition to determining whether there has been an HPRT mutation, it is now possible to identify particular sequences, with a gene, that are mutated (Thilly et al., 1982). This capability may allow for the differentiation of the mutational changes that occur spontaneously in a person's cells from those gene changes that might be induced by environmental exposures (Marx, 1989).

Markers of exposure, because of their accessibility and relative ease of interpretation, have been used more often than have markers of effect. In a number of studies markers of exposure have been used to show internal doses of such substances as lead, TCE or its metabolites, or PCBs in serum. No direct studies on persons living near hazardous-waste or Superfund sites have thus far used more sophisticated cellular and biochemical markers, such as DNA or protein adducts, to assess exposure in epidemiologic studies. However, a number of studies have detected adducts to chemicals that may also be found at such sites (see discussion of Hemminki et al., 1990, below). No epidemiologic studies have been found involving hazardous-waste sites that use biologic markers of susceptibility.

For the most part, biologic markers have not been extensively used in epidemiologic studies of hazardous-waste sites because research has not yet linked cellular and molecular biochemical tests with specific disease risks and with other biologic markers (Heath, 1983). There appears to be no impetus for performing the preparatory studies necessary to take a marker at the laboratory development stage and adequately characterize it for use in field studies of waste-site populations. This latter use requires understanding of the natural history, persistence, background levels, variability, and confounding factors for candidate markers. Also, cost considerations may be pivotal, insofar as some of the techniques involve expensive and time-consuming instrumentation. New technologies will offer some exciting options, which will be discussed further in Report 2.

The Centers for Disease Control (CDC) and the Agency for Toxic Substances and Disease Registry (ATSDR) Subcommittee on Biomarkers of Organ Damage has assessed the potential of markers for use in screening populations near hazardous-waste sites (CDC/ATSDR, 1990). The subcommittee's report discusses markers for the renal, hepatobiliary, and immune systems. It distinguishes tests that are performed routinely in clinical laboratories from those that are used in epidemiologic population studies. The criteria for the usefulness of markers will vary according to their purpose. The report concludes that the ideal marker should be relatively specific to a narrow range of toxicants and that it should be relatively absent or constant in unexposed controls. It should be possible to measure by minimally invasive means that are acceptable to the subject, and it should be inexpensive to measure, especially for intervention programs and epidemiologic studies. The ideal marker should be measurable with high sensitivity, specificity, and reproducibility, and it should yield predictive values with high probability. Changes in the marker caused by exposure to the toxicant should be larger than the normal variation in unexposed populations, and changes caused by possible confounding factors (such as diet, age, gender, and lifestyle) should be known and understood by those who interpret test results. It is important to know the extent to which a marker signals relatively recent or past exposure, the extent to which it indicates peak as opposed to integrated (chronic) exposures, and the extent to which it shows cumulative rather than noncumulative effects. Rarely does any marker meet these objectives completely (CDC/ATSDR, 1990).

BIOLOGIC MONITORING OF HAZARDOUS-WASTE
AND OTHER WORKERS

One of the first opportunities for extensive use of biologic markers will be in monitoring the health of workers at hazardous-waste sites. Even though they wear protective equipment, their exposures are qualitatively similar to those that may be encountered by residents before an area has been certified as a hazardous-waste site. Studies on these workers are relevant to the environmental epidemiologic study of waste sites. The hazardous-waste disposal industry is burgeoning (Gochfeld et al., 1990), and it is covered by an Occupational Safety and Health Administration standard that requires medical surveillance of workers. Site owners and unions already conduct health monitoring, and their experience could be applicable to groups in the community. Like community exposures, occupational exposures often will be to unknown mixtures that can react to form new substances.

The use of biologic markers of exposure generally has been limited to studies that monitor the health of hazardous-waste workers, generally for exposure to heavy metals and pesticides, and the yield of these efforts has been low to date, reflecting the evolving nature of the field (Gochfeld, 1990). Biologic markers of effect also have been identified in occupational studies (Hodgson et al., 1990). Traditional liver injury tests provide insensitive measures of overall liver function and cannot reflect specific chemical exposures. The liver is a target organ for many toxicants found at waste sites. Newer techniques that detect urinary excretion of metabolites and other specific abnormalities need to be validated, so that they can be incorporated into biologic monitoring (Hodgson et al., 1990). The interpretation of liver injury in hazardous-waste workers with potential exposure to hepatotoxins is difficult for several reasons: The true predictive value of the tests for liver injury is not known, the long-term prognosis of transient or minor elevation of liver function is undefined or poorly developed, the mathematic foundations of surveillance are poorly developed, and competing causes of nonspecific liver disease (such as viral illness, alcohol consumption, and minor exposure to hepatotoxins) are undefined (Hodgson et al., 1990).

Although other markers of effect, such as cytogenetic effects, have been used in populations near hazardous-waste sites, they have not been generally reported for workers. One impressive exception is a number of studies that use proteins that show mutated or overexpressed oncogenes in pilot studies of workers in the hazardous-waste and foundry industries. A study of 16 municipal workers engaged in hazardous-waste cleanup showed a serum oncoprotein (ras p21) abnormality not found in unexposed controls, in half the workers (Brandt-Rauf and Niman, 1988). Brandt-Rauf (1988) demonstrated the predictive utility of using protein products of oncogenes as potential markers of cancer risk. Abnormal patterns of oncogene-related protein products were detected both in the biologic fluids of individuals who had contracted cancer and in an individual who later developed a premalignant colonic polyp. At the time of the evaluation of oncogene-related proteins, all the workers surveyed were clinically healthy. Within 18 months, the individual with the abnormal ras oncogene product, who had workplace exposures to PCBs, asbestos, and pesticides and also smoked 20 cigarettes a day, had developed the colonic polyp (Brandt-Rauf et al., 1990a). The ras oncogene can be activated by two mechanisms: point mutations or overexpression of proto-oncogene. The authors speculate that asbestos exposure in this case may have produced oncogene activation by the latter process, in that asbestos fibers are capable of transfecting exogenous DNA segments, such as oncogenes and promoter sequences. Following removal of the colonic polyp, ras-encoded p21 protein was no longer detected in the patient's serum. This case points out the potential utility of oncogene protein products as markers for the early detection of cancer. Additional studies are underway to assess this possibility (Brandt-Rauf et al., 1990a).

Similar findings were obtained in a comparison of 16 municipal hazardous-waste cleanup workers handling PCBs and 17 more protected employees of a state agency, with those exposed showing higher frequencies of various serum oncogene proteins. Nine of the municipal workers had positive findings for fes, ras, or sis oncoproteins compared with two of the state workers. Some of these findings may have been attributable to smoking, but the investigators conclude than an exposure related effect was also present (Brandt-Rauf et al.,

1989). A related study of foundry workers used a new technique for detecting oncogene activation based on immunoblotting for oncogene proteins in serum. In this study, 3 of 18 foundry workers with exposures to known carcinogens, such as polycyclic aromatic hydrocarbons, exhibited abnormal expression of the proteins of the ras and fes oncogenes, in contrast to none of the unexposed workers (Brandt-Rauf et al., 1990b). This approach has promise because it uses only a small amount of serum, and appears to be a general signal for the oncogenic process (Brandt-Rauf et al., 1989).

While the risk of cancer provides a central focus for much research on markers, risks to human reproduction offer another focal point, for which much shorter time periods between exposure and evidence of a related health effect are involved (NRC, 1989). Several studies have revealed that workplace exposures to males influence their ability to reproduce, as well as the health of their offspring. After a group of workers exposed to the pesticide dibromochloropropane (DBCP) had determined that they had all been unable to father children (Whorton et al., 1977), researchers confirmed that the exposed workers had abnormal sperm morphology and motility (Babich et al., 1981). Earlier studies revealed similar effects in multiple species, including testicular atrophy (Torkelson et al., 1961).

A series of studies using refined and automated measures of sperm concentration and sperm head morphology have recently found significant effects on male reproductive capacity related to exposures to pesticides or to general environmental exposures. DeStefano et al. (1989) conducted studies of reproductive effects in Vietnam veterans and reported that those who served in Vietnam were twice as likely to have lowered sperm concentrations and significantly reduced sperm morphology, with longer axis length and head circumference. The number of children fathered in both groups were comparable. However, whether the children of Vietnam veterans may have incurred other teratospermic or genetic defects has not been determined. In this context, it is noteworthy that Silbergeld et al. (1990) report that rats exposed to low levels of lead fathered defective offspring when mated with unexposed females. Thus, male mediated exposures may allow fertilization, but nonetheless convey hazards to offspring. The possibility of germ cell mutation needs to be carefully assessed in these circumstances.

Whatever the mechanism may be, a variety of characteristics of sperm have been detected and found to change with exposures to pesticides and other chemicals, such as those encountered at hazardous-waste sites or through other channels. Markers of exposure or effect can include changes in sperm shape, concentration, pH, viability, velocity, and motility. In addition, protamine adducts have been studied in exposed animals (NRC, 1989), and adducts may also be found for other important sperm proteins. Welch et al. (1988) report that painters with exposures to ethylene glycol ethers had increased rates of sperm abnormalities, such as oligospermia and azoospermia, along with lower sperm counts. Ratcliffe et al. (1989) similarly find that workers with long term exposure to 2-ethoxyethanol, a known animal reproductive toxin, have significantly reduced sperm count, when compared to unexposed workers. Studies of pesticide exposures show similar effects in workers. Ratcliffe et al. (1987) investigated men who had long term exposures to ethylene dibromide (EDB) a now banned pesticide, known to cause reproductive dysfunction in animals. Exposed workers had significant impairments in a number of measures of sperm, including sperm count, the percentage of viable and motile sperm, and increases in the proportion of sperm with physical abnormalities (such as missing heads and abnormal tails), even though their exposures were well below the existing federal safety standard. Further work on EDB-exposed workers confirmed this finding and noted that long-term and short exposure produced distinct effects. Longer-term exposure resulted in decreased sperm motility and viability, and increased cell death, while short-term exposure slowed sperm velocity (Schrader et al., 1988).

Biologic markers of effect, such as alterations in sperm, can be used in studies of hazardous-waste workers and community residents even if the effects have not been related to specific diseases. Such markers show various routes of exposure to a multiplicity of substances and provide an indicator of total mutagenic load, which could have direct implications for reproductive or carcinogenic diseases. In this regard, such markers of effect also can be considered markers of exposure.

GENERAL ENVIRONMENTAL AND OCCUPATIONAL
HEALTH RESEARCH

A broader picture of the use of biologic markers can be gleaned by reviewing the general environmental and occupational health literature, especially the few reports that involve exposure to materials commonly found at hazardous-waste sites. Schulte et al. (1987) reviewed papers published in nine environmental and occupational health journals between 1981 and 1985. The articles are described according to trends (by year and journal) for type of markers, substances monitored, study design, biologic media sampled, and the studies' goals.

In all, 3738 articles were listed, of which 585 (15.6 percent) involved biologic monitoring. This percentage was relatively constant over the period; the highest percentage (18 percent) appeared in 1983, and the lowest (12 percent) appeared in 1985. When the articles were grouped into three categories suggested by Zielhuis (1984, 1985) it was shown that 69 percent of the studies measured a toxin, 19 percent of the studies measured a metabolite, and 12 percent measured an agent-specific nonadverse effect (a reversible biologic change that is related to a specific exposure).

Then the articles were grouped into six categories, the three previously mentioned and three others. The most frequent topics were measurements of biologic substances that were not agent-specific but that caused nonadverse biological effects. This group, exemplified by changes in routine clinical chemistries, could be termed ambiguous effects, and it accounted for 26 percent of studies. Another group of measures of health effects, such as abnormal urine cytology, made up 14 percent of the studies. A third group of studies constituted 31 papers (5.3 percent) involving genetic monitoring and 4 papers (0.6 percent) involving genetic screening. Overall, it was found that 41 percent of the studies measured a toxic substance, 11 percent measured a metabolite, and 7 percent measured an agent-specific nonadverse effect.

Approximately half of the studies involved sampling blood for biologic monitoring. There appears to be an increasing trend in the use of blood specimens for monitoring. Urine was monitored in 28.3 percent, lung tissue in 4.3 percent, expired air in 2.3 percent, hair in 2.2 percent, adipose tissue in 1.2 percent, and saliva in 1.1 percent. Other media, such as breast milk, teeth, semen, bone, feces, liver, conjunctival fluid, and skin, were 14.9 percent of the media evaluated. Each of these other media was examined in 1-2 percent of the studies. Except for blood, the trends in all other media were fairly constant.

GOAL OF BIOLOGIC MONITORING STUDIES

Bernard and Lauwerys (1986) observe that most biologic monitoring studies focus on the relationships between internal dose and external exposure rather than between internal dose and adverse effect. Schulte et al. (1987) confirmed this observation—74 percent of the studies reviewed in their paper evaluate the relationship between the level of environmental exposure and the biologic level of the toxicant or metabolite. Typical among this type of study was the correlation of lead measured in air and the concentration of lead in blood. Approximately 21 percent of studies attempt to link the results of biologic monitoring done concurrently with the assessment of a health outcome. Similarly, but to a lesser degree, approximately 3 percent of studies attempt to link historical biologic monitoring data with a subsequent health outcome. One example is a study that links past levels of mercury in urine with current evidence of neurotoxicity (Williamson et al., 1982).

In 2 percent of the studies (Schulte et al., 1987), biologic monitoring was used to supplement or confirm indirect data on exposures. For example, several studies involving biologic monitoring of heavy metals relate blood and urine levels to job classifications and length of employment or to historical air monitoring records in company personnel information (Hesley and Wimbish, 1981; Hassler et al., 1983; Piikivi et al., 1984).

VALIDATION

Few biologic markers have been validated as tools for environmental epidemiology. The validity of a biologic marker can be viewed in terms of "measurement validity" as used in epidemiology (Last, 1983). Three aspects of measurement validity have been defined: construct validity, content validity, and criterion validity. The construct validity of a biologic marker is its ability to correspond to theoretical constructs under study. For example, if kidney function changes with age, then a biologic marker of kidney function with construct validity should change as well. A biologic marker has content validity if it incorporates the domain of the phenomenon under study. For example, a DNA adduct for aromatic amines will represent exposure from various routes and from occupational and lifestyle exposures. A biologic marker will have criterion validity according to the extent to which the measurement correlates with an external criterion of the phenomenon under study. The two types of criterion validity that have been distinguished are concurrent validity and predictive validity (Last, 1983). A marker has concurrent validity if it and the criterion refer to the same point in time. For example, ambient air measures of occupational exposure to TCE could be validated against breath analysis of TCE. Predictive validity indicates the ability of a marker to predict a criterion. For example, detection of the immunologic marker HLA B27 can be validated against the appearance of ankylosing spondylitis, a degenerative joint disease.

Validation of the relationship between various components of the continuum from exposure to disease involves four levels of effort, as adapted from Gann (1986): (1) the determination of an association between a marker and a preceding exposure or subsequent effect; (2) the location, shape, and slope of the exposure-marker or marker-effect relationship; (3) the threshold of "no observed effect level" if it

exists; and (4) the positive predictive value of the marker for exposure or disease. For example, in validating a marker of exposure, the
first step would be to see whether there is an association between
exposure, such as by air, and the marker. The next step would be to
seek the nature of that relationship: How much exposure produces
how much marker? The third step is an amplification of the second.
Are there levels of exposure that might not result in the appearance
of a marker? Finally, how well does the marker indicate what exposure has occurred?

The validity of biologic markers can be assessed in terms of sensitivity, specificity, event frequency, and predictive value. The relationship
between these characteristics and the frequency with which a marker is
found is exhibited by the equation $m = bp + (1 - a)(1 - p)$; m is marker
frequency, b is sensitivity, p is disease frequency, and a is specificity
(Khoury et al., 1985). The positive predictive value (PPV) of a marker is
the probability that persons with the marker will have experienced the
event it represents. The ultimate criterion of the utility of a marker is
strong positive predictive value.

Ultimately, as discussed by Hatch and Stein (1987), an essential
requirement for a biologic marker of effect is that it should identify
from among all exposed individuals those most likely to become diseased. Ideally, we should be able to observe a considerable gradient
proceeding from left to right in the continuum between exposure and
early biologic change (Figure 7-1). If the numbers scored positive for
the left-most markers do not include those positive for altered structure and function or clinical disease, the marker is of dubious value
(Hatch and Stein, 1987).

It is useful to consider two other definitions of validity: laboratory validity and population validity. Laboratory validity is the characteristic of a marker assay or test system to be sensitive and specific
(Griffith et al., 1989). To be able to measure a marker or declare it
absent, laboratory validity depends on the characteristics of the test
(reliability, accuracy, precision) and on the biologic characteristics of
the marker. Population validity refers to how well the markers de-
pict an event in a population. It does not matter how well you can
measure a marker if there is too little to find among those being
studied (i.e., in a particular sample from a population). Hence, in
assessing the validity of a marker in a population, it is necessary to
consider the prevalence of the marker in the population and the specificity
of the test. Both affect the predictive value. Despite high test sensitivity, some markers will have little predictive value if they have a
low prevalence in the study population, unless they also have perfect
specificity.

Validation studies in humans should include determinations of sensitivity, specificity, predictive value, and the range of normal values of a marker (Schulte, 1987, 1989). Important aspects of such studies are adequate sample size; control for confounders such as age, sex, and race; and variability. It is also important that researchers understand the purpose of the marker, that is, why the marker is being considered and what aspect of the exposure-disease association it is supposed to indicate. It is also necessary to determine the extent that a marker reflects recent or past exposures, peak as opposed to integrated exposures, and cumulative rather than noncumulative biologic effects (Valanis, 1986).

Most validation studies proceed from laboratory evaluations of animals to experimental studies of small groups of humans to larger cross-sectional studies. The assessment of risk of disease or of the ability of a marker to predict disease, however, requires that temporal considerations be included in the design. Hence, retrospective or prospective studies that allow for evaluation of the presence of a marker and of a subsequent rate of disease development are necessary for true validation. Before instituting a large-scale study of the usefulness of a biologic marker, it is necessary to examine critically the initial research on the marker, including the milieu in which the research was done. Early research on tumor markers demonstrates the problems that can arise. Research on tests for tumor markers involves both the laboratory carrying out (and perhaps still developing) tests and the clinicians treating the patients. To generate mutual interest and enthusiasm, neither will have been "blind" to the findings of the other. As a result, the data available in the early stages are likely to be biased or opportunistic (Tate, 1983). To avoid this, it is important that the design of marker studies, particularly at the validation stage, be oriented toward controlling for selection or other biases and that the studies be "blinded."

The validation of biologic markers for use in epidemiologic research requires extensive laboratory work prior to testing in humans. Key to the validation procedure is agreement on what constitutes a "critical effect" (Hernberg, 1987; Perera, 1987b)—one that must occur in the progression between exposure and disease. Exposure to toxic substances results in a range of effects on biologic systems. There is a need to have general agreement on which of these effects are critical (that is, which indicate some aspect of a disease response) and which are merely adaptive. Subsequently, it is necessary to relate critical effects to dose estimates, to determine what factors affect dose and to define a level of exposure for which there is no discernible toxic effect (Hernberg, 1987; Perera, 1987b).

The U.S. Environmental Protection Agency (EPA) has commissioned the development of a decision model for biologic markers of exposure. The objective of the program is to identify and test appropriate markers for use in conjunction with other environmental data to provide better measures of exposure, and ultimately of risk, to individuals and populations (Bull, 1989; Nauman et al., 1990). The 10 steps in the process, which uses a mix of laboratory and field studies, are shown in Table 7-2. After confirmation in tests with animals, the markers will have been shown capable of reliably indicating exposure to a target chemical in a small population for which gradients of exposure are established. The final validation step will demonstrate that results are within the limits of variability defined by lifestyle, disease state, therapeutic agents, and genetic and environmental factors. This effort requires an epidemiologic design and will involve a population large enough to allow the variables to be evaluated (Bull, 1989).

MARKERS OF EXPOSURE, EFFECT, AND SUSCEPTIBILITY

This section reviews examples of the three broad categories of biologic markers—exposure, effect, and susceptibility—to identify some of the methodologic issues that pertain to using markers in epidemiologic studies of people exposed to hazardous wastes. For each type of marker, pertinent issues in the study of hazardous-waste sites will be identified. Not all of the markers discussed have been validated. In some cases, they represent potentially useful indicators. In other cases, they are included only to illustrate an issue.

Whether a marker is indicative of exposure, disease, or susceptibility will depend on the state of knowledge concerning the relationship between the marker and the conditions of exposure, disease, or susceptibility that the markers represent. The allocation of markers to one of three categories is subjective and could change.

DNA AND PROTEIN ADDUCTS, MARKERS OF EXPOSURE

DNA and protein adducts hold great promise as markers of exposure in environmental epidemiology because they allow for measurement of the amount of xenobiotic substances that interact with critical macromolecules. This is of major interest in the studies of mutagenesis and carcinogenesis in which DNA is involved. However, DNA and protein adducts also can be used to measure exposures that cause other diseases that do not have a genotoxic etiology. For example, albumin adducts could indicate a xenobiotic dose to the liver. The

TABLE 7-2   Steps in the Development of a Biomarker

Step	Action Required	Relative Importance[a]
1. Chemical Selection	Prioritize based on occurrence, significant human exposure, potential for adverse human health effects.	C
2. Conceptualization	Identify logical consequence of chemical exposure that might serve as a useful measure of exposure.	C
3. Confirmation of Concept	Experimentally confirm the validity of the basic concept.	C
4. Develop Method of Measurement	Identify method for detecting changes in biomarker at doses at or below those producing toxic effects.	C
5. Biomarker Practical for Field?	Develop plausible field methodology and develop sufficient sensitivity of biomarker to monitor existing exposures.	L
6. Establish Dose-Response Relationship	Characterize pharmacokinetics and metabolism of chemical. (Consistent relationship to systematic dose is critical; knowledge of effective dose is limiting.)	C,L
7. Identify Variables Affecting Relationship with Dose	Establish specificity of response and identify lifestyle, genetic, disease state, therapeutic, or occupational variables that modify the response.	C,L
8. Measures Toxic Effect?	Provides advantage only among biomarkers of equal ability as measures of exposure.	N
9. Validation of Applicability to Humans	Conduct pilot study in small groups of humans with defined exposure gradients to the chemical of interest.	C
10. Conduct Demonstration Study	Determine whether variation in response in larger population can be accounted for by known variables.	C

[a]C = Critical to the application of the biomarker; L = Limiting to the application of the biomarker, i.e., places limits on interpretation of results for secondary purposes, e.g., risk assessment; N = Nice to have, but not essential to the application of the biomarker.
Source: Bull, 1989.

key feature in adduct formation is that the substance binds covalently to DNA or protein.

If a macromolecular adduct is to be useful as a marker of exposure, it should meet the following criteria: Its formation should be able to be characterized by a linear dose-response curve; for single exposures over the dose range of interest, it must be stable enough to accumulate over a specific period; and it must be detectable by existing methods of analysis (Schnell and Chiang, 1990). These three requirements can be influenced by highly efficient DNA repair mechanisms. Rates of DNA repair have been shown to vary between adducts, tissues, and individuals (Perera et al., 1988). In addition, DNA adducts can be "diluted" by cell proliferation (i.e., hyperplasia), a common response to cytotoxic insult (Schnell and Chiang, 1990). Despite these limitations, DNA adduct levels for some classes of compounds have been found to correlate with genotoxic exposures (Törngvist et al., 1986a).

A study by Hemminki et al. (1990) illustrates some of the issues that must be addressed in using DNA adducts in environmental epidemiology. These investigators studied the effect of environmental pollution on DNA adducts in humans in a highly industrialized area of Poland. DNA adducts in peripheral lymphocytes were analyzed by P^{32}-post-labeling and immunoassay. Specimens were collected from three populations: coke workers who were exposed occupationally to high levels of polycyclic aromatic hydrocarbons, residents of towns around the coke ovens (local controls), and residents from rural Poland (countryside controls). Overall, local controls exhibited adduct levels and patterns similar to those of coke workers, whereas the levels in rural controls were two to three times lower. Assays were performed in duplicate, by two different laboratories, and they showed extensive interindividual variations of approximately 10-fold among local and countryside controls and approximately 150-fold among coke workers. This indicates large interindividual variations in exposure to or metabolic activation of the hydrocarbons or in the repair of DNA. Although the results were correlated, there also were interlaboratory variations. The results from one laboratory were generally twice those in the other, but the patterns were similar. Important in the type of analysis was the need to adjust the mean adduct level for age and smoking.

In addition to variability in the frequency and rate of repair of DNA adducts, there is a question of the extent to which DNA adducts in lymphocytes represent the historic exposure of an individual and the biologically effective dose. Because lymphocytes are in contact with many body tissues, they can provide an integrated measure of exposure (Perera et al., 1987; Golding and Lucier, 1990). The variable life span of lymphocytes makes the number of adducts that persist after a given amount of time extremely variable, even within the same person. However, any immune disturbance, such as a common cold, can profoundly affect the number and life span of lymphocytes, so controlling for these factors can be difficult (Golding and Lucier, 1990).

Protein adducts could be better measures of dose than are DNA adducts for some purposes. Protein adducts are not repaired and they tend to persist for the life of the protein (about 18 weeks for hemoglobin). They also accumulate in a dose-related manner (Schnell and Chiang, 1990). At least 60 compounds, including examples of most of the important classes of mutagens and carcinogens, have been shown to form hemoglobin adducts (Calleman, 1986).

The ability to monitor exposure through hemoglobin adducts is limited by the presence in some cases of high background levels that tend to mask the effects of low levels of exposure. The background levels of some human hemoglobin adducts are listed in Table 7-3. As the data indicate, the problem is greatest for methylating agents (Schnell and Chiang, 1990). Compound exposures (different chemicals and different sources of the same chemical that can produce identical adducts) from unknown sources contribute to high background levels. Additional background levels of some adducts, such as those for ethylene oxide, can be produced by endogenous metabolic reactions. The role of genetic characteristics also could affect the formation of hemoglobin adducts. Vineis et al. (1990) report that the formation of 4-aminobiphenyl-hemoglobin adducts in smokers is associated with whether they are slow or fast acetylators, which is a genetically determined metabolic characteristic.

Despite these limitations, several investigators have established a relationship between exposure to toxicants and the formation of hemoglobin adducts and DNA adducts. For example, the studies of Osterman-Golkar and Bergmark (1988) and Brugnone et al. (1986) demonstrate that the extent of in vivo hemoglobin alkylation is proportional to the concentrations of ethylene oxide in the blood, and Calleman et al. (1978) and Törngvist et al. (1986a) have shown that the amount of hemoglobin adducts is proportional to that of DNA adducts.

IMMUNE-SYSTEM MARKERS OF EFFECT

The sensitivity of the immune system to xenobiotic substances could mean that it produces biologic markers of effect that could indicate illness or other damage to health resulting from exposure to toxicants. The immune system reacts to the environment. One challenge

TABLE 7-3   Background Levels of Some Human Hemoglobin Adducts (Average Levels Expressed as nmol/g Hemoglobin or nmol/g Globin)

Adduct	Background Level	Reference
MeCys	16	Segerbäck et al. (1978)
	16.4	Bailey et al. (1981)
	13-34	Farmer (1982)
MeHis	12-42	Törnqvist et al. (1988)
MeVal	0.4-0.7	Törnqvist et al. (1988)
HOEtCys	1.5-4.3	Calleman (1986)
HOEtHis	1.41	Törnqvist et al. (1986a)
N[t]-(2-HOEt) His	0.11-0.29	Calleman (1986)
	0.53-1.6	Farmer et al. (1986)
	0.02-4.7	Van Sittert and DeJong (1985)
	0.17-1.5	Osterman-Golkar (1983)
N[t]-(2-HOEt)His	0.06-0.30	Calleman (1986)
HOEtVal	0.12-0.72	Törnqvist et al. (1986b)
	0.03-0.80	Törnqvist et al. (1986b)
	0.03-0.53	Calleman (1986)
	0.03-0.93	Farmer et al. (1986)
N[t]-(2-HOPr)His	<0.1-0.38	Osterman-Golkar et al. (1984)
ABP-Cys	<0.001	Bryant et al. (1987)
	<0.001	Perera et al. (1987)
	<0.001	Skipper et al. (1986)

"N[t]" refers to the tau nitrogen of the imidazole ring of histidine (also call "N3").
Source: Schnell and Chiang, 1990.

in using immune-system markers is to distinguish homeostatic changes from pathognomic ones (Weill and Turner-Warwick, 1981). Various investigators (Bekesi et al., 1987; Levin and Byers, 1987; Thrasher et al., 1990) have used immune-system markers to indicate biologic response to low doses of toxic substances (Burger et al., 1987). One study illustrates some of the strengths and limitations in using markers of effect in immune activation and autoantibodies in persons who have had long-term inhalation exposure to formaldehyde. Thrasher et al. (1990) compared four groups of patients with controls who had short-term periodic exposure. The patients were residents of mobile homes where formaldehyde concentrations were measured that ranged from 0.05 to 0.5 parts per million (ppm); office workers with estimated exposures ranging from 0.01 to 0.77 ppm; patients removed for at least one year from the original sources of formaldehyde exposure, where exposures had been measured at 0.14 to 0.81 ppm; and persons who were occupationally exposed but for whom no measure of exposure was given. The controls were anatomy students who had been exposed to ambient classroom concentrations of 0.43 ppm. For each group, they determined total white cells, lymphocyte and T-cell counts; T-helper/suppressor ratios; total Ta1+, IL2+, and B-cell counts; antibodies to formaldehyde-human serum albumin (HCHO-HSA) conjugate; and autoantibodies. When compared with the control group of students, the four patient groups had higher antibody titers to HCHO-HSA and increases in Ta1+; IL2+, B cells, and autoantibodies were observed.

The biologic markers used in this study in some instances lack appropriate standardization and preparatory testing for human field studies. The specificity of antibodies to HCHO-HSA has not been documented by reports of appropriate inhibition assays, and no assays have demonstrated that specific antibodies are formed after airborne exposures to formaldehyde. The assays for the autoantibodies are not sufficiently standardized to measure weak reactions reliably. There has been no independent verification of the findings of these assays.

The Thrasher et al. (1990) study illustrates the problems in assessing biologic markers of effect. First, all of the cases were self-selected; the subjects had sought medical attention because of multiple symptoms that involved the central nervous system (headache, memory loss, difficulty with completing tasks, dizziness), the upper and lower respiratory tract, and the skeleton and muscles. They also had symptoms of gastroenteritis. Three common symptoms were expressed: An initial flulike illness from which the subjects had not fully recovered, chronic fatigue, and a sensitivity to odors produced by low concentrations of chemicals. Hence, the case definition is broad and consists of a range of diverse symptoms.

Second, despite the fact that the controls were 5 to 15 years younger than the patients were (and the group contained a greater percentage of males), the investigators report no effect for age or gender, but no data are presented to support the conclusion. Studies of markers of effect are of little use when data are not provided to allow the reader to rule out confounding factors.

Similarly, no mention is made of other confounding factors, such as race; whether all assays were performed blind to the laboratory personnel; whether all assays were performed on blood collected during the same season; and whether the study subjects received more medications than did controls. Third, the study groups each had long-term exposures, whereas the students in the control group had periodic exposures that generally were as high as the exposures of one group of patients. Hence, in comparing study subjects and controls, the marker levels could have been the result of the disease status or differences in exposure, but it is not clear which was responsible. Finally, the lower titers in most cases (1:4 was the most prevalent) make these findings difficult to interpret clinically. In contrast, the patterns of these changes were consistent between groups for most of the markers and generally correlated with putative exposure to form-aldehyde. It is much better to use a collection of immune-system markers than to use single markers because no single marker will accurately reflect the state of the immune system as a whole.

ALPHA-1-ANTITRYPSIN, MARKER OF SUSCEPTIBILITY

Emphysema and other chronic obstructive pulmonary diseases (COPDs) are often studied as end points in environmental or occupational epidemiology. These conditions can result from exposure to ambient air pollution, cigarette smoke, or occupational substances, but not all similarly exposed persons will develop COPDs. A biologic marker of susceptibility, the alpha-1-antitrypsin ZZ allele, has been found to be associated with emphysema. Kueppers (1978, 1984) estimates that the risk of emphysema developing in people with the genetic ZZ homozygote is about 30 times higher than it is in the general population. The ZZ homozygote has approximately 10-15 percent the normal concentration of alpha-1-antitrypsin, and the prevalence for the trait is 1/4000 to 1/8000. The risk for individuals with the heterozygous allele is less clear. Kueppers (1978) reports that despite considerable variation, the prevalence of heterozygous MZ and FZ individuals among patients with COPD is increased. In an industrial community in northern Sweden in which the major pollutants were sulfur dioxide and chlorine from a sulfite pulp factory, persons with COPD were more likely to be heterozygotic for alpha-1-antitrypsin (MS, MZ, or MF alleles) or to have other rare allele types. Ninety-one percent of the 3466 residents of this town responded to a questionnaire about their respiratory problems and were tested for serum alpha-1-antitrypsin. Eight percent of the 3466 reported symptoms were connected with COPD (Beckman et al., 1980). Persons with the heterozygote have 55-60 percent of the normal concentrations alpha-1-antitrypsin. Other, larger controlled studies show no risk of emphysema from one allelic state, the MZ heterozygote (Cole et al., 1976; McDonagh et al., 1979). The population sizes of these two studies were small and hence there was a limitation in the ability to detect an association of heterozygotes with emphysema, which might occur in only 10 percent of heterozygotes.

Available studies do not adequately address the presence or absence of coexisting factors, such as environmental exposures that could be necessary to cause emphysema. In fact, because emphysema is a disease that has several causes, the heterozygous state—although not itself predisposing—could combine with multiple environmental factors (for example, exposure to cadmium, ozone, or cigarette smoke) to present an increased risk. Other genetic abnormalities might increase a person's susceptibility to emphysema, such as mutations in the structural gene for elastin, those that lead to increased protease activity in the alveolar macrophages, those that produce decreased antiprotease in bronchial secretions, and those that alter the structure of the chest wall (Kazazian, 1976; Koenig and Omenn, 1988).

The use of markers of susceptibility in environmental epidemiology has the potential to increase both the precision and the strength of putative exposure-disease associations by avoiding the dilution effect that occurs in populations with a large proportion of nonsusceptible persons (Brain, 1988; Hulka et al., 1990). However, certain practical limitations will affect whether determining a genetic marker in a population is warranted (Mattison and Brewer, 1988). When the prevalence of a particular genetic marker, such as with some of the alpha-1-antitrypsin alleles, is low in a population, even a highly specific test will give a relatively large number of false positives, resulting in nondifferential misclassification, that is, the inaccurate classification of groups to be compared in terms of some characteristic such as exposure (OTA, 1983). This can lead to the mistaken impression that the difference between two groups is less than it actually is. If, however, there is differential misclassification, it can bias in either direction (toward or away from a conclusion of no difference between study groups). The predictive value of a screening test will vary from 0 percent to 92 percent as the frequency of the genotype varies between 1 per 100,000 (0.001 percent) and 10,000 per 100,000 (10 percent) of the persons screened (OTA, 1983). This should be considered in the use of markers of genetic susceptibility in epidemiologic studies.

In some instances the limitation to using biological markers is the absence of markers. For example, the paucity of validated markers for reproductive events and toxic effects is likely to result in extensive misclassification with respect to reproductive performance and xenobiotic exposure (Mattison and Brewer, 1988). Since these types of studies involve both the individual (i.e., male and female) as well as couple specific factors, there is a need for sensitive measures that define the wide variation in characteristics and responses.

ETHICAL AND LEGAL ISSUES

In addition to the scientific concerns noted above, many ethical and legal issues arise in the use of biologic markers (Schulte, 1987, 1990; Samuels, 1988; Ashford et al., 1990). The major ethical issues involve what to tell individuals with "abnormal" marker results about their disease risk, and then how society should treat such people. The CDC/ATSDR subcommittee concludes that when a biologic marker is included in a study, it must be evaluated against established batteries of tests. A separate, statistically valid evaluation of the new marker must be conducted. The marker assay results produced in this evaluation should be used only for marker description and evaluation, and they should not be presented to the study subjects as individual marker assay results until all relevant data have been compiled and reviewed. Results released before the physiologic significance of the marker is thoroughly assessed could cause unnecessary public alarm and spur demand for the test before the meaning of the results is fully understood (CDC/ATSDR, 1990).

The CDC/ATSDR subcommittee also concludes that the evaluation process to find new markers should be conducted anonymously, with informed consent of the subjects and coding of specimens to delete identification of all study subjects. Before a test for a marker is considered to have completed the investigative phases, the biochemical or physical abnormality associated with the marker should be identified, and the probability that the abnormality will progress to disease and the nature of the disease should be known (CDC/ATSDR, 1990).

One suggestion for handling uncertainty about the meaning of markers with regard to health risk is to couple such research with conventional screening of high-risk groups (Schulte, 1986). This offers the opportunity at least to provide study subjects with some information (from the conventional screening) that can be interpreted with a known degree of certainty.

The societal response to people with "abnormal" levels of markers can involve ethical issues pertaining to discrimination, the need for medical follow-up, and the removal of workers or residents from areas of imminent danger (Schulte, 1987, 1990; Ashford et al., 1990). Do people with a certain biologic marker of susceptibility have the same right to be protected against discrimination as do people with other, more visible disabilities? Increasingly, these types of questions will be asked by residents and workers who live or work near hazardous-waste sites and who receive biologic monitoring as part of epidemiologic studies or routine medical surveillance.

Biologic monitoring data can also have an effect on litigation over alleged health effects that result from exposure to hazardous wastes. Ashford et al. (1990) maintain that human monitoring has the potential to bring about a change in the nature of evidence used in such cases. Typically, the evidence offered to prove causation in chemical exposure cases is premised on a *statistical* correlation between disease and exposure. Whether the underlying data are from epidemiologic studies, from toxicological experiments, or from the results of a complicated risk assessment model, they usually are *population*-based. As markers become refined, it will eventually be possible to use them to assess the probability that an individual's exposure is linked to disease.

CONCLUSIONS

The developing science of human monitoring and research on biologic markers offer methods to improve the characterization of exposure to hazardous wastes and detect relevant pathologic changes earlier. Conceivably, the data generated by various human monitoring procedures will

• Increase our knowledge of the "subclinical" effects of toxic substances, thus permitting us to track the effect of a chemical exposure over time and expanding the universe of "medical conditions" for which compensation may be provided.
• Eventually enable us to establish that a particular person has been exposed to a particular chemical (or class of chemicals).
• Eventually enable us to establish that a particular person's medical condition (or subclinical effect) was caused by exposure to a particular chemical (or class of chemicals).

Although epidemiologists could use biologic markers to reduce misclassification or to obviate the need for long periods of study, markers also could be used for purposes that are inappropriate or unethical. For example, the screening of workers for the appearance of "unvalidated" markers and the development of job placements on the basis of results have been vigorously denounced (Lappe, 1982; Murray, 1983). Screening residents who live near waste dumps also can be problematic because it can produce uninterpretable information, promote unfounded anxiety, and initiate reckless litigation—all without a strong scientific basis. Researchers and public health practitioners need to consider these ethical and legal questions before embarking on studies that use biologic markers.

A concerted effort should be made to validate biologic markers of exposure, effect, and susceptibility as applied to hazardous wastes.

This would involve interdisciplinary collaboration on a range of laboratory and field studies to ascertain not only the association between a marker with the event it indicates, but also the factors that affect the marker, the range of normal, and variability.

REFERENCES

Albertini, R. 1982. Studies with T-Lymphocytes and approach to human mutagenicity monitoring. Pp. 393-410 in Indicators of Genotoxic Exposure, B.A. Bridges, B.E. Butterworth, and I.B. Weinstein, eds. Banbury Report 13. Cold Spring Harbor, N.Y.: Cold Spring Harbor Laboratory.

Ashford, N.A., C.J. Spadafor, D.B. Hattis, and C.C. Caldart. 1990. Monitoring the Worker for Exposure and Disease: Scientific, Legal and Ethical Considerations in the Use of Biomarkers. Baltimore: Johns Hopkins University Press.

ATSDR (Agency for Toxic Substances and Disease Registry). 1989. Toxicological Profile for Trichloroethylene. Atlanta, Ga.: Agency for Toxic Substances and Disease Registry.

Babich, H., D.L. Davis, and G. Stotzky. 1981. Dibromochloropropane (DBCP): A review. Sci. Total Environ. 17:207-221.

Bailey, E., T.A. Connors, P. B. Farmer, S. M. Gorf, and J. Rickard. 1981. Methylation of cysteine in hemoglobin following exposure to methylating agents. Cancer Res. 1:2514-2517.

Beckman, G., L. Beckman, B. Mikaelsson, O. Rudolphi, N. Stjernberg, and L.G. Wiman. 1980. Alpha^1-antitrypsin types and chronic obstructive lung disease in an industrial community in northern Sweden. Hum. Hered. 30:299-306.

Bekesi, J.G., J.P. Roboz, A. Fischbein, and P. Mason. 1987. Immunotoxicology: Environmental contamination by polybrominated biphenyls and immune dysfunction among residents of the State of Michigan. Cancer Detect. Prev. Suppl. 1: 29-37.

Bernard, A., and R. Lauwerys. 1986. Present status and trends in biological monitoring of exposure to industrial chemicals. J. Occup. Med. 28:558-562.

Brain, J.D. 1988. Introduction. Pp. 1-5 in Variations in Susceptibility to Inhaled Pollutants, J.D. Brain et al., eds. Baltimore: Johns Hopkins University Press.

Brandt-Rauf, P.W. 1988. New markers for monitoring occupational cancer: The example of oncogene proteins. J. Occup. Med. 30:399-404.

Brandt-Rauf, P.W., and H.L Niman. 1988. Serum screening for oncogene proteins in workers exposed to PCBs. Br. J. Ind. Med. 45:689-693.

Brandt-Rauf, P.W., S. Smith, H.L. Niman, M.D. Goldstein, and E. Favata. 1989. Serum oncogene proteins in hazardous-waste workers. J. Soc. Occup. Med. 39:141-143.

Brandt-Rauf, P.W., H.L. Niman, and S.J. Smith. 1990a. Correlation between serum oncogene protein expression and the development of neoplastic disease in a worker exposed to carcinogens. J Royal Soc. Med. 83:594-595.

Brandt-Rauf, P.W., S. Smith, F.P. Perera, H.L. Niman, W. Yohannan, K. Hemminki, and R.M. Santella. 1990b. Serum oncogene proteins in foundry workers. J. Soc. Occup. Med. 40:11-14.

Brugnone, F., L. Perbellini, G.B. Faccini, F. Pasini, G.B. Bartolucci, and E. DeRosa. 1986. Ethylene oxide exposure: Biological monitoring by analysis of alveolar air and blood. Int. Arch. Occup. Environ. Health 58:105-112.

Bryant, M.S., P.L. Skipper, S.R. Tannenbaum, and M. Maclure. 1988. Hemoglobin adducts of 4-aminobiphenyl in smokers and non-smokers. Cancer Res. 47:602-608.

Buffler, P.A., M. Crane, and M.M. Key. 1985. Possibilities of detecting health effects by studies of populations exposed to chemicals from waste disposal sites. Environ. Health Perspect. 62:423-456.

Bull, R.J. 1988. Decision Model for the Development of Biomarkers of Exposure. U.S. EPA 600/X-89/163. Las Vegas: Environmental Monitoring Systems Laboratory, U.S. Environmental Protection Agency.

Burger, E.J., R.G. Tardiff, and J.A. Bellanti, eds. 1987. Environmental Chemical Exposures and Immune System Integrity. Princeton, N.J.: Princeton Scientific.

Calleman, C.J. 1986. Monitoring of background levels of hydroxyethyl adducts in human hemoglobin. Pp. 261-270 in Genetic Toxicology of Environmental Chemicals, Part B, Genetic Effects and Applied Mutagenesis. New York: Alan K. Liss

Calleman, C.J., L. Ehrenberg, B. Jansson, S. Osterman-Golkar, D. Segerback, K. Svensson, and C.A. Wachtmeister. 1978. Monitoring and risk assessment by means of alkyl groups in hemoglobin in persons occupationally exposed to ethylene oxide. J. Environ. Pathol. Toxicol. 2:427-442.

CDC/ATSDR (Center for Disease Control/Agency for Toxic Substances and Disease Registry Subcommittee on Biomarkers of Organ Damage and Dysfunction). 1990. Summary Report. August 27. Atlanta, Ga.

Clark, C.S., C.R. Meyer, P.S. Gartside, V.A. Majeti, B. Specker, W.F. Balistreri, and V. Elia. 1982. An environmental health survey of drinking water contamination by leachate from a pesticide waste dump in Hardeman County, Tennessee. Arch. Environ. Health 37:9-18.

Cole, R.B., N.C. Nevin, G. Blundell, J.D. Merrett, J.R. McDonald, and W.P. Johnston. 1976. Relation of alpha-1-antitrypsin phenotype to the performance of pulmonary function tests and to the prevalence of respiratory illness in a working population. Thorax 31:149-157.

CEQ (Council on Environmental Quality, Executive Office of the President). 1985. Report on Long-Term Environmental Research and Development. Washington, D.C.: Executive Office of the President.

DeStefano, F., J.L. Annest, M. Kresnow, S.M. Schrader, and D. Katz. 1989. Semen characteristics of Vietnam veterans. Reprod. Toxicol. 3:165-173.

Dorfmueller, M.A., S.P. Henne, R.G. York, R.L. Bornschein, and J.M. Manson. 1979. Evaluation of teratogenicity and behavioral toxicity with inhalation exposure of maternal rats to trichloroethylene. Toxicology 14:153-166.

Farmer, P.B. 1982. The occurrence of S-methylcysteine in the hemoglobin of normal untreated animals. Pp. 169-175 in Indicators of Genotoxic Exposure, B.A. Bridges, B.E. Butterworth, and I.B. Weinstein, eds. Banbury Report 13. Cold Spring Harbor, N.Y.: Cold Spring Harbor Laboratory.

Farmer, P.B., E. Bailey, S.M. Gorf, M. Törngvist, S. Osterman-Golkar, A. Kautiainen, and D.P. Lewis-Enright. 1986. Monitoring human exposure to ethylene oxide by the determination of haemoglobin adducts using gas chromatography-mass spectrometry. Carcinogenesis 7:637-640.

Feldman, R.G., J. Chirico-Post, and S.P. Proctor. 1988. Blink reflex latency after exposure to trichloroethylene in well water. Arch. Environ. Health 43:143-148.

Fischbein, A., M.S. Wolff, R. Lilis, J. Thornton, and I.J. Selikoff. 1979. Clinical findings among PCB exposed capacitor manufacturing workers. Ann. N.Y Acad. Sci. 320: 703-715.

Fowle, J.R. III. 1984. Workshop Proceedings: Approaches to Improving the Assessment of Human Genetic Risk—Human Biomonitoring. Report No. EPA/60019/84-016. Washington, D.C.: Office of Health and Environment Assessment, U.S. Environmental Protection Agency.

Gann, P. 1986. Use and misuse of existing data bases in environmental epidemiology:

The case of air pollution. Pp. 109-122 in Environmental Epidemiology, F.C. Topfler, and G.F. Craun, eds. Chelsea: Lewis.

Gochfield, M. 1990. Biological monitoring of hazardous waste workers: Metals. Occup. Med. 5:25-31.

Gochfield, M., V. Campbell, and P.A. Landsbergis. 1990. Demography of the hazardous waste industry. Occup. Med. 5:9-24.

Golding, J.M., and G.W. Lucier. 1990. Protein and DNA adducts. Pp. 78-104 in Biological Markers in Epidemiology, B.S. Hulka, T.C. Wilcosky, and J.D. Griffith, eds. New York: Oxford University Press.

Griffith, J., R.C. Duncan, and B.S. Hulka. 1989. Biochemical and biological markers: Implications for epidemiologic studies. Arch. Environ. Health 44:375-381.

Hakoda, M., M. Akiyama, S. Kyoizumi, A.A. Awa, M. Yamakido, and M. Otake. 1988. Increased somatic cell mutant frequency in atomic bomb survivors. Mutat. Res. 201:39-48.

Harris, C.C., A. Weston, J.C. Willey, G.E. Trivers, and D.L. Mann. 1987. Biochemical and molecular epidemiology of human cancer: Indicators of carcinogen exposure, DNA damage, and genetic predisposition. Environ. Health Perspect. 75:109-119.

Hassler, E., B. Lind, and M. Piscator. 1983. Cadmium in blood and urine related to present and past exposure. A study of workers in an alkaline battery factory. Br. J. Ind. Med. 40:420-425.

Hatch, M.C., and Z.A. Stein. 1987. The role of epidemiology in assessing chemical-induced disease. Pp. 303-314 in Mechanisms of Cell Injury: Implications for Human Health, B.A. Fowler, ed. New York: John Wiley and Sons.

Heath, C.W., Jr. 1983. Field epidemiologic studies of populations exposed to waste dumps. Environ. Health Perspect. 48:3-7.

Heath, C.W., Jr., M.A. Nade, M.M. Zack Jr., A.T.L. Chen, M.A. Bender, and J. Preston. 1984. Cytogenic findings in persons living near the Love Canal. J. Am. Med. Assoc. 251:1437-1440.

Hemstreet, G.P., P.A. Schulte, K. Ringen, W. Stringer, and E.B. Altekruse. 1988. DNA hyperploidy as a marker for biological response to bladder carcinogen exposure. Int. J. Cancer 42:817-820.

Hemminki, K, E. Grzybowska, M. Chorazy, K. Twardowska-Saucaha, J.W. Srozynski, K.L. Putman, K. Randerath, D.M. Phillips, A. Hewer, R.M. Santella, T.L. Young, and F.P. Perera. 1990. DNA adducts in humans environmentally exposed to aromatic compounds in an industrial area in Poland. Carcinogenesis 11:1229-1231.

Hernberg, S. 1987. Validation of biological monitoring tests. Pp. 41-49 in Occupational and Environmental Chemical Hazards: Cellular and Biochemical Indices for Monitoring Toxicity, V. Foa et al., eds. Chichester, Eng.: Ellis Horwood Ltd.

Hesley, K.L., and G. H. Wimbish. 1981. Blood lead and zinc protoporphyrin in lead industry workers. Am. Ind. Hyg. Assoc. J. 42:42-46.

Hodgson, M.J., B.M. Goodman-Klein, and D.H. van Thiel. 1990. Evaluating the liver in hazardous waste workers. Occup. Med. 5:67-78.

Hulka, B.S., and T. Wilcosky. 1988. Biological markers in epidemiologic research. Arch. Environ. Health 43:83-89.

Hulka, B.S., T.C. Wilcosky, and J.D. Griffith, eds. 1990. Biological Markers in Epidemiology. New York: Oxford University Press.

Jacobson, S.L., S.W. Jacobson, and H.E.B. Humphrey. 1990a. Effects of exposure to PCBs and related compounds on growth and activity in children. Neurotox. Teratology 12:319-326.

Jacobson, J.L., S.W. Jacobson, and H.E.B. Humphrey. 1990b. Effects of in utero expo-

252 ENVIRONMENTAL EPIDEMIOLOGY

sure to polychlorinated biphenyls and related contaminants on cognitive functioning in young children. J. Pediatr. 116:38-45.

Kazazian, H.H. , Jr. 1976. A geneticist's view of lung disease. Am. Rev. Respir. Dis. 113:261-266.

Khoury, M.J., C.A. Newill, and G.A. Chase. 1985. Epidemiologic evaluation of screening for risk factors: Application to genetic screening. Am. J. Public Health 75:1204-1208.

Koenig, J.Q., and G.S. Omenn. 1988. Genetic factors. Pp. 59-88 in Variations in Susceptibility to Inhaled Pollutants, J.D. Brain et al., eds. Baltimore: Johns Hopkins University Press.

Kreiss, K., M.M. Zack, R.D. Kimbrough, L.L. Needham, A.L. Smrek, and B.T. Jones. 1981. Association of blood pressure and polychlorinated biphenyl levels. J. Am. Med. Assoc. 245:2505-2509.

Kueppers, F. 1978. Inherited differences in alpha$_1$-antitrypsin. Pp. 23-74 in Genetic Determinants of Pulmonary Disease, S. Litwin, ed. New York: Marcel Dekker.

Kueppers, F. 1984. The effect of smoking on the development of emphysema in alpha$_1$-antitrypsin deficiency. Pp. 345-358 in The Role of Genetic Predisposition in Responses to Chemical Exposures, G.S. Omenn and H. Gelboin, eds. Cold Spring Harbor, N.Y.: Cold Spring Harbor Laboratory.

Lappe, M. 1982. Ethical and social aspects of screening for genetic disease. N. Engl. J. Med. 206:1129-1132.

Last, J.M., ed. 1983. A Dictionary of Epidemiology. New York: Oxford University Press.

Levin, A.S., and V.S. Byers. 1987. Environmental illness: A disorder of immune regulation. Occup. Med. 2:669-681.

Levine, R., and D.D. Chitwood. 1985. Public health investigations of hazardous organic chemical waste disposal in the United States. Environ. Health Perspect. 62:415-422.

Marx, J.L. 1989. Detecting mutations in human genes. Science 243:737-738.

Mattison, D.R., and D.W. Brewer. 1988. Computer modelling of human fertility: The impact of reproductive heterogeneity on measures of fertility. Reprod. Toxicol. 2:253-271.

McDonagh, D.J., S.P. Nathan, R.J. Knudson, and M.D. Lebowitz. 1979. Assessment of alpha-1-antitrypsin deficiency heterozygosity as a risk factor in the etiology of emphysema. Physiological comparison of adult normal and heterozygous protease inhibitor. J. Clin. Invest. 63:299-309.

Monster, A.C., G. Boersma, and W.C. Duba. 1979. Kinetics of TCE in repeated exposure of volunteers. Intl. Arch. Occup. Environ. Health 42:283-292.

Murray, T.H. 1983. Warning: Screening workers for genetic risk. Hastings Center Rep. 13:5-8.

NRC (National Research Council). 1987. Biologic markers in environmental health research. Environ Health Perspect. 74:3-9.

NRC (National Research Council). 1989. Biologic Markers in Reproductive Toxicology. Washington, D.C.: National Academy Press.

NRC (National Research Council). 1991. Human Exposure Assessment for Airborne Pollutants. Washington, D.C.: National Academy Press.

NRC (National Research Council). In press. Environmental Neurotoxicology. Washington, D.C.: National Academy Press.

Nauman, C.A., J.N. Blancato, and R.J. Bull. 1990. Decision model for exposure biomarkers. Pp. 514-525 in Proceedings of the EPA/A & WMA specialty conference, Total Exposure Assessment Methodology. Pittsburgh: Air & Waste Management Association.

Osterman-Golkar, S., 1983. Tissue doses in man: Implications in risk assessment. Pp.

289-298 in Developments in the Science and Practice of Toxicology, A.W. Hayes, R.C. Schnell, and T.S. Miya, eds. New York: Elsevier Science.

Osterman-Golkar, S., and E. Bergmark. 1988. Occupational exposure to ethylene oxide. Relation between in vivo dose and exposure dose. Scand. J. Work Environ. Health 14:372-377.

Osterman-Golkar, S., E. Bailey, P.B. Farmer, S.M. Gorf, and J.H. Lamb. 1984. Monitoring exposure to propylene oxide through the determination of hemoglobin alkylation. Scan. J. Work Environ. Health 10:99-102.

OTA (U.S. Congress, Office of Technology Assessment). 1983. The Role of Genetic Testing in the Prevention of Occupational Disease. OTA-BA-194. Washington, D.C.: U.S. Government Printing Office.

Perera, F.P. 1987a. Molecular epidemiology: A novel approach to the investigation of pollutant-related chronic disease. Pp. 61-88 in Environmental Impacts on Human Health: The Agenda for Long-Term Research and Development, S. Draggan, J.J. Cohrssen, and R.C. Morrison, eds. New York: Praeger.

Perera, F.P. 1987b. The potential usefulness of biological markers in risk assessment. Environ. Health Perspect. 76:141-145.

Perera, F.P., and I.B. Weinstein. 1982. Molecular epidemiology and carcinogen-DNA adduct detection. New approaches to studies of human cancer causation. J. Chronic Dis. 35:581-600.

Perera, F.P., R.M. Santella, D. Brenner, M.C. Poirer, A.A. Munshi, H.K. Fischman, and J. Van Ryzin. 1987. DNA adducts, protein adducts and sister chromatid exchange in cigarette smokers and nonsmokers. J. Natl. Cancer Inst. 79:449-456.

Perera, F.P., K. Herminki, T.L. Young, D. Brenner, G. Kelly, and R. Santella. 1988. Detection of polycyclic aromatic hydrocarbon-DNA adducts in white blood cells in foundry workers. Cancer Res. 48:2288-2291.

Perera, F., A. Jeffrey, R.M. Santella, D. Brenner, J. Mayer, L. Latriano, S. Smith, T.L. Young, W.Y. Tsai, K. Hemminki, and P. Brandt-Rauf. 1990. Macromolecular adducts and related biomarkers in biomonitoring and epidemiology of complex exposures. IARC Sci. Publ. 104:164-180.

Phillips, A.M., and E.K. Silbergeld. 1985. Health effects studies of exposure from hazardous waste site—Where are we today? Am. J. Ind. Med. 8:1-7.

Piikivi, L., H. Hanninen, T. Martelin, and P. Mantere. 1984. Psychological performance and long-term exposure to mercury vapors. Scand. J. Work Environ. Health 10:35-41.

Ratcliffe, J.M., S.M. Schrader, K. Steenland, D.E. Clapp, T.W. Turner, and R.W. Hornung. 1987. Semen quality in papaya workers with long term exposure to ethylene dibromide. Br. J. Ind. Med. 44:317-326.

Ratcliffe, J.M., S.M. Schrader, D.E. Clapp, W.E. Halperin, T.W. Turner, and R.W. Hornung. 1989. Semen quality in workers exposed to 2-ethoxyethanol. Br. J. Ind. Med. 46:399-406.

Rogan, W.J., and R.W. Miller. 1989. Prenatal exposure to polychlorinated biphenyls. Lancet 2(8673):1216.

Rogan, W.J., B.C. Gladen, K. L. Hung, S.L. Koong, L.Y. Shih, J.S. Taylor, Y.C. Wu, D. Yang, N.B. Ragan, and C.C. Hsu. 1988. Congenital poisoning by polychlorinated biphenyls and their contaminants in Taiwan. Science. 241:334-336.

Samuels, S.W. 1988. The arrogance of intellectual power. Pp. 113-120 in Phenotypic Variation in Populations: Relevance to Risk Assessment, A.D. Woodhead, M.A. Bender, and R.C. Leonard, eds. New York: Plenum Press.

Schaumburg, H.H., P.S. Spencer, and J.C. Arezzo. 1983. Monitoring potential neurotoxic effects of hazardous waste disposal. Environ. Health Perspect. 48:61-64.

Schnell, F.C., and T.C. Chiang. 1990. Protein Adduct-Forming Chemicals for Exposure Monitoring: Literature Summary and Recommendations. EPA 600/4-90/007. Las Vegas: Environmental Monitoring Systems Laboratory, U.S. Environmental Protection Agency.

Schrader, S.M., T.W. Turner, and J.M. Ratcliffe. 1988. The effects of ethylene dibromide on semen quality: A comparison of short-term and chronic exposure. Reprod. Toxicol. 2:191-198.

Schulte, P.A. 1986. Problems in the notification and screening of workers at high risk of disease. J. Occup. Med. 28:1-7.

Schulte, P.A. 1987. Methodologic issues in the use of biologic markers in epidemiologic research. Am. J. Epidemiol. 126:1006-1016.

Schulte, P.A. 1989. A conceptual framework for the validation and use of biological markers. Environ. Res. 48:129-144.

Schulte, P.A. 1990. Contribution of Biological Markers to Occupational Health: Keynote Address, 23rd International Conference on Occupational Health, held 22-28 September in Montreal, Canada.

Schulte, P.A., W.E. Halperin, M. Herrick, and L.B. Coinnally. 1987. The current focus of biological monitoring. Pp. 50-60 in Occupational and Environmental Chemical Hazards, V. Foa et al., eds. Chichester, Eng.: Ellis Horwood.

Segerbäck, D., C.J. Calleman, L. Ehrenberg, G. Lofroth, and S. Osterman-Golkar. 1978. Evaluation of genetic risks of alkylating agents. IV. Quantitative determination of alkylated amino acids in hemoglobin as a measure of the dose after treatment of mice with methyl methanesulfonate. Mutat. Res. 49:71-82.

Silbergeld, E., M. Akkerman, B. Fowler, E. Alberquerque, and M. Alkondon. 1990. Lead: Male Mediated Effects on Reproduction and Neurodevelopment. Paper presented at the Annual Meeting of the American Public Health Association, New York City, October 2, 1990.

Skipper, P.L., M.S. Bryant, S.R. Tannenbaum, and J.D. Groopman. 1986. Analytical methods for assessing exposure to 4-aminobiphenyl based on protein adduct formation. J. Occup. Med. 28:643-646.

Smith, M.K., J.L. Randall, E.J. Read, J.A. Stober, and R.G. York. 1990. Developmental effects of dichloroacetic acid in Long-Evans rats. Teratology 39:480.

Tate, H. 1983. Assessing tumor markers. Stat. Med. 2:217-222.

Thilly, W.G., P-M. Leong, and T.S. Skopek. 1982. Potential of mutational spectra for diagnosing the cause of genetic change in human cell populations. Pp. 453-465 in Indicators of Genotoxic Exposure , B.A. Bridges, B.E. Butterworth, and I.B. Weinstein, eds. Banbury Report 13. Cold Spring Harbor, N.Y.: Cold Spring Harbor Laboratory.

Thasher, J.D., A. Broughton, and R. Madison. 1990. Immune activation and autoantibodies in humans with long-term inhalation exposure to formaldehyde. Arch. Environ. Health 45:217-223.

Torkelson, T.R., S.E. Sadek, V.K. Rowe, J.K. Kodama, H.H. Anderson, G.S. Loquvam, and C.H. Hine. 1961. Toxicologic investigations of 1,2-dibromo-3-chloropropane. Toxicol. Appl. Pharmacol. 3:545-559.

Törngvist, M., S. Osterman-Golkar, A. Kautiainen, S. Jensen, P.B. Farmer, and L. Ehrenberg. 1986a. Tissue doses of ethylene oxide in cigarette smokers determined from adduct levels in hemoglobin. Carcinogenesis 7:1519-21.

Törngvist, M., J. Mowrer, S. Jensen, and L. Ehrenberg. 1986b. Monitoring of environmental cancer initiators through hemoglobin adducts by a modified Edman degradation method. Anal. Biochem. 154:255-266.

Törngvist, M., S. Osterman-Golkar, A. Kautiainen, M. Naslund, C.J. Calleman, and L. Ehrenberg. 1988. Methylations in human hemoglobin. Mutat. Res. 204:521-529.

Underhill, D.W., and E.P. Radford, eds. 1986. New and Sensitive Indicators of Health Impacts of Environmental Agents. Pittsburgh: Center for Environmental Epidemiology, University of Pittsburgh.

Upton, A.C., T. Kneip, and P. Toniolo. 1989. Public health aspects of toxic chemical disposal sites. Annu. Rev. Public Health 10:1-25.

Valanis, B. 1986. Environmental and direct measures of exposure. Occup. Med. 1:431-444.

Van Sittert, N.J., and G. DeJong. 1985. Biomonitoring of exposure to potential mutagens and carcinogens in industrial populations. Food Chem. Toxicol. 23:1, 23-31.

Vineis, P., N. Caporaso, S.R. Tannebaum, P.L. Skipper, J. Glogowski, H. Bartsch, M. Coda, G. Taleska, and F. Kadlubar. 1990. Acetylation phenotype carcinogen-hemoglobin adducts, and cigarette smoking. Carcinogen Res. 13:3002-3004.

Wallace, L.A., E.D. Pellizzari, T.D. Hartwell, R. Whitmore, C. Sparacino, and H. Zelon. 1986. Total exposure assessment methodology (TEAM) study: Personal exposures, indoor-outdoor relationships, and breath levels of volatile organic compounds in New Jersey. Environ. Int. 12:369-387.

Weill, H., and M. Turner-Warwick, eds. 1981. Occupational Lung Diseases. New York: Deckker

Welch, L.S., S.M. Schrader, T.W. Turner, and M.R. Cullen. 1988. Effects of exposure to ethylene glycol ethers on shipyard painters: II. Male reproduction. Am. J. Ind. Med. 14:509-526.

White, R.F., R.G. Feldman, and P.H. Travers. 1990. Neurobehavioral effects of toxicity due to metals, solvents, and insecticides. J. Clin. Neuropharmacology 13:392-412.

Whorton, M.D., R.M. Krauss, S. Marshall, and T. H. Milby. 1977. Infertility in male pesticide workers. Lancet 2:1259-1261.

Williamson, A.M., R.K.C. Teo, and J. Sanderson. 1982. Occupational mercury exposure and its consequences for behavior. Int. Arch. Occup. Environ. Health 50:273-286.

Zielhuis, R.L. 1984. Approaches in the development of biological monitoring methods: Laboratory and field studies. Pp. 373-385 in Biological Monitoring of Workers Exposed to Chemicals, A. Aitio, V. Riihimaki, and H. Vainio, eds. Washington, D.C.: Hemisphere Publishing.

Zielhuis, R.L. 1985. Total exposure and workers' health. Ann. Occup. Hyg. 29:463-475.

8

General Conclusions

ACCORDING TO A NUMBER OF recent opinion polls, the American public believes that hazardous wastes constitute a serious threat to public health. In contrast, many scientists and administrators in the field do not share this belief. On the basis of its best efforts to evaluate the published literature relevant to this subject, the committee cannot confirm either viewpoint. Regrettably, insufficient data are available for evaluating the impact on public health of exposure to substances from hazardous-waste sites. Without doubt, substances toxic to several animal species abound in hazardous-waste sites. Many sites have not been adequately assessed for content, or for potential routes of human exposure. Human health studies, while mixed in quality and persuasiveness, provide evidence that serious health effects cannot be ruled out, and have been documented to occur at some hazardous-waste sites. More and better health studies need to be conducted.

Whether Superfund and other hazardous-waste programs actually protect human health is a critical question for environmental epidemiology, at least with respect to federal and state efforts to clean up hazardous-waste sites. To answer it would require information on the scope of potential and actual human exposures to hazardous wastes and about the health effects that could be associated with these exposures. Based on its review of the published literature on the subject, the committee finds that this question cannot be answered. One recent EPA survey found that more than 40 million people live within four miles of a Superfund site. Residential proximity does not per se mean that exposures and health risks are occurring, but the potential for exposure is increased.

National decisions to clean up hazardous-waste sites have been made independently of studies about the overall impact such sites may have on public health. During the past 10 years, less than 1 percent of the estimated $4.2 billion spent each year on hazardous-waste sites in the U.S. has been used to evaluate health risks at listed Superfund sites. As a result, existing data on exposures and health effects are inadequate either to support decisions on the management of hazardous-waste sites or to allow the conduct of epidemiologic investigations of the health impact of these sites. However, recent efforts by the Agency for Toxic Substances and Disease Registry (ATSDR) and EPA have improved the information base and should be further extended.

Although billions of dollars have been spent during the past decade to study and manage hazardous-waste sites in the U.S., an insignificant portion has been devoted to the evaluation of attendant health risks. For that reason and because of technical obstacles, information about the connection between exposures from hazardous-waste sites and health effects remains inadequate.

This chapter draws on the preceding ones and recapitulates the committee's major findings about the epidemiologic study of hazardous-waste sites. Despite the lack of adequate data with which to characterize the effects of hazardous wastes on public health in general, the committee concludes that exposures from hazardous-waste sites have produced serious health effects in some populations. Table 1-1 summarizes the peer-reviewed literature on this subject. A limited number of epidemiologic studies indicate that increased rates of birth defects, spontaneous abortion, neurologic impairment, and cancer have occurred in some residential populations exposed to hazardous wastes. We are concerned that other populations at risk might not have been adequately identified.

To improve the ability to evaluate health effects associated with exposures to hazardous wastes, a number of important data gaps need to be filled and several resource constraints need to be remedied, as this report illustrates. There is a need to make health assessments a priority in the routine evaluation of hazardous-waste sites. There is also a need to create mechanisms for sharing this information as well as information from epidemiologic investigations of these sites nationwide. Accordingly, state and local health department investigations of hazardous-waste sites must be adequately sup-

ported. Better measurements or estimates are needed of human exposure from a variety of sources, including abandoned hazardous-
waste sites; other point sources, such as leaking storage tanks and
industrial operations; and from non-point sources, such as agricul-
ture, all of which can produce nonconventional pollutants (NCPs).
Monitoring of sentinel health events and increased use of disease
registries and vital statistics systems will be required to assess the
public health impacts of all of these sources of exposure.

STATE AND FEDERAL CONSTRAINTS

There are reasons to suppose that current procedures might not be
identifying the most important abandoned hazardous-waste sites, from
the point of view of public health. The congressional Office of Technology Assessment (OTA) notes that efforts to assess candidate National Priority List (NPL) sites typically relegate public health concerns to a minor role and that the process as a whole is directed at
engineering aspects of remediation rather than at the assessment of
public health risk. Because public health concerns have been given
only minor importance, many potential Superfund sites have never
been considered for inclusion on the NPL or have been dropped from
the list, even though their public health impacts have not been studied adequately.

At NPL sites where potentially critical exposures are detected, there
is no regular application of an adequate system of early assessment
of the health risks involved or of the need for interim action to protect the health of exposed populations. The failure to construct a
system for managing hazardous-waste sites that incorporates the early
assessment of health risk means that the health of nearby residents
could be imperiled. Moreover, the conditions for development of environmental epidemiology are adverse and impede the development
of useful scientific investigations of many important questions.

OTA recently concluded that the maximum number of potential
sites from which Comprehensive Environmental Release and Compensation Liability Inventory System (CERCLIS) and NPL sites are
drawn is approximately 439,000. These sites include facilities covered under the Resource Conservation and Recovery Act (RCRA) as
Subtitle C and D facilities, mining waste sites, nonpetroleum leaking
underground storage tanks, pesticide-contaminated sites, federal facilities, radioactive releases, underground injection wells, municipal
gas facilities, and wood-preserving plants, among others.

The lack of a site discovery program and of a comprehensive inventory presents a particular problem for public health. The range

and distribution of human exposure to releases from hazardous-waste sites is unknown. EPA now acknowledges that undiscovered sites could well present significant health risks, even though previously the agency had announced that most sites with serious potential for harm had been detected. Reviews in several states show that the current system of CERCLIS reporting misses potential health risks. In 1984 an evaluation of 93 sites on the California Department of Health State Superfund list showed that only 19 of the sites were on the federal NPL. Forty-six of the sites showed evidence of waste release into groundwater, and in 34 of these cases the groundwater was known to be used for drinking. Extensive or systematic sampling existed for only 22 of the sites where release into groundwater had occurred, despite the evidence of potential human exposure. Moreover, in all of the sites where there was known contamination of groundwater, more than 10,000 persons were potentially exposed.

PROBLEMS OF EXPOSURE ASSESSMENT

Exposure assessment provides critical information about potential human contact with relevant materials. Best estimates are that groundwater provides the major source of drinking water for about 50 percent of the U.S. population. In California, groundwater provides drinking water to nearly 70 percent of the population. Although current risks could be negligible, studies show that millions of tons of hazardous materials are slowly migrating into groundwater in areas where they could pose problems in the future. For instance, plumes of chemicals, including many nonconventional pollutants, are moving down the canyon from the Superfund site at Stringfellow Pits in California and could pose important problems in the future.

The public health component of the information base for decisions about site listing and remediation is inadequate, and there is no systematic tracking of deferred sites. The attendant cost has been confusion about the actual risks that hazardous-waste sites pose to human health. Clues to the potential scale of human exposure to toxic chemicals released from hazardous-waste sites are emerging, however. By mid-1990, ATSDR had completed 1151 health assessments at NPL sites. ATSDR determined that hazardous substances had been released at 85 percent of the sites and that about 15 percent of these sites merited further public health investigation.

The committee urgently recommends the development and validation of an adequate initial health assessment methodology for hazardous-waste sites. The committee recommends that initial site characterization include at least minimal information on potential exposure.

This should include sampling of tap water, estimating outgassing from showers as relevant, absorption through cooking or eating, and other residential uses, and surface soil. Epidemiology is not merely a passive science, cataloguing exposures and effects. It is an active tool for evaluating the link between potentially hazardous exposures and disease and for directing interventions to prevent further exposures. Where the evaluation of human exposures and health effects associated with hazardous-waste sites is not integrated into early site evaluation and interim remediation decisions, the real contributions of epidemiology are lost.

This is of grave concern because hazardous wastes have constituted a significant public health hazard to specific populations at specific sites, summarized in Table 1-1. Further, in 1988, ATSDR reported that conditions at about 11 percent of all 951 NPL sites constituted ongoing or probable public health concerns. During 1990, 32 percent of a specially reviewed subgroup of sites were identified as requiring some kind of protective health action. The health of the public has remained in jeopardy at many sites long after the risks could have—and should have—been identified.

As Chapter 3 reports, repositories of potentially dangerous substances can be found at a number of hazardous-waste sites. Dangerous substances also have been generated by leaking underground storage tanks, non-point sources such as agricultural pesticide runoff, automobile emissions, agricultural, mining, storage, and other activities. Information about these materials generally reflects the data requirements of environmental engineering and site remediation, rather than public health considerations. Accordingly, whether these materials pose a risk to public health cannot readily be determined in the absence of more detailed information about potential human exposures.

Improvements must be made in the ability to assess the more than 600 chemical compounds identified at hazardous-waste sites, along with the hundreds or thousands of unidentified pollutants that could enter the groundwater. The potential for exposure is of such magnitude that researchers who develop exposure assessment strategies will have to direct their attention not solely to an analysis of the contaminants at a hazardous-waste site, but to off-site migration and public exposure as well. In this context, measures of personal exposure, including the use of biologic markers and biologic monitoring as discussed in Chapter 7, along with personal sampling, although often difficult and time consuming, must receive greater scientific attention if appropriate associations are to be made between contaminants, exposures, and health effects.

Enough hazardous-waste sites have been identified where the population exposed is large and the exposures are great that it should be feasible to conduct environmental epidemiologic studies. The difficulty has been primarily with the lack of resources to conduct adequate exposure characterization or to collect sufficient outcome measures. It should be recognized, however, that for most sites the populations are too small to provide studies of sufficient power for risks to be detectable unless it is possible to combine data from a number of sites. Combining studies of small populations into meta-analyses might generate sufficient statistical power to reach conclusions, provided that the basic measures involved are comparable and that sound methods are used in all separate studies.

Several chapters explain that NCPs could be an important source of hazardous exposure. Some important pollutants are not regulated under a variety of acts, including the Safe Drinking Water Act, the Clean Air Act, and the Toxic Substances Control Act. These NCPs need to be identified and placed under appropriate regulatory control. Some preliminary toxicologic studies suggest that NCPs and so-called inert pesticide ingredients have important biologic properties of environmental persistence and mobility. More studies are needed to characterize the mixture of materials deposited as hazardous wastes and to give better estimates of their transport and fate in the environment. In the broadest sense, these unidentified, unregulated substances present a risk of unknown magnitude. The absence of evidence of their effects reflects the failure to conduct research; it should not be misconstrued as demonstrating that NCPs and "inert" pesticide components are without risk.

Where the potential for human exposure exists, exposure assessment should be conducted for important pollutants that can migrate from hazardous-waste sites. For the purposes of epidemiologic study, better characterizations of exposure are required than those usually available from engineering and hydrogeologic models and other estimates. Such models based on cursory local data often have been overemphasized while actual measurements or estimates of human exposure have gone undone. Models are only as valid as the assumptions and data on which they are based. Modeling needs to be improved both for health risks and for site assessment.

Many studies have focused on site-specific characterizations, even though pollutants do not respect boundaries. These site-specific investigations have often not proceeded to the steps of defining the populations at risk and quantitatively evaluating exposure to toxic contaminants. The characterizations of the sites more often reflect requirements of environmental engineering and site remediation than assessment of public health considerations. Whether the toxic contaminants pose a risk to the exposed population cannot be determined in the absence of more detailed information about human exposures. Instead of focusing on the toxic chemicals that have been identified at a site itself, it is necessary to develop estimates of exposure to define and assess the population at risk, including estimation of the population size and exposure-related characteristics.

AIR POLLUTION FROM HAZARDOUS WASTES

Although few studies directly assess airborne exposures to hazardous wastes, the committee finds persuasive evidence that health effects can occur from such exposures. Review of the relevant animal literature on compounds known to occur at hazardous-waste sites, along with those few epidemiologic studies of airborne exposures from sites, shows that a wide range of effects may occur, and they include serious diseases, such as cancer, neurobehavioral complaints, and constellations of self-reported symptoms. In addition, a few studies have explicitly linked airborne exposures from hazardous-waste sites to increased rates of birth defects, low birth weight, and chronic diseases in some small populations.

Lessons that have been learned in air pollution studies are relevant to epidemiologic studies of hazardous-waste sites. As with the assessment of other health effects, a crucial lesson from the recent history of epidemiologic studies of air pollution has been the critical role played by the general availability of monitoring data for criteria air pollutants. Without the extensive network of data on those pollutants for which monitoring data are routinely acquired, such as respirable particulates, epidemiologic studies of air pollution would not have been possible. Many of the pollutants of interest at hazardous-waste sites are not routinely evaluated. Exposure to hydrocarbons in urban air has not been monitored regularly since the 1970s, and there has been little work on their direct effects except in studies of the sick building syndrome and occupational studies. The committee understands that routine monitoring of ambient air around hazardous-waste sites is not generally feasible because of the number of sites, the low likelihood of detection in most cases, and the cost of monitoring. The small populations near most sites make the sites difficult to study with standard epidemiologic techniques. Nevertheless, more systematic determinations of where such specific monitoring and studies might be appropriate need to be made early in the process of identifying and describing sites for study. The methods of meta-analysis also could prove useful to the extent that examples of similar exposures at different sites could be combined.

The committee examined several cross-sectional morbidity studies of hazardous-waste sites, in which significant differences in symptoms were found between an exposed and a control population. None of these studies found differences in reproductive outcome or cancer mortality, but several documented significant self-reported symptoms including headache, irritability, and fatigue. These reports contain considerable discussion of how differences in symptom perception and recall can be avoided, but neither factor can be avoided altogether. The authors of these reports drew somewhat different conclusions from these studies, based on the degree to which they believed recall bias accounted for differences in reported symptoms. Recall bias is difficult to rule out if a community is episodically exposed to a noxious agent with a powerful odor or in other incidents of acute exposure.

Although it might be concluded that recall bias explains the symptom differences in all of the studies of self-reported symptoms, it is plausible that the symptoms complained of are more sensitive indicators of significant exposure than are more severe outcomes. The fact that disparate populations in different countries experience similar symptoms indicates that a common set of exposures may be involved. Our belief that a constellation of symptoms may be associated with airborne exposures to emissions from hazardous-waste sites relies on a number of recent studies on the sick building syndrome and other studies of neurologic symptoms in solvent-exposed workers, which have found similar effects in exposed persons in different countries. The syndrome has been firmly established for several reasons. First, a remarkable concordance has been found in the kinds of complaints made by workers in different locations and in different countries: Headaches, fatigue, inability to concentrate, and mild inflammation of the eyes and pharynx were the most common complaints. The complaints were generally more common in air-conditioned buildings, and they could not be attributed to fungi (such as Aspergillus) known to be responsible for the "humidifier fever" infection.

The sick building syndrome contains important lessons for hazardous-waste-site epidemiology. In many cases involving hazardous-waste sites the complaints are subjective and similar to those associated with the sick building syndrome. Furthermore, many of the volatile organic compounds found in modern sealed buildings, including formaldehyde, toluene, and trichloroethylene, also are common constituents of waste dumps.

Recent controlled exposure work from Denmark noted in Chapter 4 can play an important role in clarifying the specificity of reported symptoms. Symptom reports appear to be sensitive indicators of adverse health effects. The simultaneous use of air monitoring and diary records could reduce the problem of recall bias, and these methods are particularly valuable when small changes in pollutant levels cannot be detected by the subjects in a study. It has been suggested that airborne exposure to low levels of formaldehyde is followed by changes in cells that indicate that the immune system has been affected. Although the precise significance of such changes is unclear, the possibility must be considered that exposure to toxic substances from hazardous-waste dumps causes similar or related changes, as these involve similar exposures. It is likely that air emissions from hazardous-waste sites have caused a variety of symptoms that indicate low-level interference with normal function.

Asthma and other respiratory diseases are common and well-studied disturbances of the respiratory system. During the past decade, our knowledge of factors related to airway responsiveness has expanded greatly. Exposures to a wide range of substances (more than 200 are listed in one review) can change airway responsiveness or reduce the threshold for response to a specific substance. More commonly, exposure leads to a nonspecific increase in airway responsiveness as measured by inhaled histamine or methacholine aerosols. A number of studies of hazardous-waste sites document complaints of chest tightness and shortness of breath. Therefore, the possibility must be entertained that proximity to some of these sites has induced increased airway responsiveness. To our knowledge, this has not yet been specifically sought in hazardous-waste-site studies.

Although the role of ambient air pollution in asthma prevalence has not yet been determined, it seems likely that air pollution is an aggravating factor. It seems unlikely, however, that exposures from hazardous-waste sites could have played a part in the generally increased prevalence of asthma. The role of exposures from hazardous-waste sites in the development of respiratory symptoms cannot be readily evaluated.

DOMESTIC WATER CONTAMINATED WITH HAZARDOUS WASTES

As Chapter 5 makes clear, exposure from domestic water is not limited to ingestion, but includes airborne exposures from materials that can outgas during showering, bathing, or cooking, or can be absorbed through the skin. Therefore, estimates of exposure from domestic water need to be expanded to take into account the role of airborne exposures from volatile and nonvolatile substances.

We have noted that complete accounts of the possible health effects associated with human exposure to hazardous-waste sites are not generally available, both because of legal restrictions that are often placed on findings by attorneys and because of the limited government resources applied to the study of the issue. However, several factors lead us to conclude that contamination of domestic water supplies with hazardous chemicals, such as those that can be encountered at hazardous-waste sites, is injurious to human health, even though the magnitude of the risk cannot be determined. Perhaps the most persuasive evidence now derives from studies that link an increased risk of bladder cancer to exposure to chlorinated surface water contaminated with trihalomethanes (THMs). Also, both experimental and epidemiologic studies link TCE exposure to increased rates of some cardiac congenital anomalies. One large ecologic study also associates bladder cancer with exposure to contaminated drinking water from hazardous-waste sites.

Ample evidence shows an association between exposure to THMs and bladder and other cancers in test animals. Some epidemiologic studies of humans corroborate this relationship. The fact that other studies have not found an increased incidence of bladder cancer in persons exposed to toxic-waste sites could result from several factors, including the cancer's generally long latent period, the small numbers of people usually studied, the relatively pervasive exposure that occurs, and the fact that bladder cancer can have more than one cause.

In a study in North Carolina strong evidence was found that increased cancer mortality rates were associated with exposure over a period of two decades to what was estimated to be a broad range of industrial by-products and hazardous substances in domestic water supplies. In a rural area, significant clusters of cancer developed about twenty years after residents had begun drinking raw, untreated river water contaminated by hazardous wastes. The timing of the appearance of the excess in all forms of cancer corresponded to the estimated time of peak exposure to contaminated domestic water, taking into account the typical latency for cancer.

Increased rates of cancer might be anticipated in populations that have experienced solvent contamination of drinking water. Leukemia and lymphoma are of obvious concern, inasmuch as other studies have found increases linked to such occupational exposures to solvents. Unfortunately, the rarity of these diseases and the small populations usually exposed to solvents in drinking water have resulted in a dearth of studies with sufficient power to detect an increase in risk. Some researchers advocate restricting studies of clusters to those where very high rates have been found. However, the number of heavily exposed individuals that might be expected to show an increase in risk of fivefold or more is generally so small that for cancers as rare as leukemia or lymphoma such risks would be difficult to detect. Meta-analysis, which allows the appropriate pooling of relevant studies to increase the statistical power for detecting an effect, could offer some solution. This will be discussed further in the committee's next report on research opportunities in environmental epidemiology.

A limited number of reports in the peer-reviewed scientific literature have linked spontaneous abortion, low birth weight, and birth defects to the consumption of contaminated domestic water supplies. Studies in Santa Clara County, California, have been inconclusive as to the cause of a cluster of birth defects observed there. Two distinct studies in Love Canal, New York, however, link low birth weight to exposure to hazardous wastes. In Tucson, Arizona, the rate of congenital cardiac anomalies was three times higher in children of persons who consumed water contaminated with TCE. Such effects should continue to be monitored because there is far less difficulty with the latent period for reproductive effects than for cancer. Human population studies in Arizona and laboratory studies of animals provide evidence that cardiac abnormalities can develop after exposure to TCE. Recent reports of increasing trends in cardiac anomalies should be carefully evaluated, as improvements in case finding may be involved, along with real increases.

There also is evidence that neurologic, hepatic, and immunologic function can be damaged by exposure to domestic water contaminated with toxic chemicals. The long-term consequences of the abnormalities detected, however, are largely unknown and must be the subject of further research, on which the committee will comment in more detail in its next report.

SOIL CONTAMINATED WITH HAZARDOUS WASTES

Although direct ingestion of contaminated soil poses a risk chiefly to toddlers and children, as noted in Chapter 6, adults also could be at risk if they eat food grown in contaminated soil, or fish that have absorbed contaminants, or if they otherwise come into regular contact with contaminated soil through their work or personal habits. Sophisticated methods have been devised for improving assessments of soil exposures. These take into account peak, average, or cumulative exposures, to determine relationships between exposure and disease. Refined methods need to be applied in epidemiologic studies to improve the ability to estimate exposures from soil. These should include detailed metabolic studies of ingested plants, adequate characterization of chemical transformation, and better measurements of residues.

One area that should not be neglected entails estimating exposures from consumption of fish that bioconcentrate lipophilic materials from sediment and water. Site assessments should use more realistic exposure measures, including direct studies of contaminants at the tap for domestic water supplies and estimates of consumption of contaminated foods and fish. In addition, efforts should be made to include relevant soil, food, and airborne measurements, so that integrated exposure assessments can be made.

Current public health burdens from hazardous-waste sites appear to be small, but the future risk could be greater insofar as many of the substances involved are highly persistent and other materials already in the groundwater or soil can migrate or be transported into areas where exposure potential is greater. For instance, some of these materials in soil, such as chromium and other heavy metals, can contaminate large and populous sections of urban areas and remain persistent, as noted in Chapter 6. Similarly, lead is found at most Superfund sites and also contaminates some sections of urban areas; it is a nondegradable, persistent substance. Even for these materials, plausible routes of human exposure must be carefully assessed. Occurrence only increases the potential for risk. In some cases, unnecessary or inappropriate remediation can create more of a hazard than would be caused by leaving such materials undisturbed.

CONCLUSIONS

Although the effect on large populations of very low levels of toxic pollutants is unknown, action must be taken now to protect public health in the future. Threats of contamination of groundwater merit serious preventive policies. A substantial risk of contamination of groundwater is not being averted by current remediation practices, according to a number of assessments. It should be recognized that if exposure becomes general and almost uniform through contamination of groundwater, current epidemiologic techniques might not be able to ascertain any related health effects. There is now an opportunity to begin studies in areas where groundwater pollution has remained high and localized. There also is an important opportunity for prevention that could forestall major public health problems in the future.

A number of research techniques should be extended to the study of health effects linked with hazardous wastes, including the use of "sentinel health events" as additional indicators of environmental contamination. Such indicators are most useful when they identify causes of morbidity and mortality that are uniquely or predominantly associated with specific and preventable exposures. Some illnesses, such as methemoglobinemia, which results from exposure to excessive amounts of nitrate in water, indicate hazardous environmental exposure, even when they occur as single cases. Other diseases indicate potential environmental exposures when they occur at elevated rates among larger populations, such as bladder cancer among non-smokers or chronic respiratory disease among children. The committee believes that further studies of acute symptoms, if combined with exposure measurements, are likely to reveal that reported symptoms are not completely explained by recall bias. The current data base clearly indicates the importance of continued study in this area. Surveys of the similar constellations of subjective symptoms reported by persons exposed in different countries to hazardous wastes indicate that such symptoms collectively can represent sentinel health events associated with such exposures. The further development and application of this approach to environmental surveillance holds particular promise for the epidemiologic investigation of populations exposed to hazardous wastes.

A six-part environmental epidemiology program needs to be developed to inform policy decisions about risks to public health presented by hazardous-waste sites.

• Establish an active and coordinated system of site discovery for hazardous-waste sites, based in EPA and providing technical assistance to federal and state programs. An aggressive site discovery program, in combination with improved assessments and triage of sites for interim and final remediation, will restore the original congressional intent to protect the public from hazardous-waste-site exposures.

• Define a revised approach to site assessments that integrates public health determinations of population exposures, health effects, and the necessity of interim and final remediation or other actions into a continuum of site evaluation. Establish protocols and criteria for the revised preliminary assessment of all sites, with triggers for interim remediation or other action such as relocation, and require that all sites undergo a revised preliminary assessment within one year of discovery.

• Establish a comprehensive national inventory of hazardous-waste sites that will track the status of all sites through assessment and remediation or closure. Use the inventory to ensure that sites are not deferred or placed in closure status without a revised preliminary assessment as described above.

• Rigorously evaluate the data and methodologies used in site assessment, including the characterization of potential and actual releases to groundwater, surface water, air, and soil that result in human exposure; and the methodologies for estimating the size and make-up of populations exposed to hazardous-waste site emissions. Use this information in preliminary assessments and in deciding how to protect the public health. Evaluate compliance with public health recommendations for the protection of exposed populations and site remediation.

• Improve and expand research to fill data gaps in environmental epidemiology to illuminate the distribution and severity of exposures, risks, and health effects associated with hazardous-waste sites. Establish an extensive program of applied research, including exposure registries linked to priority substances, and further the development of surveillance methods such as community health data bases, biologic monitoring, and sentinel events.

• Direct ATSDR and other relevant agencies to expand cooperative agreements with states and develop a comprehensive program of technical assistance for state and local agencies. Federal and state agencies, such as ATSDR and the National Institute of Environmental Health Sciences, also should provide increased support for university-based research in environmental epidemiology.

The legislative mandates, policies, and programs of the federal and state agencies that currently manage hazardous-waste sites are inadequate to the task of protecting public health. Although evidence suggests that specific populations near specific hazardous-waste sites are exposed to substantial risks, the distribution and frequency of these exposures cannot be ascertained, because the needed data have not been gathered.

A decade after implementation of Superfund, and despite congressional efforts to redirect the program, substantial public health concerns remain, and critical information on the distribution of exposures and health effects associated with hazardous-waste sites is still lacking. Whether for the purposes of environmental epidemiology or for the protection of public health, the nation is failing to adequately identify, assess, or prioritize hazardous-waste-site exposures and their potential effects on public health. Our next report will contain a review of selected state health department reports on this subject and of case studies of legal decisions that have evaluated epidemiologic evidence not otherwise available in the published literature. On the basis of this review, we will recommend important research initiatives in the field.

Until better evidence is developed, prudent public policy demands that a margin of safety be provided regarding potential health risks from exposures to hazardous-waste sites. We do no less in designing bridges and buildings. We do no less in establishing criteria for scientific credibility. We must surely do no less when the health and quality of life of Americans are at stake.

Index

ATSDR assistance, 92–93, 97, 259,
269
federal cooperation with, 7, 8, 69–
70, 75, 78, 85, 92–93, 97, 259, 268,
269
funding, 85, 92–93
groundwater contamination, 92,
110–113, 259
health departments, information
from, 2
legislation, 60, 86
NPL sites, 103
regulations, 2, 5–8, 60
remediation efforts, 86, 92
research, 93
risk assessment, 86
site assessment, 69–70, 76, 86, 92,
268
see also Demography; *specific states*
Statistics and statistical approaches,
42, 256
biologic markers, 220, 236–239, 247,
248
confidence intervals, 32, 42
disease registries, 37, 45–47, 70, 181–
182, 188
effect size, 32
exposure data, limitations, 126–131
exposure registries, 8, 75, 97
multivariate, 182
national site inventory, 6, 8, 76–77,
93, 94, 96, 268–269
number of sites, 9
power, 36
recall bias, 11, 12, 33, 135, 164–165,
263–264, 268
significance assessment, 2, 32–34,
38–39, 43, 185
volume of waste generated, 1–2, 26,
60, 102
see also Error of measurement
Superfund Amendment and
Reauthorization Act (SARA), 46,
62, 65-66, 80
Superfund sites, 1, 5, 6, 10, 13, 15, 19,
61–86 , 92
air pollution, 161
biologic markers, 224–225
lead, 212–213

legislation for, 45, 46
National Priority List (NPL), 7, 9,
64, 66, 67–68, 70, 71–74, 75, 77, 79,
80, 81, 83, 93, 95, 103–105, 108–
109, 119, 144–146, 187, 211, 258,
259, 260
population proximate to, 2, 26, 67,
68, 103, 114–116, 137–138, 257
remediation, 80–83
site discovery funding, 77
torts, 43
Surface water, 8, 20–21, 179, 180, 182
see also Water pollution
Surrogate measures, 120, 124, 131–142
Sweden, 160
Symptomatology, 4, 31, 70, 130, 137,
263
airborne toxins, 164–165, 170, 173
diary records, 12, 166–167, 170, 173,
264
nonspecific, 135–136
recall bias, 11, 12, 33, 135, 164–165,
263–264, 268

T

Taiwan, 184, 208, 224
Taxonomy, *see* Classification
Technical assistance, 7, 8, 268, 269
Tennessee, 18, 141, 214
Testicular cancer, 215
Tetrachlorethane, 166, 188
Time factors
causation and, 40, 35, 36, 40–41
exposure assessment, 102, 116, 132,
134
see also Longitudinal studies;
Retrospective studies
Time series analysis, 29, 173
Torts, *see* Litigation
Total Diet Study, 214
Total Exposure Assessment
Methodology, 117, 124, 128
Toxic Substances Control Act, 45, 261
Toxicokinetics, 123
Trichloroethane (TCA), 133–134, 181
Trichloroethylene (TCE), water
pollutant, 13, 14–15, 18, 118, 139–
140, 142, 194, 197, 265, 266

282 INDEX

biologic markers, 18, 224–225, 229, 230, 236
Trihalomethanes (THMs), 13, 180, 181–184, 184, 265

U

United Kingdom, 41, 44, 159
United Nations Environmental Program, 27
Urban areas, 77, 160, 172, 179, 185, 212, 262, 267
Urine, 224, 225, 235, 236
Utah, 167, 168, 172

V

Vietnam, 215, 233
Vinyl chloride, 11, 38, 160–161, 205
Volatile organic compounds (VOCs), 13, 14–15, 18, 118–119, 123, 128, 131–134, 140–142, 158, 179, 196, 263
  see also specific compounds
Volatilization, 15, 18, 117, 140–141, 179, 195, 264

W

Water pollutants, 9–10, 13–15, 19, 125, 158, 179–199, 264–266
  animal studies, 194
  birth defects, 14–15, 180, 189–197, 265
  cancer, 13–14, 110, 180, 181–189, 198, 265–266
  case-control studies, 13–14, 180, 183–184, 187, 188–189, 191

causal inference, 180, 186
CDC, 193–194
children and, 185–186, 190
chlorination, 13–15, 180, 182, 183–184, 195, 225–226
chronic diseases, general, 180, 194–195
cross-sectional studies, 194–195, 196
demographic factors, 5, 10, 61, 259
descriptive studies, 13, 14, 180
dose-response assessment, 184, 194
EPA, 179, 185–186
exposure analysis, 131–134, 135, 139–142
fish, bioaccumulation, 15, 16
immune system, 15, 199
individual studies, 181
liver disease, 184, 185, 195–196, 199
morbidity and mortality, general, 14, 181–189
neurotoxic effects, 14, 15, 18, 189, 197, 199
reproductive toxicology, 14, 185, 189–195
TCE, 13, 14–15, 18, 118, 139, 140, 139–140, 142, 194, 197, 224–225, 229, 230, 236, 265, 266
volatilization, 15, 18, 117, 140–141, 179, 195, 264
  see also Groundwater; Surface water
Weight, see Body weight
Women
  cancer, 14, 140–141, 183
  kidney disease, 195
  see also Gender differences
World Health Organization, 27, 212